Does This Sound Like You?

You've lost weight dozens of times, only to gain it back and sometimes, more. You are tired of deprivation diets that don't let you eat the foods you love. You've tried to stay "on track," but monotony, boredom or rigidity throw you "off track."

If this description fits you, you've probably been one of the people victimized by quick-fix, unbalanced fad diets.

Now, you're in for a treat. *The Cooper Clinic Solution to the Diet Revolution* allows you to eat all the foods you love and lose weight in a balanced, healthy way.

Congratulations!

By opening this book, you already have taken a step to improve your health and well-being! If you are like most Americans, you have struggled with your weight and are looking for a way to get fitter, not fatter every year. Studies indicate we are consuming 150 more calories a day than 25 years ago, and those 150 calories can lead to an extra 15 pounds a year! Moreover, every year after age 25, we lose muscle mass, which slows down metabolism. Fortunately, we can replace that muscle through physical activity and prevent a metabolic slowdown, as well as weight gain.

We *can* get a grip on weight in this country! It's a matter of being better informed—drawing on accurate information, the research of scientists and the experience of expert-losers to apply learned lessons that lead to success. It requires a new mind-set, open-mindedness and a willingness to take one step at a time using the simple strategies and solutions laid out for you in these pages.

Use this book as a step-by-step tool to guide your actions and decisions daily. Go that extra mile some days; take a mini-step another day. Following the steps outlined for you—at your own pace—will lead to your success.

Ready? Set. Begin!

About the cover: Plate displays two extra-lean tenderloin medallions (2-ounces each), and 1/2 cup each of roasted potatoes, sugar snap peas, and steamed carrots. This depicts balanced eating.

For your best health and weight management, STEP UP TO THE PLATE!

What Others Are Saying . . .

"Whether you want to know more about how to successfully take off excess weight or live a healthy, balanced life, this book can make the difference."
—Dr. Kenneth Cooper, MD, MPH,
Founder, President & CEO
Cooper Aerobics Center
Dallas, TX

"Georgia Kostas is a highly respected nutrition professional. Her common sense, motivational approach combines state-of-the-art science with admirable practicality. If more people followed the guidelines so persuasively outlined in this book, we would be fitter and less fat!"
—James M. Rippe, M.D., Director
Center for Clinical and Lifestyle Research
Tufts University, Boston, MA

"Simplify your life! This fun and dynamic tool makes adapting a healthier lifestyle easier than you think. Packed with practical tips, this book takes the mystery out of healthy eating and weight management. I recommend it to consumers and health professionals. It's a win-win for all!"
—Antigoni Pappas, M.B.A., R.D.

"This book is an invaluable component in my personal and group fitness training practice. Combined with an appropriate exercise prescription, this comprehensive, sensible weight management program is easy to follow and very effective in helping my clients and students reach their wellness goals, including weight loss, and management of hypertension and high cholesterol. I am an R.N., A.C.S.M. certified health fitness instructor, A.F.A.A. certified fitness practitioner and A.C.E. certified group fitness instructor. Since I am not a registered dietitian and therefore not licensed to prescribe diets to my clients, I feel confident prescribing this book. It really covers all bases!"
—Olea De Fore, R.N., A.F.P., Personal Trainer,
Owner, The Fitness Nurse

"Busy people love this book! It gets you moving immediately in the right direction."
—Eric Smith, Health Educator

"Most complete, sensible approach I've seen."
—Leni Reed, M.P.H., R.D.

"This book is like the Bible; you can open it up anywhere and it speaks to you. Our clients have found this book to be a valuable resource during our Skills for Lowfat Living Program. The simple, step-by-step approach helps them meet their goals by providing useful suggestions for permanent behavior change.
—Kathy Oppenheim, M.S., C.D.E.
Wellness Coordinator, Columbia LifeCare Center

"I've lost a lot of weight using this book and have managed to keep it off. I would recommend this approach to anyone who is tired of getting rid of the same 10 pounds each year."
—Edna Ground, patient

"This is the only nutrition book you'll ever need! I recommend it to all my clients."
—Kathy Duran, R.D., L.D.
Nutrition Director, Cooper Wellness Program

"This book is like putting a plate full of food in front of a hungry dieter."
—Vinton Taylor Murray, Writer

" I use this book as my food Bible. I have lost 40 lbs. and will lose 60 more. My mind's set."
—D. Marceille, reader

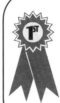 *Utilizing this book under the direction of Linda Steakley, R.D., Huntsville Medical Center won a national award for the best hospital-based weight-loss program in the country!*

GEORGIA G. KOSTAS, M.P.H., R.D., L.D.

The Cooper Clinic Solution to the Diet Revolution

Step Up to the Plate!

Good Health Press ♦ 6702 Park Lane ♦ Dallas, TX 75225

ISBN No. 978-09635969-2-5

Library of Congress Card Catalog Number 00-193269
the cooper clinic solution to the diet revolution:step up to the plate!/
by Georgia G. Kostas
1. weight loss   2. low-fat diet   3. exercise   I. Title

TO ORDER BOOKS & HANDOUTS:

- **For books, volume discounts and**
- **reproducible masters and pages as handouts (in hard copies, CD's or e-handouts)**

Contact or order online:
(214) 587-4241 or fax (214) 363-0539, or
web: www.georgiakostas.com, or
see book order form p. 301

Publisher: **Good Health Press**
6702 Park Lane
Dallas, TX 75225
www.georgiakostas.com
Editor: **Carol Chapman Stertzer**
Layout/Book Designer: **Wendy Rice, WR Enterprises**
Cover Designer: **Jay Colt Weesner**
Cover Photographer: **Pat Haverfield, Haverfield Studios**
Cover Food Stylist: **Gail Greene, AIWF, ASCP, Les Dames d'Escoffier**
Cartoon Illustrator: **Bruce Peschel**

PLEASE NOTE

Fitness, diet and health are matters which necessarily vary from individual to individual. Readers should consult with their own physician about personal needs before starting any diet or exercise program, and especially if one is on any medication or is already under medical care for illness.

Use of this book by individuals, health professions or organizations as a teaching tool does not reflect an endorsement by the author or The Cooper Clinic of the instructor's or the organization's program or practice.

For additional copies, refer to the order form in the back of this book.

DEDICATION

*to **Dr. Kenneth H. Cooper**,*

founder and chief executive officer of the Cooper Clinic,

who had led this nation in the preventive medicine and fitness movement,

and is my mentor, colleague and friend,

inspiring me with his example, dedication and support

to love teaching others how to achieve optimal health

through diet, physical activity, emotional well-being and faith.

A Special Thanks

First and foremost, I wish to acknowledge with gratitude, Dr. Kenneth H. Cooper, Dr. Larry Gibbons and all the Cooper Clinic physicians whose practice of preventive medicine incorporates nutrition, exercise, weight management and emotional well-being as the basis of optimal health. This philosophy enables those seeking a healthy lifestyle to find needed direction.

Two extraordinary individuals made this book happen. I'd like to thank my editor and dear friend, Carol Stertzer, for her invaluable help in the preparation of this book. She was extremely sensitive to what I was trying to accomplish and always there with advice, fresh ideas and encouragement when I needed it most. To Wendy Rice, book designer, a very special thanks for her beautiful and creative interior design. I can never thank them enough for their patience, kindness, persistence and commitment to the completion of this project.

I am also most grateful to the following individuals who contributed to the professional typesetting and layout work — Debby Hanry, Rebecca Lillard, Kim Wise, Shariyun Thompson-Brown, Haley Harper, Lisa Russell, Floyd Black. Thank you to Jay Weesner, cover designer and illustrator, and to Bruce Peschel, cartoonist/illustrator. A very special thank you to Demetrios Lahiri for his insightful input, enthusiasm and consulting on various aspects of the book's production. My many thanks to Colette Cole, who designed the exercise plans and followed this project closely for 15 months. Her counsel, encouragement, persistence and friendship helped me more than she'll ever know. In this most recent edition, I thank also nutrition graduates Janice Turner and Megan Pattison for their creative ideas and tedious updating that helped me tremendously. Without this wonderful teamwork, this book could never have become a reality.

I am also grateful for the team of outstanding registered dietitians/nutritionists with whom I work. They apply these strategies with patients every day, contributing to transformed lives and success stories.

Lastly, and most importantly, I am deeply grateful for my dear friend and colleague, Kim Goldstrohm, R.D., who helped author the original version of this book as a class manual called *The Balancing Act.* This book later evolved into *The Balancing Act Nutrition & Weight Guide.* *The Cooper Clinic Solution to the Diet Revolution* is the latest, updated version.

How I Lost 200 Pounds With Georgia's Plan

Three years ago, I walked out of my doctor's office and into a nearby gym, finally ready to sign up. I was in bad shape in so many ways. More than 200 pounds overweight, I had hit rock-bottom and was ready to make a change.

As part of my gym membership, I received two free consults with a personal trainer. To help me in the area of proper nutrition, my trainer suggested a book he recommended to all of his clients: *The Balancing Act Nutrition & Weight Guide* by Georgia Kostas, M.P.H., R.D. (*The Cooper Clinic Solution to the Diet Revolution* is her newly updated version of this book.)

I had read excerpts from popular weight-loss books such as *Mastering the Zone*, but they were too complicated for me. Taking weight-loss drugs never appealed to me. Honestly, I felt stuck—afraid that I would never take off the weight.

Georgia's book was a godsend. I took it home and devoured it. It was reader-friendly and made sense. I loved the workbook style. In addition, Georgia offered five simple weight-loss plans and provided oodles of menus and recipes to help people like me learn to cook healthfully. I learned all about concepts such as portion control and the "P-C-F Balance."

After looking over the plans, I found one that suited me. The best thing was that I could purchase "normal" foods at the grocery store—I didn't have to spend a lot of money at health-food stores that were clear across town. Each day for the next ten months, I built my diet around 1,000 calories. After the first week, it didn't take much time at all to plan my meals. I soon discovered that as long as I kept it simple, I could plan my day in less than ten minutes. When I traveled, I planned my meals before I went.

The Balancing Act became my "nutrition Bible." I wouldn't deviate from it for anything. On a trip to San Antonio, Texas, shortly after I began changing my way of eating, I managed not to gorge on Mexican food. Instead of gaining weight, I lost seven pounds while I was there.

Physical activity also became a way of life for me. In the past, I had never done cardio work faithfully. I believe the combination of eating healthfully, doing cardio exercise every day and training with weights three times a week had a profound impact on my weight loss. I also began to feel better than I had felt in years. My headaches and leg cramps began to go away, and I didn't feel as fatigued. My blood sugars stabilized and I felt like a new woman.

At about the six-month mark, I hit a plateau. For a couple of weeks, I got the blues because I thought I was doing everything right. Several people told me: "Your system is having to re-gear and figure out what you're doing." I kept on the plan, and soon, more weight began coming off.

By this time, people at the gym, family members and other acquaintances were asking me how I did it. On numerous occasions, I loaned *The Balancing Act* to friends in need of good advice. Georgia had become somewhat of a "coach" in my home, and I wanted to "share" her with others.

I reached my goal in the fall of 1998 by taking off more than 200 pounds. Following Georgia's plan and making time for daily activity saved my life and gave me back my self-confidence. No longer do I have to ask for seatbelt extenders on airplanes. Shopping for clothes isn't a chore. Picking up something I've dropped is not an impossibility. Thanks to this book, I have a new outlook on life.

If I can follow a workbook without personal guidance, anyone can do it. The effort it takes is minimal—and the rewards are everlasting.

Noel Smith, Dallas, Texas

Table of Contents At-a-Glance

Table of Contents Detailed

Foreword

I believe you picked up this book for a good reason:

- You've tried other "diets" that lasted for a season; now you're ready for a complete lifestyle change.
- You want to shed a few pounds and have more energy.
- You need an up-to-date refresher course based on sound principles of nutrition.
- You're not getting any younger and realize you need to make changes before it's too late.

Whatever the reason, seize the moment! Every day, there's new proof that healthy eating contributes in some way to a better quality of life. In recent years, we've seen the following examples:

- A study at Tufts University revealed that a balanced diet is the most important factor in maintaining a healthy immune system.
- People who eat at least five servings of fruits and vegetables a day have a 30% lower risk of the most common type of stroke compared to those who eat less. Eating fruits and vegetables also can lower your risk of developing heart problems, cancer and other diseases. Further, health professionals know that eating plant foods can help you achieve your desired weight.
- Eating fruits and vegetables with the antioxidants lutein and zeaxanthin (found in broccoli, corn, squash, spinach and kale) are believed to reduce the risk for age-related macular degeneration, the leading cause of blindness in people over 65 years of age.
- Researchers have found that soy may fight cancer, menopausal symptoms, heart disease and osteoporosis.

While many people associate my message with physical fitness and "aerobics" (a term I coined in 1968), I have focused on nutrition in many of my own books. Nutrition is a budding science, and I believe many more dietary discoveries are on the way.

The Cooper Clinic Solution to the Diet Revolution is one of the most comprehensive books you'll find on making lifestyle changes. It presents a safe, effective solution to the obesity epidemic that leads to an estimated 300,000 deaths a year and affects 66% of our adult population. We know that being overweight has been associated with greater risk of heart disease, high cholesterol and blood pressure, diabetes and stroke.

Whether you want to know more about how to successfully take off excess weight or live a healthy, balanced life, this book can make the difference. Georgia Kostas, M.P.H., R.D., packs each page with practical insights. As the former Director of Nutrition at the Cooper Clinic in Dallas, Georgia has counseled thousands of clients, taught groups of all different types and worked with preventative health professionals for more than 25 years. She has seen what works and what doesn't and knows the most effective steps a person can take to achieve optimal health through nutrition.

While Georgia shares a wealth of nutrition information, she doesn't ignore other areas necessary for achieving balance: stress management, relaxation techniques, cardiovascular fitness, strength training and more. You have much to gain by delving into this book—and nothing to lose (but a few unwanted pounds, of course).

Studies show that over half of all diseases in the United States result from an unhealthy lifestyle. I encourage you to take responsibility for your own health. You've conquered at least the first step by picking up this book! I trust that the message presented in these pages will guide you in your own walk to wellness. May you experience success as you make the journey.

Kenneth H. Cooper, M.D., M.P.H., Founder, President and CEO
The Cooper Aerobics Center, Dallas, Texas

Letter From the Author

Dear Friends,

The connection of food and weight has fascinated me since I was 10 years old. It was then that I realized that I was plump and my twin sister was called "Twiggy" for a reason! We ate the same meals and snacks at the same time; yet our bodies handled the calories and consequences differently. For years we were the same height, but I always carried the extra 5 pounds.

As I grew older, I adopted my parents' fundamental belief that "food is health." The desire to study nutrition was a natural outcome of accepting this philosophy and believing in the personal practice of preventive medicine. In college, I discovered that the "nutrients" talked about in nutrition classes were the same "biochemicals" discussed in biochemistry. Science had validated "food is health."

*It seemed fitting to pursue a career in nutrition. After reading Dr. Kenneth Cooper's first book, **Aerobics**, in 1977, I was convinced that working in a preventive medicine clinic (preferably his) was the ideal way to teach others about the benefits of diet and exercise in promoting health and preventing disease. I wrote Dr. Cooper and soon afterward, joined his clinic. Since then, for 25 years, I worked daily with individuals wanting to enjoy better health and fitness through improved eating and exercise. Most wanted to find the most effective way to lose weight and keep it off—for life. The reality is, they could!*

In these pages, I bring to you effective strategies and solutions that have worked for many of my patients. What have I learned?

1. *Lifelong weight loss is achievable.*

2. *It involves a change of lifestyle, attitude and thinking about food and fitness . . . with:*
   - *attention to mindful eating, portion size, health and meal times*
   - *a desire to move more daily with gratitude for being able to move*
   - *lifelong self-accountability . . . rather than a short-term, quick-fix mind-set.*

3. *It takes a sensible, realistic plan of eating and exercising daily . . . five choices are in this book:*
   - ***Plan A: Healthy Choices**—a lifestyle approach to comparing and making better food choices.*
   - ***Plan B: Select-a-Plan**—a more structured approach to jump-start your program using:*
     - *Food Groups (Option 1)*   ◆ *Mix and Match Meals (Option 3)*
     - *Sample Menus (Option 2)*   ◆ *Calories (Option 4)*

Mindful eating is the basis for weight success; mindless eating leads to weight gain. What do I mean by "mindful eating?" Be aware of your circumstances, options, vulnerabilities and obstacles that impact your eating. Base your meals and snacks around ground rules. Develop a pattern of repeated habits that enable "automatic" weight management over time.

The concepts and actions needed for you to step out and begin are at your fingertips. By following the steps outlined in this book, you will achieve success, safely and permanently. Take this knowledge and run with it!

All my best to you as you embark on this life-changing journey!

Ginger G. Kostas

Nutrition Consultant, Speaker, Author,
Founder & former Director of Nutrition, Cooper Clinic

How to Use This Book

Use this book as your personal daily counselor or "coach."

1. IDENTIFY what foods, snacks, habits, etc., lead to extra calories in your life.

2. READ FIRST the sections in this book pertinent to your primary needs or challenges (just scan the Table of Contents).

For example, do you need help with:

- ❏ Fast-food choices (Appendix C)
  - ❏ Snacks (p. 120-123)
  - ❏ Chocolate (p. 126)
  - ❏ Ice cream (p. 126)
  - ❏ Cheese (p. 124-125)
  - ❏ Breakfast ideas (p. 89-90)
- ❏ Eating out: restaurant choices (p. 174-183)
- ❏ Eating in: balanced menus (p. 71-85)
- ❏ Eating on the run: quick-fix meals (p. 88-96)
- ❏ How to cut fats in foods (p. 113-115)
- ❏ Your "game plan" – choosing the food plan that best fits you (p. 53, 57)

- ❏ Fitting in exercise (p. 141-142, 151)
- ❏ How to add muscle, lose fat and "rev up" metabolism (p. 16)
- ❏ How to maximize energy and minimize hunger (p. 47-48)
- ❏ Reasonable portions (p. 51, 201)
- ❏ How to "rate your plate" (p. 8-9)
- ❏ Habits that make weight control easier ("skill-power", not "will-power") (p. 19)
- ❏ How to slow down your eating pace, saving thousands of calories and hundreds of pounds over your lifetime (p. 202)

Try the strategies suggested. Decide which works best for you…and use them daily!

3. WRITE DOWN what you eat each day for 30 days. This "ups" your awareness, alertness and action. Recording is your 100% guarantee of weight loss and is the #1 top-rated tool for successful weight loss. Record your activity daily, too…This will motivate you to move more!

4. PLAN AHEAD. Have the right foods on hand – at home, work, eating out, etc. THINK QUALITY and PORTIONS. Have a "game plan" for food and activity daily.

5. SEEK SUPPORT of family, friends, activities, restaurants, reading, etc., to keep you "on track."

6. REFLECT AND REVIEW daily: What worked well or didn't? Commit to what will work tomorrow.

7. ENJOY YOUR SUCCESSES DAILY. Keep moving forward. . .one step at a time.

Getting Started

Do you want to arrange your closet by *season*, not by *size*? Do you want to eat a fudge brownie, enjoy a cool ice cream cone on a hot summer day, eat Mexican food or a hamburger…and still be healthy and lose weight?

You can! This book shows you how.

I promise that I'm not talking about any gimmicks or magic potions. Typical unbalanced "diets" have done people more harm than good. Despite four decades of national focus on weight loss, the average American weighs 8 pounds more than a person of the same age 10 years ago. Consumer surveys indicate that over 50% of Americans are overweight today, as opposed to 25% in the late 1970's, and the statistics grow every year. An estimated 45% of women and 25% of men in the U. S. report they are "dieting" to lose weight. People are dieting more, yet weighing more than ever.

In a world where we are tempted to move less and consume more (especially with larger portions, more meals out and snack opportunities everywhere), can we tip the scales in our favor and permanently lose weight?

Yes, if we change old eating and living habits, establishing new ones for a lifetime. Otherwise, our efforts will be in vain. We have proof that trendy "diets" don't work in the long run; nor do powders, pills, shakes, bars, prepackaged meals or other gimmicky approaches. These methods may result in short-term weight loss, but with time, the weight usually returns because old patterns of living return. Often, the "post-diet" weight is greater than before the diet began and afterward, even harder to lose. This is because the body's composition changes with weight regain (more fat, less muscle), which slows down metabolism (your body's rate of calorie-burning). Regained weight is often redistributed around the "middle," which increases one's risk of heart problems, high blood pressure and diabetes.

Very low-calorie "quick fixes" do not work either. Eating too few calories can actually lead to bingeing, uncontrolled eating, muscle loss and a slowed-down metabolism.

Now, for the good news: You really can eat foods you enjoy—even brownies, ice cream and burgers—and still lose weight. You simply need:

- a practical system for food selection, balancing high-fat foods with low-fat foods
- a sensible fitness routine that "revs up" your metabolism so you can burn more body fat
- "skill-power," not "will-power"—routine habits for life.

Counseling more than 20,000 men and women for 20+ years has taught me that the key to successful weight loss is a "no gimmick" approach that puts you in charge. You choose what you eat and where—at home or out. No special foods are required. *The Cooper Clinic Solution to the Diet Revolution* (an update to *The Balancing Act Nutrition & Weight Guide*) outlines strategies that have been used successfully by Cooper Clinic patients and class participants. What strategies work?

WHO SUCCEEDS

At the Cooper Clinic, we've found that people who are most successful in losing weight:

1. **Enjoy eating a healthy mix of all foods**, balancing low-fat, high-fiber foods with higher-fat choices and developing strategies for eating favorite foods in reasonable amounts.

2. **Exercise moderately and consistently** to boost metabolism, decrease appetite, burn more body fat and feel energized.

3. **Practice "I'm in charge," sensible eating habits** and the lifestyle that promotes one's chosen weight.

4. **Shift thinking to "lifestyle" and "lifetime."** This shift away from the "on again, off again" dieting mentality sets you free and enables you to maintain a more productive life focus.

5. **Work toward moderation, balance and variety** with food choices and exercise.

6. **Set realistic goals.** Since you didn't gain overnight, you can't expect to lose overnight.

7. **Have a meaningful purpose** for losing weight and keeping it off for good.

8. **Write down a daily description of food consumed and daily exercise.** Records build awareness and motivate action. (One client was amazed to discover she was eating thousands of calories while cooking, preparing and clearing her family's plates!)

Have you heard of the "80/20" rule? I believe it can be applied to a healthy lifestyle. It means that if you make healthy choices 80% of the time, you can eat "fun foods" 20% of the time and still stay healthy and achieve your weight goals. For example, if you eat that brownie with its 250 calories and 10 fat grams, you can still lose weight. How? By using low-fat salad dressing on your salad and skipping the croutons. Or, by holding the extra tablespoon of butter on your baked potato and by drinking a glass of water instead of a 12 oz. regular soda. Either way, by making these simple trade-offs, you can enjoy the brownie, guilt-free. Chances are, you won't miss the croutons, fat-laden dressing, butter or soda. You've simply traded (and balanced out) the calories and fat.

How the "Balancing Act" Works
Using the "80/20" Rule

Example 1: *Balance the fat across the day*

	BREAKFAST	LUNCH	DINNER		*OPTIONS
	1 fruit	hamburger (1/4 lb.)	Chinese stir-fry dinner		
	1 c. cereal	small fries*	or low-fat frozen		Omit fries
	1 c. fat-free milk	1 fruit	dinner		
		1 diet drink	1 fruit		
TOTALS:	300 Calories	700 calories	350 calories	= 1350 calories vs.	1030 calories
	0 Fat	36 grams fat	8 grams fat	= 44 grams fat vs.	28 grams fat

Example 2: *Balance the fat within the meal*

	BREAKFAST	LUNCH	DINNER		*OPTIONS
	1 bagel	fast-food grilled	2 slices cheese pizza		
	1 banana	chicken sandwich	huge salad with fat-free		
	8 oz. fat-free	(no mayo)	dressing		
	fruit yogurt	small fries*	4 oz. fat-free frozen		Omit fries
		diet drink or water	yogurt		
TOTALS:	350 calories	550 calories	500 calories	= 1400 calories vs.	1180 calories
	0 fat	20 grams fat	17 grams fat	= 37 grams fat vs.	25 grams fat

Add a brisk 2-mile walk (30 minutes) and burn 200 calories. You'll net 1,150 calories the first day (Example 1) and 1,200 calories the second day (Example 2). Anyone can lose weight this way!

700 calories (45 chips or cake a la mode) *without* making a trade-off. The best trade-off? Either burn off extra calories through exercise…or cut back a little throughout the week by making sensible choices daily. Perhaps your goal is to take off 10 pounds in a year. Eliminating a mere 100 calories a day will get you there.

One man who lost 120 pounds in one year following the steps outlined in this book said,

> *"I set up this program just as I would a business. Taking certain steps daily led to my success. I wrote down what I ate daily to be accountable to myself. I preplanned meals and set up an appointment with myself daily to exercise at a set time and take a nature walk."*

Raynelle Briggs, a lovely woman I recently met in person, told me her success story of using the eating and exercise guidelines of this book and losing 100 pounds in 13 months, then 122 pounds total in 30 months. Over the first 12 months, she lost weight consistently by consuming 1,300 calories per day and "casually adding walking." Then the next six months, she lost nothing, even though she ate the same way and walked once or twice weekly. Willing to keep making lifestyle changes, she increased her walking and began riding her bike several times a week. Twenty-two pounds gradually came off over the next 12 months and she met her goal!

After losing 100 pounds, Raynelle e-mailed me this message:

> *"I wanted you to know that I feel this book is the most complete and healthy approach to weight loss I have ever read—and I have read a lot! I have lost 115 pounds over the past two years using the steps in this book. I calculated my target weight, base weight, etc., and have increased my exercise. I feel healthy! I just wanted you to know how highly I recommend this program. It really has made a difference in my life. No tricks, no gimmicks, no quick fixes…just advice that genuinely works. Thank you."*

Whether you want to lose 5, 25, 50 or 100+ pounds, the same methods work!

With the informative tips and strategies found in these pages, you will discover the ultimate keys to your best health and weight—developing the lifestyle skills for your own *"balancing act solution."* Take one step at a time. You'll see results that will last for a lifetime!

Step 1
Step Up to the Plate!

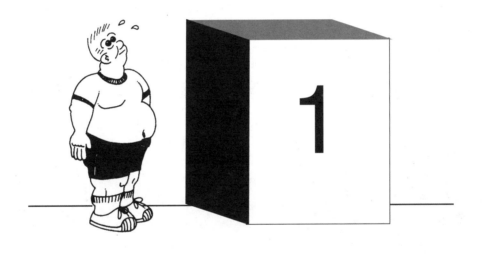

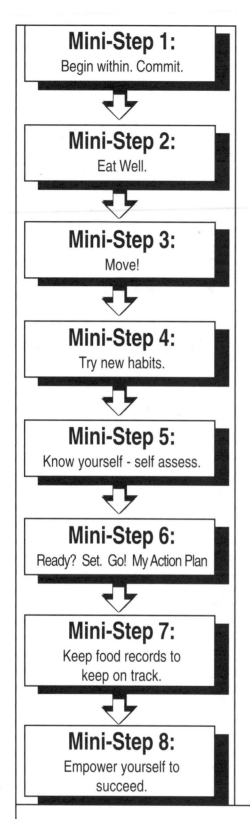

Mini-Step 1:	Begin within. Commit.
Mini-Step 2:	Eat Well.
Mini-Step 3:	Move!
Mini-Step 4:	Try new habits.
Mini-Step 5:	Know yourself - self assess.
Mini-Step 6:	Ready? Set. Go! My Action Plan
Mini-Step 7:	Keep food records to keep on track.
Mini-Step 8:	Empower yourself to succeed.

Step 1

Eating well is a major component of healthy living and weight management. Of course, more than food is involved! Many studies conducted at The Cooper Institute and other renowned organizations have demonstrated the impact of exercise *and* behavioral change on health and weight. Throughout this book, we will focus on the healthy habits one needs to develop and enjoy a better quality of life and easier weight management. Step 1 lays an important foundation, so I encourage you not to jump ahead before you cover the pages in this chapter. Some of the nuggets you'll walk away with include:

- a visual understanding of what a balanced plate looks like
- a formula to determine your calorie needs, based on your desired weight and activity level
- tips on how to feel satisfied while cutting back on calories
- the low-down on some of today's popular diets
- my "Ten Golden Rules for Healthy Eating & Weight Loss" and the five easiest steps to take you there
- ways to overcome roadblocks, so lifestyles can change
- success tips from expert losers

Make sure you complete the Self-Assessment questionnaire on p. 23 - 25. This will help you see what factors have contributed to your being overweight and will help motivate you to establish new habits for life!

ACTION STEPS

① Forget about quick-fixes. Focus on the long-term behaviors needed to eat more healthfully and exercise regularly.

② Identify and make changes gradually. Have a positive attitude. Enjoy yourself!

③ Establish your overall game plan and ways to overcome barriers to change.

④ Keep food, exercise and weight records.

⑤ Find activities you enjoy to build muscle and burn fat.

Think Healthy

This book shows you how to eat right, exercise efficiently and create the lifestyle habits that promote a permanent, healthy weight. As a result, you'll look and feel your best. But first, there are a couple of points to grasp as you prepare to become a healthier you.

Give Up the Belief in a "Quick - Fix"

Later in this section, you will read more about the pitfalls of "miracle diets" that entice Americans to spend $20 billion each year pursuing leanness and youthfulness. These quick-fix diet programs don't work long-term because they do not produce lasting solutions. Beyond the negative physiological impact of repeatedly losing and regaining weight, the psychological impact can be devastating. Shift gears now to avoid the disappointment and frustration that can be so demoralizing.

Why Most Quick-Fix Diets Fail

- New behaviors, healthy eating habits, good food choices and smart "trade-off" eating **cannot be learned** if you are relying on fad diets, special products, etc. Nutrition-wise, "food replacements" cannot replace meals; nor are they habit replacements.
- Standardized programs become boring and **too rigid** to follow long-term. By choosing your own personalized, varied eating plan, you'll enjoy your meals and "stay with the program" for lifetime success.
- Your **metabolism slows down**. Fast weight loss means muscle loss. Losing weight slowly and exercising regularly helps your body burn more body fat, retain muscle, boost your metabolism, speed weight loss and keep the weight off.
- **Medical complications** can arise from diets that are too restrictive, low in calories, or unbalanced.

Remember: There is no miracle cure or "magic potion" to melt fat away.

 Eating right + Exercise + Sensible lifestyle habits = A HEALTHY WEIGHT

Commit Yourself to Unlearning Old Habits and Relearning New Ones

Eating is one of our most complex behaviors. Eating behaviors are deeply entrenched and learned through a lifetime of family, ethnic, cultural and religious customs. Fortunately, just as we learn how to eat, we can *relearn* to eat. New behaviors enable us to attain and maintain a desired weight. To get started, don a fresh attitude and commit to change.

What Experiences and Attitudes Influence Your Eating Habits?

If you grew up with the following thoughts and sayings, you will need to develop a new mind-set, discarding ideas that simply have no merit.

- "Clean your plates. Children in far-off lands are starving."
- "Eat your vegetables and clean your plate before you can have dessert."
- "A fat child is a healthy child."
- Food may be served as rewards. Food may be equated with love.
- Food is associated with social life.
- Food is comfort; a tranquilizer; a "companion."

What Types of Ads Influence Your Eating Behavior?

Marketing executives do their best to persuade you to try and buy their product. Don't let them make your buying decisions for you. You know your body and eating habits better than anybody else. Beware of the following gimmicks:

- discount coupons, mailers
- all-you-can-eat promotions
- tantalizing magazine and newspaper ads
- colorful billboard adds
- enticing food packaging
- exciting menus and recipes

Learning new eating behaviors and how to make informed food decisions is a gradual process that becomes ingrained over time. Repeating behaviors becomes "habit." Make your habits work *for* you . . . not against you. Create habits that work!

Key Points:

- **Small, permanent lifestyle changes are better than large, temporary ones.**
- **Small, permanent weight losses are better than large, temporary ones.**

Are you ready to become more energetic, vibrant, productive and stress-resistant? Step 1 involves the right mind-set, followed by good nutrition, an exercise routine and healthy habits. Be informed!

  © 2009, *The Cooper Clinic Solution to the Diet Revolution* by Georgia G. Kostas, M.P.H., R.D., L.D., Dallas, Texas

Attitude Check

A positive attitude is important as you make life-changing decisions that will impact not only you, but others around you. Examine your motives. Focus on developing a realistic approach by acting on principles listed below: ☑

- ☐ Set realistic target weight (see chart on p. 36).
- ☐ Set realistic weight-loss goals of 2-4 pounds/month (women), 4-8 pounds/month (men).
- ☐ Let go of a "quick-fix" mode and think long-term.
- ☐ Anticipate eating events, meals out, etc. Visualize how you'll handle them. Be prepared.
- ☐ Be motivated by how great you feel.
- ☐ Acquire a "take charge," "action oriented" approach to weight loss rather than a passive "victimized" approach.
- ☐ Stay positive and upbeat. Practice positive self-talk; counter negative thoughts immediately!
- ☐ Don't let a slip-up make you give up. Get back on track. A "yield" or "stop" is not a "dead-end!"
- ☐ Re-identify yourself as a physically active person—a recreational athlete.
- ☐ Avoid "all or none" thinking. Blend high-fat food choices with low-fat food choices for balance.
- ☐ Aim for progress, not perfection.
- ☐ Think one day at a time.
- ☐ Surround yourself with support: motivational reading, encouraging family and friends, etc.
- ☐ Keep reminding yourself it's never too late to change.
- ☐ Think before you eat.
- ☐ Take charge of your eating and your life!
- ☐ Keep it simple.
- ☐ Don't deprive yourself.
- ☐ Recognize that *small changes count*. **Yes, they add up—and they last.**

BOTTOM LINE
1. Make small changes.
2. Make changes you can successfully do.

Eating for Health

Healthy eating is all about **balance!** The right balance promotes your best health and weight.

THE BALANCING ACT
Overeating or underexercising upsets your caloric balance. Extra pounds result.

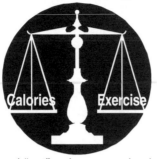

Complex Carbohydrates (C)
(Plant Foods) Grain/starch, Vegetables & Fruits

Proteins (P) + Fats (F)

LOOK AT YOUR PLATE!
P-C-F Balance satisfies appetite, reduces hunger & sustains energy between meals.

Adjust your calories "in" and "out" to lose or maintain weight.

☐ Shade those you currently do
☑ Check those you will try

Food Balance & Variety

1. Vary foods consumed daily to maximize nutrient variety.
   - ☐ Select 3-5 plant foods and 3-5 colors per meal (colors denote nutrients).
   - ☐ Choose fresh, wholesome, unprocessed foods.
   - ☐ Divide your plate (as pictured above) to balance your meals, overall diet and portions.
2. Strive daily for this optimal nutrient balance:

NUTRIENT	% OF CALORIES	WHAT / HOW MUCH TO EAT DAILY
LEAN PROTEIN	10 to 25%	☐ 4-8 oz. fish, poultry, lean meat, dried peas or beans & ☐ 2-3 c. fat-free or low-fat milk or yogurt
COMPLEX CARBOHYDRATE	45 to 65%	☐ 5-10 fruit and vegetables, at least 2 raw, plus. . . ☐ 5-8 starches, at least 3 wholegrains
HEALTHY FAT	20 to 35%	☐ 3-8 tsp. added fats (margarine, oil, dressing, nuts) ☐ Eat only baked or broiled foods, not fried
WATER		☐ 4 glasses (1 quart) minimum plus 1 quart other fluids

For Energy and Appetite Control

1. ☐ Mix protein-carbohydrate-fat at each meal (P-C-F Balance) to feel full and "last longer" between meals.
2. ☐ Eat every 3-6 hours. Establish consistent eating patterns. Consume 3 meals and 1-2 snacks daily. Do not skip meals. Eat breakfast (to eat less and better all day).
3. ☐ Eat slowly in a relaxed environment. Enjoy every meal, snack or bite.

Healthier Selections

CHOOSE LEAN PROTEIN

- ☐ fish - 2+ times per week
- ☐ ≤ 12 oz. lean meat cuts per week
- ☐ beans - 4 times per week

EAT MORE FIBER RICH COMPLEX CARBS

- ☐ fruit
- ☐ vegetables
- ☐ potatoes
- ☐ peas/beans
- ☐ lentils
- ☐ corn
- ☐ popcorn
- ☐ wholewheat bread & cereals
- ☐ bran
- ☐ brown rice
- ☐ cracked wheat
- ☐ oatmeal
- ☐ grits
- ☐ kashi

EAT MORE FIBER

- ☐ Eat at least 8 fiber foods daily to:
  - regulate blood sugar & cholesterol levels
  - help feel more satisfied &, therefore, eat less per meal
  - aid digestion
  - aid prevention of digestive problems and colon cancer

LIMIT CHOLESTEROL & SATURATED FAT

- ☐ egg yolks & organ meats
- ☐ fatty meats (sausage, cold cuts, bacon, ground beef)
- ☐ high-fat dairy products (whole milk, sour or sweet cream, cheese, ice cream, butter)
- ☐ fried foods
- ☐ pastries, baked goods
- ☐ commercial snack foods

Eat Less Total Fat

- ☐ fried foods
- ☐ butter & margarine
- ☐ mayonnaise
- ☐ salad dressings
- ☐ sauces
- ☐ nuts (1-3 Tbsp. / day)
- ☐ avocados
- ☐ granola
- ☐ crackers/chips
- ☐ dips
- ☐ fast foods
- ☐ convenience foods
- ☐ commercial pastries
- ☐ commercial snack foods
- ☐ high-fat meats (bacon, sausage, cold cuts, hot dogs, marbled beef, lamb & pork, burgers)
- ☐ high-fat dairy products (whole milk, sour or sweet cream, cheese, ice cream, butter)

1 Tbsp. fat (3 tsp.) = 100 calories!

Omit 2 Tbsp. of fat per day & you'll lose 20 pounds a year!

Choose Healthier Fats

Polyunsaturated
(with Omega-6's)

- ☐ Vegetable oils - safflower, corn, sunflower, soybean
- ☐ soft tub trans-free magarines
- ☐ nuts, seeds
- ☐ non-hydrogenated peanutbutter

Polyunsaturated
(with Omega-3's)

- ☐ Seafood, especially salmon, tuna steak, sardines, bass, haddock
- ☐ canola oil
- ☐ flaxseeds
- ☐ flax oil
- ☐ walnuts

These lower lipid (cholesterol and triglyceride) levels.

Monounsaturated

- ☐ olive oil, olives
- ☐ peanut oil, peanuts
- ☐ canola oil
- ☐ avocado
- ☐ almonds
- ☐ nuts, seeds

Less: Saturated

- ☐ dairy foods (with butterfat)
- ☐ meats
- ☐ "hydrogenated" (trans) fats in commercial baked goods and fried foods
- ☐ butter
- ☐ chocolate
- ☐ coconut
- ☐ palm oil

These raise lipids.

Less is Best! Limit:

☐ SUGAR

Limit to 1-3 sweets a week.

Sugar sources: table sugar, honey, jam, jelly, soft drinks. desserts, candy, cookies, cakes, pastries, processed foods and beverages, sweetened juices and fruit, sugar-coated cereals and peanutbutter. Most desserts are rich in sugar, fat and calories.

☐ SODIUM

Limit your sodium to 2400 mg (1 tsp. salt) to 4000 mg daily.

Main sources: salt, pickles, olives, luncheon meats, hot dogs, ham, bacon, sausage, cheeses, processed foods, fast foods, packaged snack foods (chips, crackers, pretzels), canned soups and vegetables, sauces (chili, barbecue, soy, steak), pizza, commercial bakery products.

☐ CAFFEINE

Limit to 200 mg daily (two 6-oz. cups of coffee).

Caffeine is a stimulant found in coffee, tea and cola drinks. Replace caffeine with water.

☐ ALCOHOL

Limit alcohol as your doctor directs. At most:
Men: 0-2 drinks per day
Women: 0-1 drink per day
A drink is 1 1/2 oz. liquor, 4 oz. wine, 1 light beer, 12 oz. regular beer. Each contains 100-150 calories. Alcohol sabotages weight loss efforts by slowing down the burning of fat stores. On an empty stomach, alcohol impairs judgement. Drink with food!

In Summary - Create Your Own Balancing Act!

- ☐ Enjoy the pleasure of eating healthy foods that taste great using these guidelines!
- ☐ Be physically active. Exercise aerobically 5 times per week (30-45 minutes) & strength train 2-3 days per week (20-30 minutes). Fitness adds health & energy, suppresses appetite & helps you feel & look your best!

Step Up to the Plate!

Here's what a healthy plate looks like!

A healthy, balanced meal is 20-35% fat, 45-65% carbohydrate and 10-25% protein. This means, on your dinner plate, cover **3/4ᵗʰ plate** with **plant foods** (complex carbohydrates such as vegetables, fruit, grains/ starches, beans), choosing, for example, equal portions of carrots, green beans and rice. Limit **protein** to **1/4ᵗʰ** of your plate (i.e., 3 oz. of fish, chicken, lean meat).

"HOME PLATE"
Follow the "3/4ᵗʰ Plate Rule"
(as depicted on book cover)

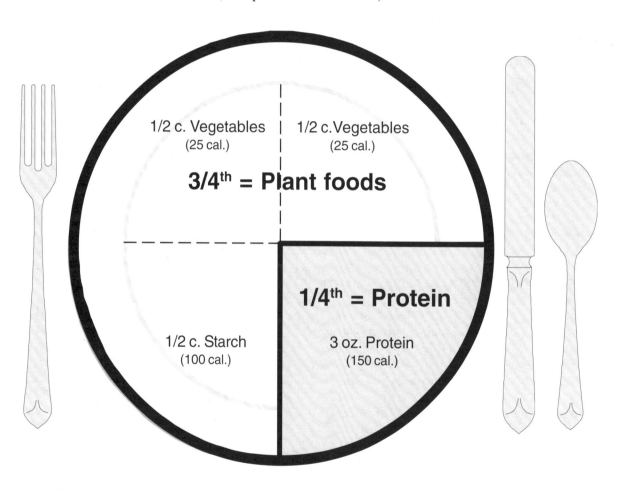

1/2 c. Vegetables (25 cal.) | 1/2 c.Vegetables (25 cal.)

3/4ᵗʰ = Plant foods

1/4ᵗʰ = Protein

1/2 c. Starch (100 cal.)

3 oz. Protein (150 cal.)

Balance Your Diet By . . .

- eating 1/4 protein, 1/4 starch, 1/2 vegetables on your plate.
- blending higher fat with lower fat foods per meal or per week.
- eating 8-9 high-fiber foods a day (3 fruit, 3 vegetables, 3 wholegrains/beans).
- keeping fat at ≤ 50 grams a day (in 6 oz. protein and 1-3 Tbsp. oil/fat).

Standard Base Plates for Weight Loss

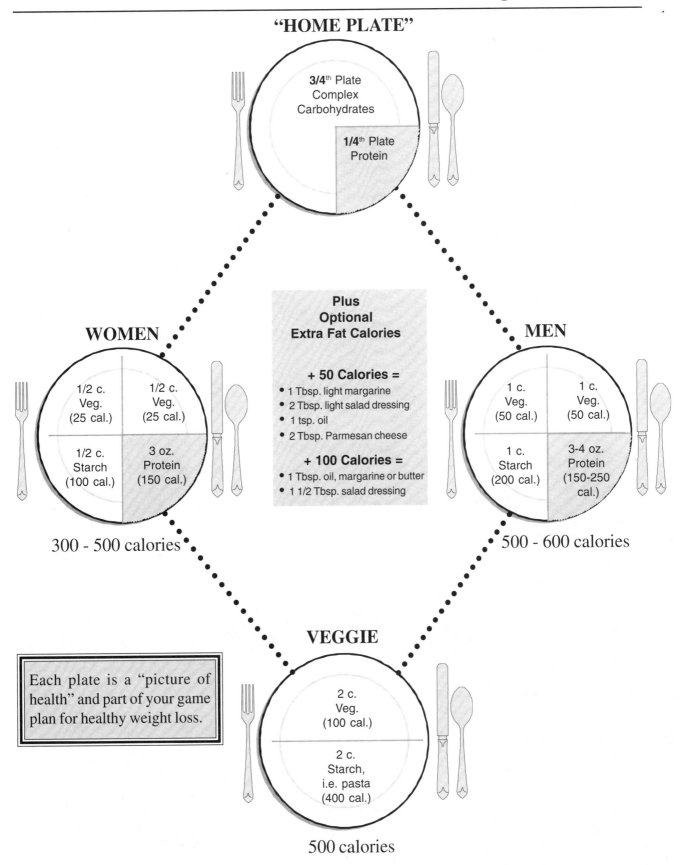

"HOME PLATE"

3/4th Plate
Complex
Carbohydrates

1/4th Plate
Protein

WOMEN

1/2 c.
Veg.
(25 cal.)

1/2 c.
Veg.
(25 cal.)

1/2 c.
Starch
(100 cal.)

3 oz.
Protein
(150 cal.)

300 - 500 calories

**Plus
Optional
Extra Fat Calories**

+ 50 Calories =
- 1 Tbsp. light margarine
- 2 Tbsp. light salad dressing
- 1 tsp. oil
- 2 Tbsp. Parmesan cheese

+ 100 Calories =
- 1 Tbsp. oil, margarine or butter
- 1 1/2 Tbsp. salad dressing

MEN

1 c.
Veg.
(50 cal.)

1 c.
Veg.
(50 cal.)

1 c.
Starch
(200 cal.)

3-4 oz.
Protein
(150-250
cal.)

500 - 600 calories

Each plate is a "picture of health" and part of your game plan for healthy weight loss.

VEGGIE

2 c.
Veg.
(100 cal.)

2 c.
Starch,
i.e. pasta
(400 cal.)

500 calories

Winning Strategies for Your "Game Plan"

Since 3,500 calories = 1 pound of fat, here's how to lose 1-2 pounds a week			
CALORIES Food + Exercise	CALORIES Daily	CALORIES Weekly	LOSE Weekly
↓ 250 + ↑ 250 =	500	3500	1 pound
↓ 750 + ↑ 250 =	1000	7000	2 pounds

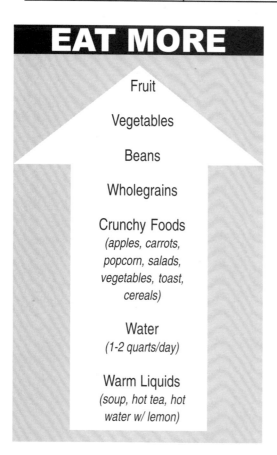

EAT MORE

Fruit

Vegetables

Beans

Wholegrains

Crunchy Foods
(apples, carrots, popcorn, salads, vegetables, toast, cereals)

Water
(1-2 quarts/day)

Warm Liquids
(soup, hot tea, hot water w/ lemon)

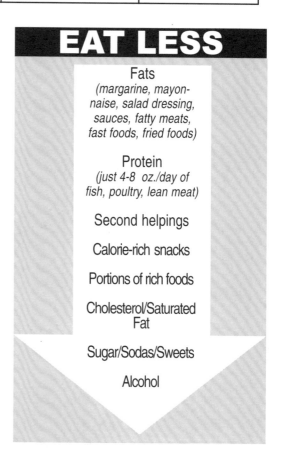

EAT LESS

Fats
(margarine, mayonnaise, salad dressing, sauces, fatty meats, fast foods, fried foods)

Protein
(just 4-8 oz./day of fish, poultry, lean meat)

Second helpings

Calorie-rich snacks

Portions of rich foods

Cholesterol/Saturated Fat

Sugar/Sodas/Sweets

Alcohol

5 Basic Tips for Weight Loss

1. Don't wait too long to eat. It's best to eat every three to six hours, using the P-C-F Balance (p. 47-48).

2. Eat foods that last—add a little protein at each meal.

3. Eat only 1/2 of entrée when ordering out, and double up on veggies for more fiber, vitamins, minerals, antioxidants…and less fat, cholesterol and calories.

4. Eat the "3/4th plate" way—for balance and correct calories (500-700 calories).

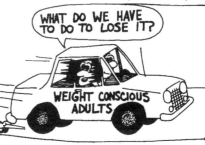

5. Drink more water: 16 oz. when you get up, 16 oz. at lunch, 16 oz. afternoon, 16 oz. dinner.

Ten Golden Rules
for Healthy Eating & Weight Loss

1. **Eat often** . . . every three to six hours (with the P-C-F balance) to:

   - Keep energy high
   - Keep appetite low
   - Lessen stress
   - Feel your best

   - Prevent overeating
   - Make better food decisions
   - Keep blood sugar stable, longer
   - Feel enthusiastic

2. **Follow the "3/4th Plate Rule."** When plant foods comprise most of your lunch/dinner plate, you automatically consume meals with the correct portions and balance. (Choose equal amounts of two vegetables and one starch, and 3-4 oz. protein.)

3. **Choose quality: eat a high-fiber, low-fat diet.**
   - **Fiber**: Double your fruit and vegetables daily . . . eat 5+ servings a day (two fruit, three vegetables). Choose eight to nine plant foods daily (2+ fruit, 3+ vegetables, 3+ wholegrains, beans).
   - **Fat**: A little fat at each meal delays hunger. Choose 1-3 tsp. per meal. *Note: Fiber fills you up. Fat lasts. Both delay hunger.*

4. **Plan ahead.** Think before you eat. Make healthy eating convenient. Keep foods and snacks on hand.

5. **Have a game plan** - a system for eating right that fits your day's schedule.

6. **Set ground rules for yourself** - eating out, portions, snacks, meal timing, etc.

7. **Move more daily.**

8. **Get hooked on healthy habits.** Small changes produce big results.

9. **Write it down.** Records raise awareness, action, accountability.

10. **Don't let a slip-up make you give up.** Keep going!

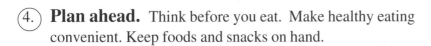
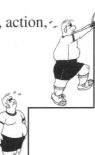

Five Easy Steps
to Healthier Eating & Weight Loss

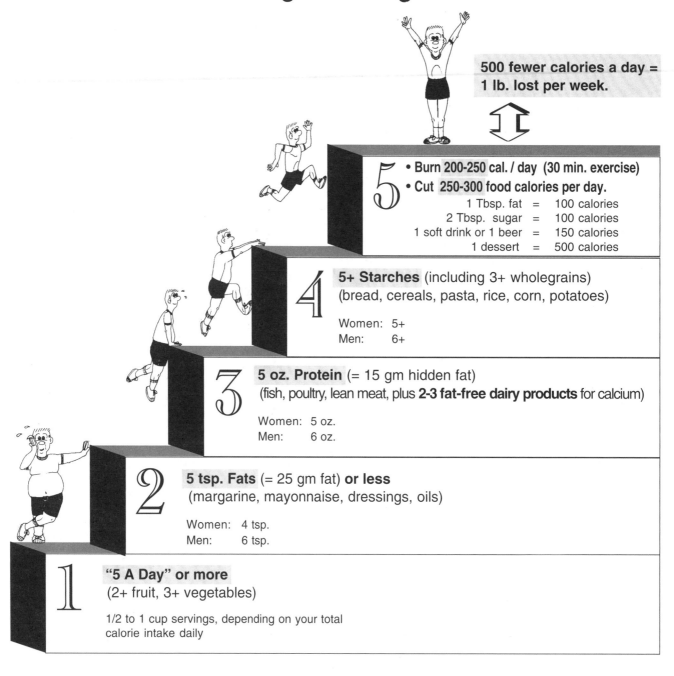

500 fewer calories a day =
1 lb. lost per week.

5
- Burn **200-250** cal. / day (30 min. exercise)
- Cut **250-300** food calories per day.

1 Tbsp. fat	=	100 calories
2 Tbsp. sugar	=	100 calories
1 soft drink or 1 beer	=	150 calories
1 dessert	=	500 calories

4
5+ Starches (including 3+ wholegrains)
(bread, cereals, pasta, rice, corn, potatoes)

Women: 5+
Men: 6+

3
5 oz. Protein (= 15 gm hidden fat)
(fish, poultry, lean meat, plus **2-3 fat-free dairy products** for calcium)

Women: 5 oz.
Men: 6 oz.

2
5 tsp. Fats (= 25 gm fat) **or less**
(margarine, mayonnaise, dressings, oils)

Women: 4 tsp.
Men: 6 tsp.

1
"5 A Day" or more
(2+ fruit, 3+ vegetables)

1/2 to 1 cup servings, depending on your total
calorie intake daily

Take Five Steps to Better Health!

Balancing Eating With Exercise

In recent years, studies have shown that most people who successfully lose weight and keep it off for at least five years not only change their eating habits, but they incorporate some sort of regular physical activity into their lifestyle. I encourage my patients to find activities they will do at least several days a week. In addition to helping them lose or maintain their weight, exercise has the power to boost one's spirits and help prevent some diseases such as cardiovascular disease.

Have Realistic Expectations

Don't expect the pounds to fly off you when you begin healthier habits. Instead, **a successful weight-reduction program involves a gradual weight loss of ½ to 2 pounds a week**, which allows you to:

- maintain nutritionally balanced meals
- lose body fat, not muscle
- produce big results
- maintain your weight loss

> *Cooper Clinic studies show that women realistically lose 2-4 pounds/month, men 5 per month.*

Calories Count

You can make calorie-cutting easier by adding exercise and cutting back on portions. Let me show you specifics:

- To lose **½ pound** per week, decrease your daily calories by **250**.
- To lose **1 pound** per week, decrease your daily calories by **500**.
- To lose **2 pounds** per week, decrease your daily calories by **1000**.

Calorie Cuts	
Example:	**Calories Omitted per Day**
⇒ Reduce 8-oz. meat portion to 4-oz.	280
⇒ Reduce salad dressing to 1 Tbsp. (not 3 Tbsp.)	200
⇒ Snack on a crunchy apple instead of 1/2 c. peanuts	270
⇒ Walk 52 minutes per day (2 1/2 miles per day)	250
Total Calories Saved Daily =	**1000**
In seven days, lose two pounds!	

3500 CALORIES = 1 POUND

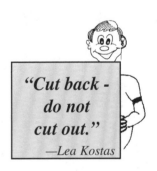

"Cut back - do not cut out."
—Lea Kostas

Small Changes...Big Results!

At first, trying to shed pounds can seem difficult. But truly, it's easier than you think:

! An extra 100 calories, such as a large apple, 20 peanuts or 1 Tbsp. margarine, each day adds up to 36,500 calories in one year. **That's 10 extra pounds!**

! Walking 30 minutes daily burns 200 calories per day and 73,000 calories a year. **That's 20 pounds** lost a year!

! Omit 300 calories a day (100 from each meal), and **you'll lose 30 pounds in a year!**

You don't have to be an athlete to benefit greatly from physical activity. Exercise:

- Burns calories and helps maintain weight loss
- Promotes fat-burning and decreases body fat
- Speeds metabolism (calorie-burning)
- Improves physical fitness and muscle tone
- Increases cardiopulmonary health

- Suppresses appetite
- Minimizes stress
- Maximizes energy
- Enhances mental health
- Enhances emotional well-being

Lose 10 Pounds in 10 Weeks!
A simple 3-step solution:

① **Trim off 300 calories from your daily diet. Options:**

		Calories Omitted
◆	Omit 1 Tbsp. mayonnaise, oil, butter	100
◆	Omit 1 Tbsp. salad dressing	50-100
◆	Drink 8 oz. fat-free milk instead of whole	100
◆	Cut back on snacks and high-calorie drinks	150+
◆	Drink 6 oz. of orange juice instead of 12 oz.	100
◆	Eat 4 oz. of lean meat/poultry instead of 6 oz.	100

⇨ choose 300 / day

② **Walk 2 miles in 30 minutes, five times a week:** 1000/week*

= 1400 cal. / week

③ **Lift weights for 40 minutes, twice a week:** 400/week*

⇩

200 / day (average)

Based on a person weighing 150 lbs. If you weigh more, you'll burn more calories.

For mathematicians:

Consuming 300 less calories a day and burning 200 daily means omitting 500 calories a day . . . or 3500 a week . . . and 3500 calories = 1 lb. lost!

The Perfect Balance

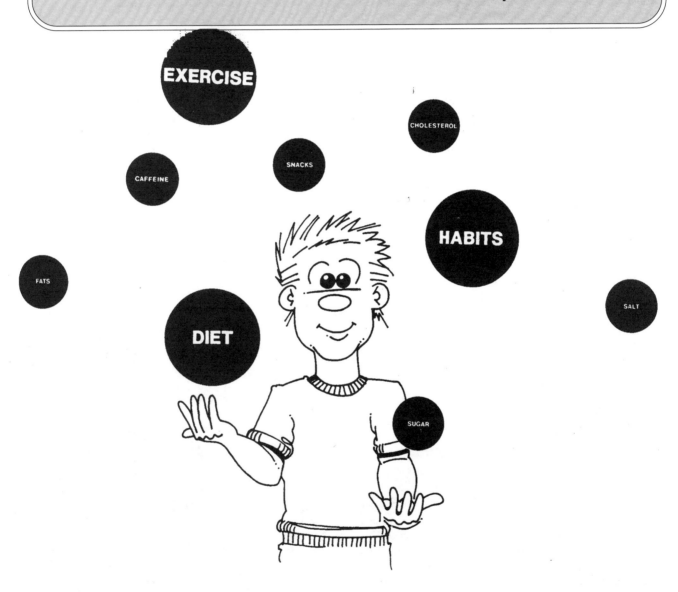

A HEALTHY WEIGHT = eating right + exercise + sensible lifestyle habits

combined with

desire . . . determination . . . consistency

EXERCISE

CHOLESTEROL

SNACKS

CAFFEINE

HABITS

FATS

SALT

DIET

SUGAR

EAT RIGHT! GET FIT! LOSE WEIGHT! FEEL GREAT!

Body Composition & Metabolism

You must change your body composition to change your weight for life. Your body composition says much more than the numbers on a scale. I encourage you to **focus on body composition as your primary weight objective**. The more muscle you have, the more permanent your weight loss. Muscle speeds metabolism (calories you burn daily), so that you burn more body fat and leave it off.

> **Total Weight = Fat + Lean Body Mass (muscle, bone, water)**

Exercise: A Prerequisite for Maintaining or Gaining Muscle & Metabolism

Each year, as part of the aging process, we lose muscle and gain fat. This process slows down metabolism and, consequently, one gains body fat and weight. The only way to prevent or reverse this process is to exercise. For best results, I recommend both **aerobic exercise**, which helps keep the muscle and lose the fat, along with **weight training**, which helps build muscle. Why both?

- If you lose weight without exercise, you lose approximately 50% lean tissue and 50% fat. If you cut back on fat calories *and* exercise, the majority of the pounds you lose are fat, not lean tissue.
- An extra pound of muscle burns an extra 30 to 50 calories a day. That adds up!
- The more muscle you have, the more you can eat to maintain weight because your metabolism is higher. An extra 5 pounds of muscle can burn an extra 250 calories per day!

A Word on Body Composition & Metabolism*

You can be the same height and weight and have different body compositions at different times in life, and therefore, have different calorie needs. The more muscle you have, the more you can eat to maintain weight because your metabolism is higher.

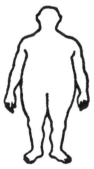

200 Pounds
150 pounds lean body mass
50 pounds fat (25%)
needs **2000** calories per day
(200 lbs. x 10 calories per lb.)

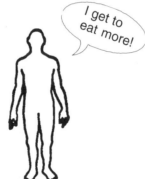

I get to eat more!

200 Pounds
175 pounds lean body mass
25 pounds fat (12.5%)
needs **3000** calories per day
(200 lbs. x 15 calories per lb.)

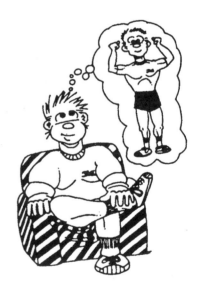

> Your most appropriate percent body fat and weight are based on your age, health status, fitness level, body build and other individual factors. Check with your physician or dietitian for your most appropriate body fat and weight. The Cooper Clinic recommends: **MEN:** 10-20% (avg: <20%)   **WOMEN:** 18-27% (avg: <24%)

*The best ways to measure body composition are with underwater weighing and skinfold measurements done with calipers at seven body sites. A trained expert is a must. Check with your local YMCA or physician's office.

Get Moving!

How active are you? You cannot improve your body composition, fitness, fat-burning potential, metabolic rate, and enjoy lasting fitness and weight-loss results unless you exercise regularly and strive to live an active lifestyle.

The American College of Sports Medicine and The Cooper Clinic recommend:

- aerobic exercise 30-45 minutes, 4-5 times a week to **lose body fat**.
- strength training (i.e., weights) 20-30 minutes, 2-3 times a week to **build muscle**.
- burning 200-300 calories a day, as the above allows.
  (This type of routine builds muscle and burns fat.)

Set Some Goals

Work up to burning approximately 250 calories a day as follows:

Activity	Calories Per Hour	Time Needed to Burn 250 Calories
Walking, 4 mph (15 min. per mile)	415	42 min.
Tennis (doubles)	405	37 min.
Aerobic Dance	405	37 min.
Downhill Skiing	475	32 min.
Skating (moderate)	475	32 min.
Swimming, crawl (50 yd/min.)	545	28 min.
Jogging, 5 mph (12 min. per mile)	540	28 min.
Biking, 13 mph	545	28 min.
Stair-climbing (machine)	545	28 min.
Jogging, 7 mph (8.5 min. per mile)	780	20 min.
Handball, Squash	815	19 min.

NOTE: *These figures are for a 150-pound person. If you weigh more, you'll burn more calories in the same time; if you weigh less, you'll burn fewer calories.*

■ *See p. 154 - 155 for calories burned from various exercises at various body weights and to develop your own best exercise and fitness program.*

Bottom line: Keep moving!

it Assessment

Another important step in a successful weight-loss program is being able to identify your eating habits. When you become familiar with your own behaviors, you can more easily make lifestyle changes. Complete the form below to identify key habits that contribute to your overeating. Be honest and mark the habits that you need to modify. Work toward new ways of eating.

ASSESSMENT OF EATING HABITS

FACTOR	EATING BEHAVIOR - DO YOU:	YES	NO
Meal Time	1. eat at irregular meal times daily?		
	2. eat unpredictably from day to day?		
	3. eat fewer than three meals a day?		
	4. skip meals?		
	5. snack excessively between meals?		
Length	6. eat rapidly? (less than 20 minutes a meal)		
Place	7. eat in more than one room at home?		
	8. eat in more than one place in your kitchen?		
	9. eat standing up or lying down?		
	10. eat while involved in other activities (i.e., reading, writing, watching TV, working)?		
Environment	11. eat more food when alone? If "yes," why?		
Social	12. eat more with others? If "yes," why?		
Mood	13. eat under stress?		
	14. eat in response to moods? Which ones?		
Amount	15. take second helpings?		
	16. feel guilty if you leave an "unclean" plate?		
	17. add more "extras" - butter, jam, salad dressing, gravies, sauces?		
Type of Food	18. frequently (daily) eat high-calorie foods (fried foods, creamy foods, desserts, soft drinks, alcohol)?		
	19. eat fewer than five fruits and vegetables daily?		
	20. drink less than 6-8 glasses of fluids daily?		

A "yes" answer to any of these questions identifies behaviors to retrain for successful weight loss. *Which must you focus on for maximum benefits?* (Rank them and focus on one at a time.) This book will outline strategies in each section to help you establish new habits.

Helpful Habits

You must change your habits to change your weight—your eating habits, exercise patterns and your way of thinking about food, moods and physical activity. This means making a few lifestyle changes...for life! Focus on one to two key habits per week, as listed below.

Top Ten Habits

1. **Eat three meals at regular times daily.** Do not skip meals or change your eating patterns each day. Skipping meals leads to overeating or bingeing. Feel more energetic and speed your metabolism by eating every three to six hours. This also reduces appetite.

2. **Eat slowly.** Take at least 20 minutes for meals, 10 minutes for snacks. You will feel more satisfied with smaller food quantities and eat less than those who eat fast. It takes 20 minutes for the brain to sense the stomach's signal, "I'm full!"

3. **Eat in one place. Sit down. Enjoy! Eat mindfully.** Be aware of unconscious eating in front of the TV, at the movies, while reading or studying, driving, cooking or standing. Eat sitting only. When you are involved in an activity while eating, you can be distracted from really tasting or enjoying your food; consequently, it is easy to overeat (almost an unconscious act!). Savor each bite. Taste and chew slowly. Involve your senses...the aroma, flavor, texture, mouth-feel, crunch of each bite.

4. **Be alert to what affects your eating behavior,** especially social eating (people, places, special occasions), moods, time of day, etc. Avoid or be cautious in situations that encourage overeating. Choose quality, low-fat, low-calorie foods. Don't stand next to the food table, etc.

5. **Plan ahead** to ensure quality food choices and eating strategies for restaurants, parties, weekends, etc. With the right foods present, meals and snacks are healthier. Plan daily. Avoid restaurants such as all-you-can-eat buffets, where it's easy to overindulge. Write down what you'll eat before eating!

6. **Keep food out of sight.** Make problematic foods inconvenient or unavailable. Keep low-calorie foods convenient. Put raw vegetables and fruit in the front of your refrigerator. Serve food from the stove, not in bowls on the table.

7. **Control emotional eating.** Resolve emotion with motion. Don't reach for food to make you content or relaxed. Do something: move or communicate. Food is not the answer.

8. **Add pleasure** to your life in ways other than with food. Reward yourself for changing habits.

9. **Support your efforts at controlled eating** by putting yourself in supportive situations. Don't let weak "dieters" weaken you! You are not on a "diet!"

10. **Control the type and amount of food you choose.**

How To Change Habits

Improving one's life involves change—inside and out. Change may begin within and direct outer (behavioral) change. Or, change may begin outwardly with behavioral changes that later lead to inner changes (motivation, self-esteem, etc.). Either way, the desired outcome results.

Change is energized by a synergy of mind, spirit and will. One activates the other, or all three act together to motivate behavior change.

How will you establish new habits?

Take These 4 Steps - The 4 A's:

Awareness ♣
♣ What, where, when, why you eat. Keep records daily—to be aware constantly. ♣ A

Action ♥
♥ Take small steps in a consistent direction. Practice, practice, practice! ♠ A

Accountability ♠
♠ Report to yourself, a significant other, a health professional. ♠ A

Auto-pilot ♦
♦ Automatically assume the habits and choices that enable healthy eating and weight management. ♦ A

Stages of Change:

"I know what to do...I just can't seem to do it." Sound familiar? Your mental readiness progresses through stages, moving you forward to make changes. You can help yourself move from one stage to the next. See more on this in Appendix E. Which stage are you in today?

The stages of change include:

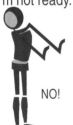

(1.) **Resistance:** "I'm not ready."

NO!

(2.) **Semi-ready:** "I'm thinking about it." "I need to change but don't know how."

ON YOUR MARK!

(3.) **Getting ready:** "I want to change." "I'm preparing for action." (I have the correct foods at home, walking shoes, action plan, etc.)

GET READY! GET SET!

(4.) **Ready:** "I take action daily to eat well and be active...I've been doing this for 4 months."

GO!

(5.) **Routine:** "This new lifestyle is *me*!" "It's been 6 months now and I'm still with it."

KEEP GOING!

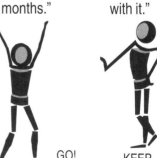

Based on Dr. J. O. Prochaska's Behavioral Model of Stages of Change:
① Pre-contemplation
② Contemplation
③ Preparation
④ Action
⑤ Maintenance

⇒ *See Appendix E for details.*

Factors That Enable Change:

1. Establish the right mind-set—a positive attitude; commitment and discipline; recognition that gradual changes are lasting changes.
2. Eat mindfully: enjoy the texture, aroma, color and taste of each bite; eat slowly.
3. Plan ahead/think ahead/have a game plan daily (keep account of what you eat before you eat it).
4. Plan purposeful physical activity daily.

Initiating Change:

1. Identify your trouble spots (habits, sweets, snacks, favorite restaurants, etc.). Establish solutions.
2. List your barriers to change. Create solutions.
3. Take one step at a time.
4. Solicit support. Be accountable to self and others. Counsel with an expert.
5. Persevere.

How To Overcome Barriers To Change:

What are your barriers to change? Strategize what will overcome the barriers. Examples:

BARRIER	STRATEGIES & SOLUTIONS
Time (grab-and-go eating style)	• Think ahead by taking portable, healthy food with you. • Select healthier fast-food alternatives such as sandwich shops, grocery store salad bars, cafeterias, soup bars, etc.
Convenience	• Plan ahead. Take cooked chicken breasts home to add to frozen vegetables for a stir-fry. • Know 4-5 quick-fix meals for daily last-minute cooking.
Knowledge	• Learn which foods are the most healthful choices at your favorite restaurants and which snacks are best. • Read labels at the grocery store so you can make better selections.
Attitude	• Remember that making change is worth it! Little changes add up to big results. • You don't have to "give up" a favorite food. Simply eat it in much smaller amounts.
Habit	• Know your pitfalls. If you typically eat a big container of popcorn at a movie, for example, eat before going to the theater so you will not be hungry.
Portions	• Be aware that the typical restaurant meal contains 2,000 to 2,500 calories. • Lose the "bigger is better" mentality. Know how to transform meals out to 500-700 calories. • Set "ground rules" for portions, and follow your plan.

Continued

BARRIER	STRATEGIES & SOLUTIONS
Emotions	• Understand the role food plays and find other sources of fun, relaxation, comfort, etc. • Choose lower-calorie options. Use motion to resolve *emotions*.
Stress	• Learn new ways to lessen stress and respond to it healthfully.
Self-deception	• No excuses! Recognize portions and healthy choices.
Boredom	• Eat at least five foods per meal. • Seek variety.
"All-or-none" attitude	• Avoid the word "diet." Instead, work on a system that enables portion management, moderation and an "all foods fit in" approach.
Speed-eating and not chewing enough	• Slow down! You will feel more "full" if you chew your food well. In addition, eat more fiber-rich foods for "fill-up value" and health (i.e., fruit, vegetables, wholegrains, beans). Chew and crunch!
"Light" foods are not satisfying	• Eat the "real" thing (in a reasonable amount). Often, it is more satisfying than eating more of a lighter food.
Your additional barriers _____ _____ _____	• Your solutions: _____ _____ _____

   © 2009, *The Cooper Clinic Solution to the Diet Revolution* by Georgia G. Kostas, M.P.H., R.D., L.D., Dallas, Texas

Self-Assessment: Know Thyself

Do you understand how your past eating and "dieting" habits have affected you up to now? To prevent repeating past patterns, complete this form. What have you learned?

Weight History

1. What do you consider a good weight for yourself? _____ Current weight: _____
2. What is the most you have weighed? _____ at what age? _____
3. What is the least you have weighed? _____ at what age? _____
4. Have you lost or gained weight recently? _____ How much? _____ Time frame? _____
5. Is your spouse overweight? _____ Children? _____ Parents? _____ Siblings? _____
6. Are you overweight right now? _____
7. How long have you been overweight? _____

Related Factors

8. What do you see as your reason(s) for being overweight or overeating?

   ___ type of food   ___ depression   ___ job   ___ lack of time
   ___ portions   ___ emotions   ___ fats (fried foods) ___ unplanned meals
   ___ alcohol   ___ anger   ___ sugar/sweets   ___ no support
   ___ lack of exercise   ___ boredom   ___ fast foods   ___ conflicts
   ___ snacks   ___ nervousness   ___ soft drinks   ___ inconsistent meal
   ___ travel or eating out ___ stress   ___ desserts   times
   ___ habits   ___ fatigue   ___ meat   ___ lack of food knowl-
   ___ socializing   ___ quit smoking   ___ "extras"   edge
   ___ watching TV, sports, ___ relaxation/comfort ___ convenience   ___ enjoy food
       movies   ___ escape

9. Are you dissatisfied with the way you look at this weight? _____

   Why do you want to lose weight?

   ___ appearance   ___ improve physical fitness
   ___ pressure from family/friends ___ health
   ___ feel better   ___ physician/nutritionist's advice
   ___ clothes fit better   ___ other: _____

10. How do others influence your weight loss goals? Give their names.

INFLUENCE	NAMES	HOW
Positive	_____	_____
Negative	_____	_____
None	_____	_____
Other	_____	_____

11. What is your biggest challenge regarding weight loss?

Dieting History

12. List diets and/or weight-loss plans you have followed in the past.

TYPES	SHORT-TERM RESULTS	LONG-TERM RESULTS
1. _____	_____	_____
2. _____	_____	_____
3. _____	_____	_____
4. _____	_____	_____

 Which worked best?_____ Why? _____

13. What do you wish to achieve now? _____

14. Is it more difficult for you to lose weight or maintain weight? _____

Eating and Exercise Patterns

16. List vitamin/mineral/dietary supplements with the amounts you take daily:

 _____ _____ _____

 _____ _____ _____

17. How many meals a day do you eat? _____ Skip? _____ Which ones?_____

18. How many times a day do you snack? _____ Types?_____

19. Where do you eat your meals (M) and snacks (S)? *(For example: _M_ kitchen, _S_ den)*

 _____ kitchen _____ dining room _____ TV room

 _____ den _____ bedroom _____ other:_____

20. How many meals do you eat out each week? _____

 Where? ____restaurant ____fast food ____deli ____cafeteria ____other: _____

21. Who prepares your meals at home?_____

22. What is your eating pace? ____fast ____slow ____moderate

23. List foods in which you overindulge (your problem foods):

 _____

24. Do you exercise? _____ If yes, describe below:

	SAMPLE	FILL IN	FILL IN
Form of exercise (jog, swim, stationary bike, etc.)	*Walk*		
Length of Workout (minutes)	*40 minutes*		
Distance per workout	*2 miles*		
Number of workouts per week	*4*		

© 2009, *The Cooper Clinic Solution to the Diet Revolution* by Georgia G. Kostas, M.P.H., R.D., L.D., Dallas, Texas

25. Do you smoke? _____ If yes, how many (cigarettes) do you smoke daily? _____

26. Do you drink alcohol? _____ Amount daily: _____ beer _____ liquor _____ wine

Your Health

27. Present medical conditions:
    _____ heart disease   _____ liver disease   _____ ulcer
    _____ diabetes   _____ kidney disease   _____ gastrointestinal problem
    _____ high blood pressure _____ cancer (type)_____ _____ hiatal hernia
    _____ overweight   _____ elevated cholesterol   _____ diverticulosis
    _____ gallbladder disease _____ elevated triglycerides _____ diverticulitis
    _____ other _____

28. Rate your health: _____ excellent _____ good _____ fair _____ poor

29. Do you feel this is a good time for you to begin your eating and exercise program? _____
    Have you checked with your doctor and received his or her OK? _____

30. If your overeating is linked to moods, emotions or unknown causes, have you worked with a professional counselor to help with this aspect of overeating?_____
    We recommend counseling when habits are difficult to change and compulsive overeating and weight and food preoccupation continue.

31. Describe a day's eating with comments about variations you may have. **Please be accurate and specific!**

SAMPLE		
BREAKFAST	*8 oz. orange juice* *1 egg, scrambled in* *1 tsp. margarine*	*2 pieces whole wheat toast with* *2 tsp margarine + 1 Tbsp. jam* *1 c. coffee + 1 Tbsp. cream*
BREAKFAST		
LUNCH		
DINNER		
SNACKS		

What did you learn about your eating style and habits? _____

Feeling Satisfied

One of our greatest fears with weight loss involves satiety. Will I feel "full" and "satisfied" as I make lifestyle changes—and, more specifically, will I feel happy and able to succeed? The fear is, I'll feel "hungry" and "deprived"—or "unhappy" and "upset."

These feelings are legitimate. Let me explain how you can feel full and satisfied while calorie-cutting.

1. **Choose "lingering calories"** (calories that last).
    - **a little protein at each meal -**
      1 oz. low-fat cheese, turkey slice, chicken; cottage cheese, yogurt, milk; roast beef, Canadian bacon, lean meat, tuna; egg, egg white; beans, etc.
    - **a little fat at each meal -**
      "Hidden" (as in meat and cheese) or "added" (as in light mayonnaise, margarine, cream cheese or salad dressing; nuts).
    - **fiber at each meal -**
      Wholegrain or bran cereals, 100% wholewheat bread, corn tortillas, oatmeal, brown rice, dense breads with seeds; nuts; beans and bean soup; fruit and vegetables (apples, carrots, green beans, melon, etc.); popcorn
    - **protein-carbohydrate-fat (P-C-F) balance at each meal -**
      Carbs for short-term; protein for moderate energy; and fat for long-term fuel. This combination delays hunger and adds energy continuum for five to six hours.

2. **Eat often.**
    - Meal frequency (eating every three to six hours) keeps you "full" and "satisfied."
    - Do not skip meals or deprive yourself.

3. **Eat slowly. Make a meal last.**
    - 20 minutes after eating anything, you'll feel full.
    - Never go for seconds until letting 20 minutes pass.

4. **Take little bites for more bites.**
    - They slow you down.
    - They keep you eating longer.
    - They keep you mindful of eating.
    - Try eating a scoop of ice cream or frozen yogurt or cereal with a baby spoon or Baskin Robbins sampling spoon—the serving will never end!

5. **Use smaller plates, spoons, forks, glasses, bowls.**
    - Your food appears like more and is psychologically more satisfying.
    - You'll eat less!

6. **Go for color.**
    - Adds nutrition and nutrient variety and sensory variety.
    - Provides psychological satisfaction/sensory appeal.
    - We eat with our eyes.
    - Select three to five colors per meal.

7. **Crunch and chew more.**
   - Jaw satisfaction (fatigue!) translates to fullness.
   - Add carrots to a lunch sandwich.
   - Make salads crunchy (water chestnuts, celery, bell pepper, etc.)
   - Choose dense, coarse bread packed with seeds (sunflower, flaxseed, sesame, poppy, etc.)

8. **Fill up with volume.**
   - 16 oz. water at each meal or between meals.
   - Hot, decaffeinated tea or coffee before eating.
   - Hot soup with meals or pre-meal (1 c. tomato soup = 100 calories!)
   - Hot lite cocoa as snack.
   - Hot liquids especially "fill" us and "last."
   - Drink 64 oz. water per day for optimal hydration, energy, health.
   - Fruit and vegetables are 90% water and very filling.
   - ½ cantaloupe or a whole grapefruit or 2 c. grapes or strawberries = only 100 calories
   - 4 c. popcorn or 1¼ c. Cheerios = 100 calories
   - 2 c. veggies = 100 calories

9. **Spice it up.**
   - Hot, spicy foods "fill" us. Tantalizing flavors make the taste buds say "stop."
   - Use picante sauce, cilantro, red pepper flakes, pickles, Creole seasoning, Mexican flavors (chili powder, cumin), garlic, onion, poblano or chili peppers, jalapenos, etc.

10. **Get enough calories.**
    - Eating too little rebounds and triggers overeating.
    - Eating too little signals "deprivation" or "fatigue," triggering overeating.

11. **Tune in to yourself. Ask yourself, "Am I eating for hunger or emotions?"**
    - Apply the **HALT** principle: Am I **H**ungry? **A**ngry? **L**onely? **T**ired?
    - Then make a conscious food selection, or talk out a problem. Other helps: Take a walk, seek out a friend's companionship/communication or take a nap. Walking your dog or playing with a pet may resolve several HALT moods.

12. **Choose substantive calories.**
    - **For equal calories, sometimes you feel more satisfied within from:**
      4 oz. regular yogurt vs. 8 oz. light yogurt
      3 oz. lean beef filet vs. 6 oz. seafood
      1 "real" chocolate chip cookie vs. 4 "light" ones
      2 Tbsp. "real" dressing vs. 4-5 Tbsp. light dressing
    - **More does not mean better...**
      A lot of a little is still a lot of a little, which adds up!
      Would you rather have 10 fat-free chocolate chip cookies for 500 calories or 2 Mrs. Field's cookies for the same number...You choose!
    - **Bottom line: Calories are calories.**

Diets That Don't Work

The federal government has issued U.S. Dietary Guidelines that recommend eating sensibly and moderately, cutting back calories, and exercising to lose weight safely. Weight loss results from eating less and/or exercising over time. As research has shown, diets do not work for the long haul.

Unfortunately, desperate dieters turn to the abundance of books with misinformation and gimmicks that promise magical, quick weight loss. "Dieting" schemes come and go, and there is one to suit every taste, budget and misconception. Have you seen any of the following?

Hollywood Eighteen Day Diet	The Egg Diet
Banana Diet; Grapefruit Diet	High-Protein
Crenshaw Super Beauty Diet	Never Say Diet
Easy No-Flab Diet	Dallas Diet
Three-Day Prune Diet	Doctor's Diet
"Spring Shape-Up"	Beverly Hills Diet
No-Aging Diet	Liquid Diets
Cabbage Soup Diet	Etc.

What's Wrong With Them?

- These diets do not teach eating strategies or sensible meal planning.
- They are poor preparation for a lifetime of eating ahead.
- They can be dangerous because they often severely restrict calories and restrict or eliminate foods that supply essential nutrients for good health and nutritionally balanced meals.

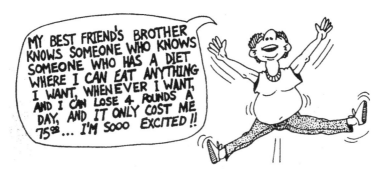

Bottom Line:

- A *balanced diet* provides protein, carbohydrates, fats, vitamins and minerals for sound nutritional health. All foods can fit in.
- An *unbalanced diet* overemphasizes one food group or single nutrient at the expense of others, or restricts a few specific foods.

Low-Carbohydrate / High-Protein Diets

High-protein diets such as the Atkins Diet, Scarsdale Diet, Stillman Diet, etc., come and go in popularity. So many people have tried a high-protein diet that *Time* magazine has even devoted a cover story to the topic! Day after day I hear about people's experiences with the high-protein diet. Some have been burned; others are convinced that it "works" . . . for awhile. If you're unfamiliar with the diet, let me explain what it is and why I cannot recommend it.

Rules of the Diet:

In essence, here's how the high-protein diet works:
1. Eat all you want, any time, of the foods that have no carbohydrates (steak, fish, chicken, eggs, cheese, spareribs, lobster Newburg, etc.). These foods are high in protein and fat.
2. Limit amounts of carbohydrate foods such as starches, certain vegetables, fruits, wholegrains.
3. Avoid sugar and starches (potatoes, bread).

Claims:

Atkins — A no-carbohydrate diet stimulates a fat-mobilizing hormone that helps to burn body fat.

Stillman — Protein molecules are so large that extra energy is required to digest them.

Reality:

- You decrease body fat through exercise and reduced calorie intake, not a high protein intake.
- Energy (fat) does not just "disappear" (unless you have cosmetic surgery!).
- A very high-protein diet is usually unbalanced. By restricting wholegrains and fresh produce, it does not provide all needed nutrients, fiber, antioxidants and plant phytochemicals.
- It is high in total fat, saturated fats and cholesterol, low in fiber—increasing one's risk of heart disease, cancer and digestive problems.
- It does little or nothing to alter overall eating behavior for long-term weight maintenance.
- The rules are too rigid and monotonous to follow over a long period.
- The diet results in abnormal fat breakdown due to inadequate carbohydrates . . . ketones form, causing ketosis.
- The state of ketosis is unhealthy and, if continued over a long period of time, may damage the liver or kidneys. Side effects of ketosis include temporary dizziness, headache, weakness, diarrhea, nausea, low blood pressure, dehydration, fatigue, sleeplessness.
- More water loss than fat loss occurs with the high-protein diet.
- Water loss may lead to dehydration and/or electrolyte imbalance.
- Studies show the diet is effective short-term, but after 6-12 months, weight gain returns. It is healthier and more effective to choose a plan one can maintain for life.

> *Bottom line: The high-protein diet is neither safe nor effective long-term.*

Liquid Diets

Liquid diets have been popular from time to time . . . they are simple! I do not endorse "one food" diets. Often, liquid diets are very low calorie or excessive in protein.

Rules of the Diet:

- Take daily doses of "liquid nutrition" or "liquid protein." Limit your carbohydrates and calories.

Claims:

- "Quick weight loss" with freedom from having to choose, plan and manage food intake.

Reality:

- These diets do nothing to alter eating habits permanently. "Normal" eating is resumed, weight is regained, one's metabolism slows down.

- Muscle is lost from quick weight loss. Fat is gained.

- Real food is needed to lose weight permanently.

- Serious health hazards may result from prolonged use: irregular heart beat and heart damage, kidney and liver damage, diarrhea, low blood volume, dehydration, nausea, hair loss, nervous disorders, abdominal cramps, even death. Bingeing disorders and food cravings often follow very low-calorie liquid diets.

> *Bottom line: Risky!*

High-Carbohydrate Diets

Along with high-protein diets, some people will go to the other extreme and try very high-carbohydrate, low-fat diets such as the Rockefeller, Watermelon, Quick Inches-Off diets, and those that are 80% carbohydrate, 10% fat, 10% protein.

Rules of the Diet:

- Consume mainly high complex carbohydrates. Reduce sugar, saturated fat and protein.

Reality:

- A balanced vegetarian-type, low-fat diet has advantages. If unbalanced and protein-deficient, a high-carbohydrate diet may lead to protein, iron, calcium and Vitamin B12 deficiencies.

- Carbohydrate foods will not have "staying power" unless mixed with protein and fat. Constant hunger leads to over-eating.

> *Bottom line: Hard to sustain*

Single Food Diets

Diets under this umbrella include the Grapefruit, Rice, Banana, Ice Cream, Cabbage Soup Diets, etc.

Rules of the Diet:

- One or a few foods that are said to have magical properties are permitted. For example, on the Grapefruit diet, the saying is that "grapefruit contains enzymes that help increase the fat-burning process," so dieters should eat 1/2 grapefruit at the start of every meal.

Claims:

- Easy to remember; no calorie counting.

Reality:

- There are no special foods that "melt" fat away or make foods less fattening.

- A limited diet results in vitamin and mineral deficiency, and is too boring to follow.

> *Bottom line: Unsafe long-term*

High-Fiber, Combination Diets

Rules of the Diet:

- Combine foods properly to allow the enzymes in foods and those in your body to effectively digest food and make it less fattening. As new foods are introduced in the Beverly Hills Diet, you may eat as much as you want as long as you eat foods separately. (For example, fruit should be eaten alone or it gets "trapped" by other foods in your stomach.)

- In the Beverly Hills Diet: For the first 11 days, eat fruit only; second week: vegetables and breads are introduced; third week: lobster; fourth week: regimen of bran.

- In the Fit for Life Diet, only fruit can be consumed in the morning; milk and milk products cannot be consumed; certain foods cannot be eaten together.

Claims:

- When certain foods are combined, your body cannot digest them and they turn to fat. Combine foods properly for most efficient digestion.

Reality:

- The more foods are combined at meals, the better the absorption and utilization of nutrients.

- There is no magic combination of foods to make them less fattening. Undigested food is eliminated from the body, not stored as fat. All foods are digested as soon as they pass through the digestive system.

- Single food diets can lead to serious illnesses and death. Large quantities of fruit may lead to severe diarrhea with water loss, causing potassium deficiency and an irregular heart beat. Fever, muscle weakness, a rapid pulse and fatal drop in blood pressure may develop.

> *Bottom line: Ineffective, misleading*

Other Attempted Methods for Weight Control

- Acupuncture
- Diet pills
- Gastric stapling
- Ear patches
- Starvation
- Hypnosis
- Jaw-wiring
- "Fat burners"
- Intestinal bypass surgery
- Spas
- Shellfish shells

> ***Bottom line: Stick with what works and is safe: sensible, balanced eating of all foods, regular activity and the right mind-set. All foods fit in!***

With so much information bombarding us about weight loss and looking good, it gets tough to know what's fact and what's fiction. A healthy food plan for weight loss should contain the following:

- A **balanced variety** of food on a daily basis.

- **Ample calories** (1,200-1,800/day) to prevent muscle loss and a slower metabolism.

- **Close to 30% fat** calories (meaning 20-50 fat grams daily).

- **45 to 70% complex carbohydrate calories to energize you and to prevent muscle loss.** This means at least 10 fruits, vegetables and starches daily.

- **Re-education** toward new eating habits for life-long weight maintenance.

- **The P-C-F Balance** (protein-carbohydrate-fat) at each meal. This helps to maximize energy, minimize stress and limit "empty-calorie" snacks by stabilizing your blood sugar. (See p. 47-48 for details.)

- **Smaller servings of calorie-dense foods** – foods with fat, sugar, alcohol, meat products and cheese.

How to Rate a Weight-Loss Diet

If you see a program that sounds good, see if it checks out by asking the following questions:

- *Is the diet based on proven principles of nutrition?* Is it well-balanced nutritionally? Does it eliminate one or more of the basic six food groups? Or, does it claim that one food or food group will promote weight loss? Be careful. A well-balanced diet includes foods from all six food groups* *and* is safe.

- *Is the diet based on a "secret" no one has discovered?* Does it promote extremely rapid weight loss of more than three pounds per week? Are unlimited amounts of food promised? Remember, there are no miracles for losing weight and keeping it off!

- *Could you eat like this for the rest of your life?* Does the diet allow for individual preferences, practice and taste? Rigid diets that tell you what and when to eat and give no nutritional information are doomed to fail.

- *Is the author credible?* Check degrees and work experience. Distinguish between "nutritionist" and R.D. (registered dietitian), "doctor" or M.D. The national credentialed professionals are known as "R.D.'s" and "M.D.'s."

- *Has the author supported "success" claims?* Was the diet tested on a sufficient number of overweight people and the results objectively compared to the results of a similar group of people following another weight-reducing diet? Were the results published? If the answer is *no*, consider the claims to be questionable. Congressional rulings in 1992 require that any claims be substantiated with published research.

*Basic six food groups: milk, meat/protein, fruits, vegetables, grains/starches, fats.

Calculate Your Calorie Needs

You must eat sensibly to control your weight and promote your best health. Always eat at least 1,300 calories a day (women) or 1,600-1,800 calories a day (men) for healthy weight loss. You'll be more likely to lose body fat, feel energetic and not slow your metabolism. Moreover, you won't "starve" and binge. By following these guidelines, you'll be able to embrace these eating principles for life. How many calories a day are right for you?

① Start With Your Target Weight

What Should You Weigh?

- The more accurate method of determining your target weight is by body composition (using skinfold measurements and/or underwater weighing). Your target weight is calculated from your percentage of body fat vs. lean tissue (muscle). The percentage of body fat for men should not exceed 19% and women, 23%. A reliable health or fitness facility in your area can measure your body fat.

- Or, refer to p. 36 for Height/Weight Charts and BMI Charts.

- Or, calculate your target weight with this simple formula:

   Women: 100 + (inches over 5 ft. x 5 lbs.) = target weight
   Men: 106 + (inches over 5 ft. x 6 lbs) = target weight
   Add or subtract 10% for a large or small frame, respectively.
   For example, if you are a 5'6" woman:
   100 + (6" x 5) = 100 + 30 = 130 = target weight

- My target weight is _____

② How Many Calories Can You Eat to Lose Weight?

Step 1:

Calculate Your Baseline Calorie Needs at Your Current Weight

Current weight in pounds x 12 calories per pound = **baseline calories per day**
For example: 130 pounds x 12 calories per pound = **1560 calories per day**
(Note: Most people need 10-15 calories per pound):

Ages 20-30	weight x 13-15
Ages 30-40	weight x 12
Ages 40-50	weight x 11
Ages 50+	weight x 10

My Baseline Calorie Needs are:

_____

Step 2:

Choose How to Lose Weight

Since 3,500 calories = 1 pound body weight:
- Omit 1,000 calories per day to lose 2 pounds per week.
- Omit 500 calories per day to lose 1 pound per week.
- Omit 250 calories per day to lose 1/2 pound per week. Through exercise alone:
   ⇒ *Walk 1 mile briskly in 15 minutes to burn approximately 100 calories.*
   ⇒ *Walk 2.5 miles in 37 minutes, or jog it in 25 minutes to burn 250 calories.*
Combine diet and exercise for maximum results!

Step 3:

- Use the Exercise Chart below to calculate the calories you expend weekly.
- Determine the calories you burn daily (an average):

minutes of exercise each week	x	calories burned per minute	÷	7 days in a week	=	average calories burned daily

Example One: **Your Usual Exercise**
- Walk 5 times a week x 40 minutes (2 miles) each time = 200 minutes weekly
- 200 minutes weekly x 5 calories per minute = 1,000 calories weekly
- 1,000 calories a week ÷ 7 days in a week = **140 average calories burned daily**

Example Two: **Extra Exercise**
- Strive to burn 200-300 calories/day for optimal weight loss.
- Here's how:
  ⇒ Walk 5 times a week x 60 minutes (2.5 miles) each time = 300 minutes weekly
  ⇒ 300 minutes weekly x 5 calories per minute = 1,500 calories weekly
  ⇒ 1500 calories a week ÷ 7 days in a week = **215 average calories burned daily**
- If you walk/run 15 miles weekly, as Dr. Cooper recommends for cardiovascular health, you'll burn an average 200-300 calories per day.

Calories I burn daily: _____

EXERCISE CALORIES

This chart shows approximate exercise energy expenditure.* To compute more specifically by rate of calories burned per pound of body weight, see p. 154-155.

5 Calories Per Minute	7 Calories Per Minute	10 Calories Per Minute
walking, 3 mph	walking, 4 mph	stationary jogging
cycling, 5.5 mph	cycling, 9.5 mph	cycling, 12 mph
volleyball	stationary cycling	jogging, 6 mph
table tennis	tennis, singles	skipping rope
dancing slow step	dancing fast step	calisthenics (heavy)
domestic work	swimming, 30 yd/minute	swimming, 45 yd/minute
golf (no cart)	skiing (water)	snow skiing
bowling	Badminton, singles	paddleball
light gardening	heavy gardening	squash, handball
	skating (ice, roller)	climbing stairs
	horseback riding (trot)	(up and down, approx. 35 steps per minute)

For a 150-pound person. Add or subtract 10% of calories for each 10 pounds you are above or below 150 pounds.

Step 4:

Calculate Calorie Needs Daily to Lose Weight

Example: OMIT 500 CALORIES A DAY TO LOSE 1 POUND A WEEK:

1. **Adjust FOOD Only:**

Baseline calories	=	1560
subtract 500 calories		- 500
Eat daily:	=	**1060 calories**

2. **Adjust FOOD and add your usual EXERCISE to baseline calories:**

Baseline calories	=	1060
add your exercise cal.		+140
Eat daily:	=	**1200 calories**

   OR

   Add your EXTRA EXERCISE to baseline calories:

Baseline calories	=	1060
plus extra exercise cal.		+215
Eat daily:	=	**1275 calories**

- I recommend adding extra exercise to your baseline calories because you can eat more. Further, 215 calories of exercise daily promotes a leaner body composition and speeds metabolism and fat-burning...all keys to optimal success!
- If you wish to lose faster (1 1/2 to 2 pounds a week), add more exercise and/or decrease calories consumed. Never eat fewer than 1,300 calories per day (women) or 1,600 calories per day (men).

Baseline Calorie Needs + Exercise Calories Burned = CALORIE REQUIREMENTS

What Calorie Intake Maintains Your Target Weight? _____

SUMMARIZE YOUR GOALS

1. My current weight: _____ lbs. My target weight:_____ lbs.
2. My current baseline calorie needs daily: _____ calories.
3. Subtract calories I will omit daily to lose _____ lbs/wk: (-_____) calories.
4. Add exercise calories (average) I will burn daily: (+_____) calories.
5. Calories I will eat daily to lose weight: _____ calories.
6. I will reach my TARGET WEIGHT in _____ weeks.

Recommended Height & Weight *

Women

Height Feet Inches	Small Frame	Medium Frame	Large Frame
4' 10"	102-111	109-121	118-131
4' 11"	103-113	111-123	120-134
5' 0"	104-115	113-126	122-137
5' 1"	106-118	115-129	125-140
5' 2"	108-121	118-132	128-143
5' 3"	111-124	121-135	131-147
5' 4"	114-127	124-138	134-151
5' 5"	117-130	127-141	137-155
5' 6"	120-133	130-144	140-159
5' 7"	123-136	133-147	143-163
5' 8"	126-139	136-150	146-167
5' 9"	129-142	139-153	149-170
5' 10"	132-145	142-156	152-173
5' 11"	135-148	145-159	155-176
6' 0"	138-151	148-162	158-179

Weights at ages 25-59 based on lowest mortality. Weight in pounds according to frame (in indoor clothing weighing 3 lbs.; shoes with 1" heels).

Men

Height Feet Inches	Small Frame	Medium Frame	Large Frame
5' 2"	128-134	131-141	138-150
5' 3"	130-136	133-143	140-153
5" 4"	132-138	135-145	142-156
5' 5"	134-140	137-148	144-160
5' 6"	136-142	139-151	146-164
5' 7"	138-145	142-154	149-168
5' 8"	140-148	145-157	152-172
5' 9"	142-151	148-160	155-176
5' 10"	144-154	151-163	158-180
5' 11"	146-157	154-166	161-184
6' 0"	149-160	157-170	164-188
6' 1"	152-164	160-174	168-192
6' 2"	155-168	164-178	172-197
6' 3"	158-172	167-182	176-202
6' 4"	162-176	171-187	181-207

Weights at ages 25-59 based on lowest mortality. Weight in pounds according to frame (in indoor clothing weighing 5 lbs.; shoes with 1" heels).

* Source: Metropolitan Life Insurance Height/Weight Tables, 1996

Body Mass Index (BMI)**

The Body Mass Index (BMI) more accurately determines a healthy body weight. It is a ratio of height to weight, and indicates body fat (and related disease risk).

BMI	Weight Assessment	Heart Risk
<25	healthy	minimal
25-29.9	overweight	moderate
≥30	obese	high

Calculate your BMI:

$$\left(\frac{\text{Weight (in pounds)}}{\text{Height (in inches)} \times \text{Height (in inches)}} \right) \times 703$$

Are You a Healthy Weight? (This chart gives you the BMI for various heights and weights. Weight is measured with underwear, but not shoes.**)

Ht. \ BMI	21	22	23	24	25	26	27	28	29	30	31
4' 10"	100	105	110	115	119	124	129	134	138	140	148
5' 0"	107	112	118	123	128	133	138	143	148	153	158
5' 1"	111	116	122	127	132	137	143	148	153	158	164
5' 3"	118	124	130	135	141	146	152	158	163	169	175
5' 5"	126	132	138	144	150	156	162	168	174	180	186
5' 7"	134	140	146	153	159	166	172	178	185	191	198
5' 9"	142	149	155	162	169	176	182	189	196	203	209
5' 11"	150	157	165	172	179	186	193	200	208	215	222
6' 1"	159	166	174	182	189	197	204	212	219	227	235
6' 3"	168	176	184	192	200	203	216	224	232	240	248

** Source: National Institute of Health, 1998

Treat Yourself

Developing new eating and exercise habits, as well as a new mind-set, takes time! Set goals, and reward yourself along the way. You deserve it!

REWARD YOURSELF WHEN YOU:

✓ Exercise regularly

✓ Practice new eating habits

✓ Follow your meal plan

✓ Lose 5 pounds, 10 pounds, etc.

✓ Take any step for health!

Pleasures can help reduce stress, boredom, loneliness, anger, anxiety, nervousness and moodiness. More importantly, rewarded behaviors tend to be *repeated* behaviors. Just don't use food as a reward!

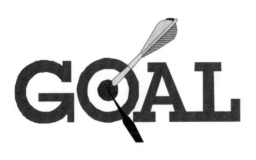

Mark the ways in which you REWARD YOURSELF				
Activity	None	A little	Much	Very Much
1. Watching television				
2. Listening to radio/CDs				
3. Playing cards				
4. Doing crossword puzzles				
5. Reading books, magazines				
6. Dancing				
7. Sleeping late				
8. Shopping				
9. Buying new clothes				
10. Buying kitchen appliances				
11. Buying CDs				
12. Buying books/magazines				
13. Telephoning a friend				
14. Calling a friend long distance				
15. Visiting friends				
16. Taking a relaxing bath or shower				
17. Attending sporting event				
18. Attending movie				
19. Attending play or concert				
20. Playing recreational sport (golf, bowling, etc.)				
21. Aerobic exercise				
22. Participating in team sports				
23. Participating in organizations				
24. "Pampering" yourself (manicure, facial, pedicure, massage)				
25. Personal time				
26. Camping				
27. Traveling				
28. Hiking				
29. Gardening				
30. Hobbies (painting, drawing, needlework, carpentry)				
31. Playing with pet				
32. Other _____				
_____				

My Overall Game Plan

I am committing myself to these specific health goals:

- I will eat _____ calories per day for ____ weeks.
- I will exercise ____ times a week for ____ weeks.
- I will modify these eating behaviors:

  _____ _____ _____ _____
  _____ _____ _____ _____

- I will burn an average of ____ calories per day.
- I will lose ____ pounds in ____ weeks.

- I will enjoy these rewards: _____ when I _____
  _____ when I _____
  _____ when I _____

I will utilize these strategies: ☑

1. Eat Fewer Calories:

- ☐ Consume less alcohol, soft drinks, sweets, junk food, _____.
- ☐ Control portions by skipping seconds, serving smaller first portions or _____.
- ☐ Eat more nutritious, high-fiber foods such as fruit, vegetables, wholegrains,_____.
- ☐ Eat less "extras" such as sauces, toppings, butter, dressing, _____.
- ☐ Eat less fat such as _____.
- ☐ Other: _____.

2. Burn More Calories

(See calculations on page 1-34.)

Activity	Calories/Minute	Minutes/Week	Calories/Week
_____	_____	_____	_____
_____	_____	_____	_____
_____	_____	_____	_____

TOTAL CALORIES WEEKLY ÷ 7 = _____ calories/day

3. Establish New Lifestyle Skills

- ☐ Plan meals in advance.
- ☐ Consistently practice new eating habits.
- ☐ Take charge of my environment by _____.
- ☐ Involve myself in activities that build my self-esteem: _____.
- ☐ Build and utilize an effective support team. My key supports are _____,
  _____ _____, _____, _____.
- ☐ Respond to stress without food by _____.
- ☐ Other:_____.

Signed _____ Support Person _____ Date _____

Progress Check

1. ☐ Am I eating better?

2. ☐ Am I finding ways to be more active?

3. ☐ Am I exercising more?

4. ☐ Am I eating slowly?

5. ☐ Am I pre-thinking meals and food events?

6. ☐ Am I choosing healthier snacks?

7. ☐ Am I eating more veggies?

Two First Ladies, Two First-Rate Techniques

Two women I particularly have admired through the years are Jacqueline Kennedy Onassis and Nancy Reagan. Their strategies to maintaining their weight:

1. Eating just half of everything served on their plates.
2. Removing plate "cues." The waiter removed their partially eaten dinner plates after 30 minutes of eating.

Plate techniques work!

Success Tip:

People who write down their goals are more likely to reach their goals.

Success Tools

Tool #1 Food Records

Studies show that people who keep food and exercise records daily are more successful with changing eating patterns and losing weight. I encourage you to keep accurate food records each day. Record *everything* you eat and drink, even if you overeat. It is best to write down what you'll eat right **before** you eat. This mental pre-thought will help you select the best choices. Include the following:

- *time* you eat
- *how long* it takes to eat
- the exact *place*
- with *whom*

- *mood or activity* while eating
- the *amount*
- *how the food is prepared*

Then list which best fits your goals—fat grams, calories, food groups, etc.

DAILY TOTAL

___	Milk	_____
___	Veg	_____
___	Fruit	II
___	Bread	I
___	Meat	I
___	Fat	JHT I

Sample

DAILY FOOD RECORD
(Write one food on each line.)

Date __Monday, October 1_____

Time/ Min. Eating	Place / With Whom	Mood / Activity	Amount	Food - How Prepared	Food Group or Calories	Fat Grams
7:15 am 10 min.	kitchen table / alone	nervous	8 oz. 1 2 tsp.	orange juice egg, scrambled margarine (egg, toast)	2 fruit 1 meat 2 fat	0 5 10
			1 slice 2 strips 1 c. 2 tbsp.	wholewheat toast bacon coffee cream	1 bread 2 fats free 2 fat	1 10 0 10

(Records show: **D** id **I** **E** at **T** hat?)

Tool #2 Exercise Records

Post your Exercise Log to remind yourself to exercise five days a week.

Sample

MONTHLY EXERCISE LOG

Sunday	Monday	Tuesday	Wednesday	Thursday	Friday	Saturday	Weekly Totals	Cal. Totals*
	Walk 2 miles (40 min.)	Beginner aerobic dance class (60 min.)	Walk 2 miles (40 min.)		Stationary bike, Vigorous 5 miles (30 min.)	Pleasure bike ride (60 min.)	Walk - 4 miles Dance - 1 hour St. Bike - 30 min. Outdoor bike - 60 min.	400 + 400 + 200 + 600

Goal = 1400 calories a week or 200 a day (average).
Note: See pg. 34 and 154 - 155 for calorie calculations.

Note: See Appendix A for blank food and exercise records and charts.

Tool #3 Weight Charts

Post your weight record in a prominent place and record your weight **weekly**. Weigh at the same time and day each week, using the same scale. Day-to-day fluctuations in weight are typical due to fluid shifts, activity level, etc. Look for an overall downward trend. Note: It is normal to gain water weight when losing body fat. Expect a weight gain (from water) on the scales at some point, even when you are doing everything consistently to lose. Hang in there! The water will go away with time.

WARNING: Don't get caught up with numbers! Work on *habits*. Record weight **weekly**, not daily.

WEEKLY WEIGHT GRAPHS

Sample

Starting Weight _____172_____   Date _____Sept. 1_____

Desired Weight _____130_____   Date _____June 23_____

Week No.	Date	Weight	Weight Change	Total Weight Change
0	Sept. 1	172		
1	Sept. 8	171	-1	-1
2	Step 15	170 1/2	-1/2	-1 1/2
3	Sept. 22	169	-1 1/2	-3
4	Sept. 29	168	-1	-4
5	Oct. 6	167	-1	-5
6	Oct. 13	168	+1	-4
7	Oct. 20	166	-2	-6
8	Oct. 27	166	0	-6
9	Nov. 3	164	-2	-8
10	Nov. 10	162	-2	-10
11	Nov. 17	161 1/2	-1/2	-10 1/2
12	Nov. 24	160	-1 1/2	-12
13				
14				

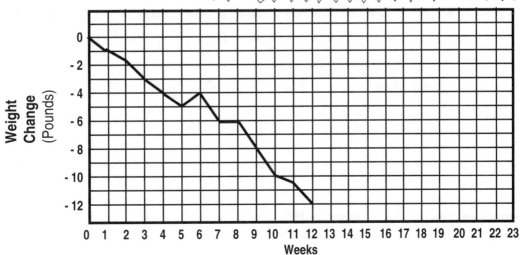

Tool #4 Climb the Step-by-Step Ladder to Success

✧ Note where you stand weekly.
✧ Plan smart moves.
✧ Keep climbing!

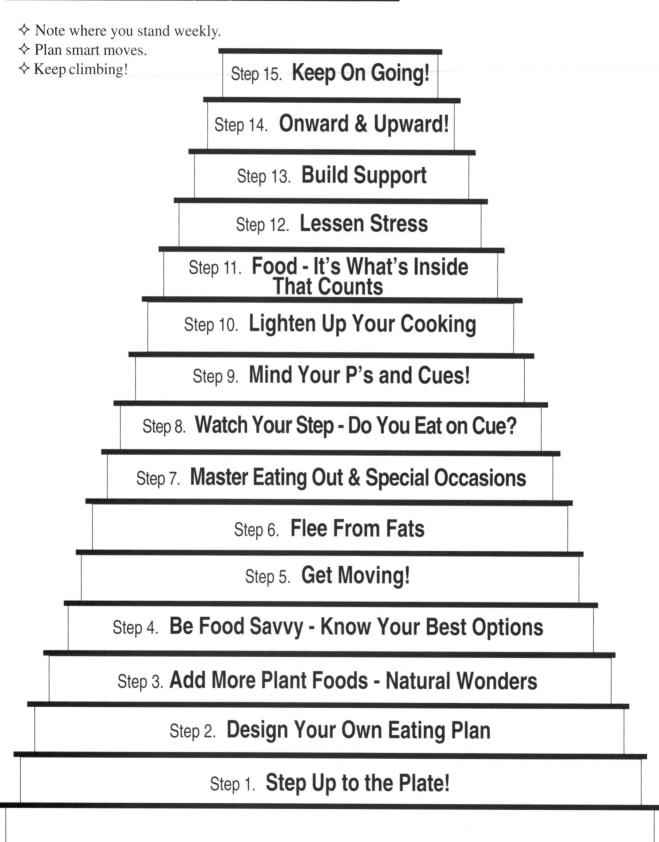

Step 15. **Keep On Going!**

Step 14. **Onward & Upward!**

Step 13. **Build Support**

Step 12. **Lessen Stress**

Step 11. **Food - It's What's Inside That Counts**

Step 10. **Lighten Up Your Cooking**

Step 9. **Mind Your P's and Cues!**

Step 8. **Watch Your Step - Do You Eat on Cue?**

Step 7. **Master Eating Out & Special Occasions**

Step 6. **Flee From Fats**

Step 5. **Get Moving!**

Step 4. **Be Food Savvy - Know Your Best Options**

Step 3. **Add More Plant Foods - Natural Wonders**

Step 2. **Design Your Own Eating Plan**

Step 1. **Step Up to the Plate!**

Empower Yourself to Succeed
Secrets of Successful Losers

To be successful, create your own strategies and utilize the "secrets of success" reported by those who have successfully lost weight and kept if off for 2 or more years. The following tips and strategies are based on research by Judith Stern, Ph.D. (University of California, Davis), Kelly Brownell, Ph.D. (Yale University), John Foreyt, Ph.D. (Baylor College of Medicine), and The National Weight Loss Registry (University of Pittsburgh), as well as my own patients!

Here's what we've learned so far:

✓ **Set your own "ground rules"** for weight loss and maintenance. **Design your own eating plan**, based on "low-fat, high-fiber" eating. Include foods you enjoy and know realistically you'll eat.

✓ **Exercise** three to five times a week. An active life is absolutely essential to keep metabolism up and pounds off.

✓ **Keep food and exercise logs.** They boost your awareness. Tracking helps you stay on track.

✓ **Surround yourself with support** (individuals, groups, places, events that motivate and reinforce the good habits and lifestyle you wish to continue).

✓ **Stay accountable**. Join a group, see a qualified nutritionist (registered dietitian) periodically, weigh-in at your doctor's office, weigh yourself at home daily or weekly.

✓ Keep in mind your **personal incentives** to lose weight and keep it off.

✓ Never think of yourself as "dieting." **Focus on "healthy eating."**

✓ **Don't let a slip-up make you give up.** Get back on track if you do have an "off" day. The longer you delay, the harder it is to resume new habits. Despite a few speed bumps, keep moving forward!

✓ **Focus on these key words**: *healthy eating, long-term, proactive, guilt-free, no deprivation.*

✓ **Develop problem-solving strategies** and "back-up plans." Be prepared.

✓ **Take baby steps**. Go slow. Take one step at a time.

✓ **Think "I can do it"! Have a positive expectation.**

✓ **Enjoy and realize the benefits** of a healthy lifestyle.

✓ **Set realistic goals.**

✓ **Don't delay. Have a "do it now" attitude.**

> ### There is nothing you can't do
> ### if you want to.

Success Tips

Success is yours when you:

- **Develop a game plan,** and stick with it daily. **Plan ahead.**
- **Be AWARE, take ACTION and be ACCOUNTABLE** (three A's of change).
- **Commit** to a new lifestyle of health and fitness.
- **Become food savvy.** Be proficient at reading labels.
- **Assert yourself** and your program. **Be responsible**—for nutritious meals and regular exercise.
- **Become sensitive and responsive to your thoughts and feelings that hinder weight loss.** Act! Don't turn to food as comfort or a substitute for resolving something important.
- **Learn to eat for your body's needs** and not for emotional comfort.
- **Be enthusiastic** about your new endeavor. **Reward yourself.**
- **Be patient.** It takes practice to learn and maintain new habits.
- **Believe in your goals** and in yourself. **Expect success.**
- **Experience new sensations of success** . . .
  - ⇒ **New routines. A new mind-set.** Portable snacks and lunches. Less impulsive eating!
  - ⇒ **A sense of "fullness"** when you slow down, chew more, drink more water and eat P-C-F.
  - ⇒ **Less stomach capacity . . .** you will feel full after 3 cups per meal instead of 4.
- **Enjoy and savor the results**—feeling better, looking better, having more vitality.

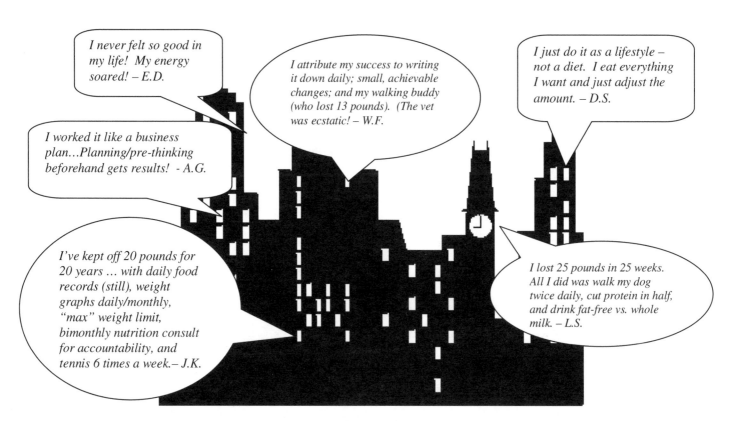

I never felt so good in my life! My energy soared! – E.D.

I attribute my success to writing it down daily; small, achievable changes; and my walking buddy (who lost 13 pounds). (The vet was ecstatic! – W.F.

I just do it as a lifestyle – not a diet. I eat everything I want and just adjust the amount. – D.S.

I worked it like a business plan...Planning/pre-thinking beforehand gets results! - A.G.

I've kept off 20 pounds for 20 years ... with daily food records (still), weight graphs daily/monthly, "max" weight limit, bimonthly nutrition consult for accountability, and tennis 6 times a week.– J.K.

I lost 25 pounds in 25 weeks. All I did was walk my dog twice daily, cut protein in half, and drink fat-free vs. whole milk. – L.S.

Remember, it's the "little things" you do that count the most.

Step 2
Design Your Own
Eating Plan

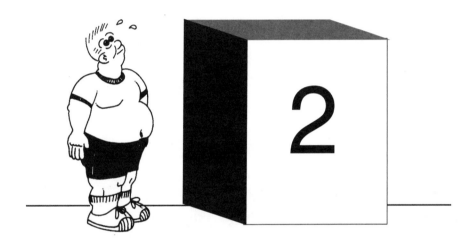

Step 2

The principles in this step will help you rethink your eating patterns, develop an eating plan and lay a solid foundation for lifetime eating habits. I realize that "one plan doesn't fit all." That's why I present five options, all of which have the same basic goal: to help you eat balanced meals in portions that will enable you to either lose or maintain weight. The benefit is that you can create your own eating plan based on the approach that you are able to follow most easily. Here are the approaches:

Plan A - "Basic Healthy Choices" Approach

- Designed for people who don't want a plan involving calorie-counting or other specifics. It is based on the Pyramid Guide for healthy eating and focuses on the "3/4th Plate Rule."

Plan B - "Select-A-Plan" Approaches:

1   **Select by Food Groups**—Plan your meals by eating a set number of servings daily from each of six food categories.

2   **Select by Menus**—Follow two weeks of sample menus at 1,300 or 1,600 calories. This is for the person who wants ideas to jump-start his/her program.

3   **Select by Mix-and-Match Meals**—Works best for people who eat on the run. Based on fuss-free, quick meals, this system offers structure, flexibility, convenience and planned meal ideas . . . at specific calorie/fat ranges.

4   **Select by Calories**—Choose meals and snacks based on calories. This is designed for the person who likes numbers, precision and no questions regarding success.

Decide which approach works best for you. Try at least two or three; then decide!

Mini-Step 1:

Understand the basics:
- P-C-F (to decrease hunger)
- Fats (seen and unseen)
- Portions

Mini-Step 2:

Choose your favorite eating plan (p. 53 & 55) by:
- "Healthy Choices"
- Food Groups (make a plan)
- Menus (your choice)
- Meals (you mix and match)
- Calories (simplify the count)

Mini-Step 3:

Test 3 approaches then select the best fit for you.

Mini-Step 4:

Acquaint yourself with the:
- Food Group Quick List, p. 62.
- Simplified Calorie Counter, p. 97.
- Fat Scale, p. 50.

These are tools for life!

ACTION STEPS

①   Apply the P-C-F concept at each meal to regulate your appetite and maximize your energy.

②   Choose your own eating plan following one of the five approaches that works best for you. Record "My Daily Eating Plan" (see p. 61). Pre-think all meals.

③   Acquaint yourself with food groups, portion sizes, hidden fats and how to get the most food for the calories.

Eating Plan Basics

Know what you need for healthy eating; then create a plan for weight loss around these principles. No *one* weight-loss plan works best for everyone. The best method for weight management is a personal system that fits your lifestyle, needs and goals; is healthy; and includes your favorite foods in specific amounts. As you design your personal plan, be sure to note the following criteria for success.

All Successful Plans Include:

- **A specific eating plan**, tailored to fit your needs, that is practical and livable.
- **An exercise program** that burns fat and adds muscle to speed up your metabolism.
- **Behavioral strategies** that put you in control.
- **A lifetime commitment** to total well-being and a healthy weight.

All Healthy Eating Plans Include:

- **food variety** for optimal nutrition
- **low-fat, high-fiber** foods for health
- **P-C-F** meals for balance, composed of:
  ⇒ 10-25% **Protein (P)**
  ⇒ 45-65% **Complex Carbohydrates (C)**
  ⇒ 20-35% **Fat (F)**
  (See table below)
- **regularly spaced meals** for appetite control
- **foods you enjoy**
- **enough calories** to boost energy, control appetite, prevent fatigue (1300+ calories/day)
- **a blend of higher-fat, lower-fat foods** to include your favorites
- **a plan you can live with for life**

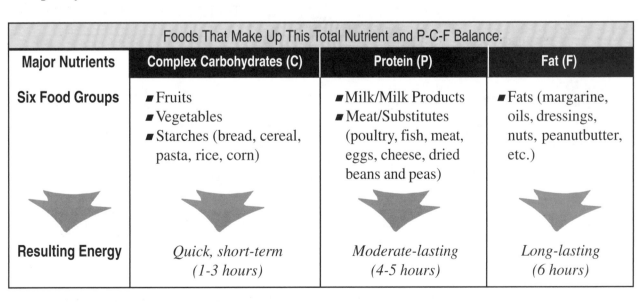

Foods That Make Up This Total Nutrient and P-C-F Balance:			
Major Nutrients	**Complex Carbohydrates (C)**	**Protein (P)**	**Fat (F)**
Six Food Groups	▪ Fruits ▪ Vegetables ▪ Starches (bread, cereal, pasta, rice, corn)	▪ Milk/Milk Products ▪ Meat/Substitutes (poultry, fish, meat, eggs, cheese, dried beans and peas)	▪ Fats (margarine, oils, dressings, nuts, peanutbutter, etc.)
Resulting Energy	*Quick, short-term (1-3 hours)*	*Moderate-lasting (4-5 hours)*	*Long-lasting (6 hours)*

You'll optimize your nutrition and maximize your weight loss if you plan your eating around the principles above.
Your next steps: (1) Select P-C-F meals.   (2) Focus on fat first.   (3) Prioritize portions.

P-C-F Balance

The **P-C-F** (**P**rotein-**C**arbohydrate-**F**at) **Balance** at three meals daily will boost your weight control efforts by regulating your blood sugar levels, keeping your energy high and appetite low. As a result, you will enjoy:

- more energy and alertness
- a finer sense of well-being
- less stress
- fewer "sugar cravings" between meals

- better food choices and decisions
- more enthusiasm
- less hunger
- a sense of control over eating

For Optimal Blood Sugar Control:

- Eat P-C-F at each meal
- Eat every three to six hours
- Add snacks, if needed

Comparison of Blood Sugar Changes from Food		
Food	**Blood Sugar Changes Over Time**	**Impact**
SUGAR (soft drinks, candy, sugar, jam, etc.)	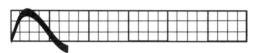 *Normal blood sugar range (80-100 mg%)*	Sugar causes a rapid rise, then fall, in blood sugar, lasting 15-30 minutes.
COMPLEX CARBOHYDRATES (C) (fruits, vegetables, beans, whole grains, starches, plant foods)	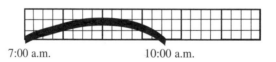 7:00 a.m. 10:00 a.m.	Complex carbohydrates (C) raise blood sugar at a steady, short-term rate, over 1-3 hours.
PROTEIN (P) + CARBOHYDRATES (C) (milk, cheese, fish, poultry, meat, eggs, beans) + carbs	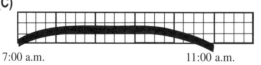 7:00 a.m. 11:00 a.m.	Carbs (C) with Proteins (P) raise blood sugar gradually, over 4-5 hours.
FATS (F) + CARBOHYDRATES (C) (margarine, mayonnaise, salad dressing, peanutbutter, oil, etc.) + carbs	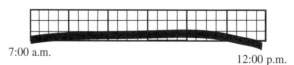 7:00 a.m. 12:00 p.m.	Carbs (C) with Fats (F) sustain blood sugar over an extended period of time, 4-6 hours.
P-C-F COMBINATION (i.e., turkey, bread, fruit, light mayonnaise at lunch)	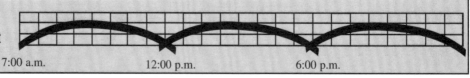 7:00 a.m. 12:00 p.m. 6:00 p.m.	

© 2009, *The Cooper Clinic Solution to the Diet Revolution* by Georgia G. Kostas, M.P.H., R.D., L.D., Dallas, Texas

Focus First on Fats

Fat calories seem to promote weight gain more readily than other calorie sources. Cut fat, and you cut calories. Fat calories also contribute to body fat, raise cholesterol levels, and increase one's risk of cancer, heart disease and diabetes. If you want to stay healthy, feel fit, lose weight and keep the weight off, you guessed it: *focus first on fats.*

How Much Fat Should You Eat?

Although most Americans eat 100-150 grams of fat daily, most nutrition experts agree that we should consume half this much, meaning only 20-35 grams of fat per 1,000 calories, or 20% to 35% of one's total daily calories.

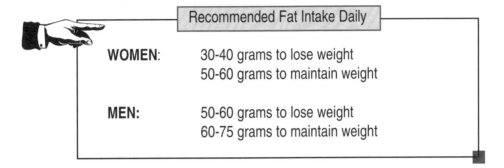

Recommended Fat Intake Daily

WOMEN: 30-40 grams to lose weight
50-60 grams to maintain weight

MEN: 50-60 grams to lose weight
60-75 grams to maintain weight

How To Do It

How Do You Stay Within This Fat Limit?

Read labels and use this guide.

Daily Food to Eat	Fat Grams
4-6 oz. lean meat, fish, poultry	4-18
3-6 tsp. (1-2 Tbsp.) fats/oils	15-30
5-7 starches/breads/cereals	0-7
3+ fruit	0
3+ vegetables	0
2-3 fat-free milk products	0
TOTAL	**20-55**

See Step 4 for more information on fat grams in foods.

Fat (in grams) to Eat by Calorie Intake:

Calories	% Calories from Fat		
	20%	**25%**	**30%**
1000	20g	25g	30g
1200	25g	30g	40g
1500	30g	40g	50g
1800	35g	45g	60g
2000	40g	50g	65g
2200	45g	55g	70g
2500	50g	65g	80g

Note:
fat = 9 calories/gram
carbohydrates = 4 calories/gram
protein = 4 calories/gram

Warning

Do not eliminate fat completely (although it would be difficult to do so). Fat-free eating may lead to constant hunger and overeating. A little fat provides "staying power," giving longer-term energy and less hunger.

Where's the Fat?

- Use this Fat Scale to scale down your fat intake.
- Choose foods primarily from columns 1, 2, 3 and occasionally from columns 4, 5, 6.

Healthy Fat Guidelines:

30-50 g fat per day (women)
50-70 g fat per day (men)

25 grams

1 hamburger
(1/4 lb.)
3 oz. Prime Rib
3 oz. Brisket
1/2 c. macaroni
& cheese
20 Mexican
restaurant
chips
3 slices 13"
pizza

20 grams

3 oz. ground
beef
1 taco
2 slices 13"
pizza
1 fried chicken
sandwich
1 pkg. peanut-
butter crackers
1 scoop ice
cream
1 slice pie
1 slice cake
1 chocolate
candy bar

15 grams

3 oz. corned
beef
3 oz. fried
chicken
1 hot dog
1 small French
fries
1 Danish roll
1 large biscuit
1 small crois-
sant
1 lunch bag
chips
3 c. buttered
popcorn
1 Tbsp. oil

10 grams

3 oz. beef filet
3 oz. eye of
round
3 oz. top sirloin
1 c. whole milk
1 oz. (slice)
cheese
1 Tbsp. salad
dressing,
margarine,
mayonnaise,
peanutbutter
2 Tbsp. nuts/
seeds

5 grams

3 oz. turkey
3 oz. chicken
3 oz. fish
1 oz. low-fat
cheese
1 slice bacon
2 pancakes
1 tsp. oil,
margarine,
mayonnaise
2 Tbsp. sour
cream
5 olives

0 grams

fruit/juice
vegetables
beans
bread
bagels
cereals
oatmeal
rolls
tortillas
rice
grits
pasta
potatoes
corn
graham crackers
oyster crackers
popcorn
pretzels
soup (broth or
tomato based)
fat-free milk
fat-free yogurt
fat-free cheese
fat-free hot
cocoa
1 scoop fat-free
frozen yogurt

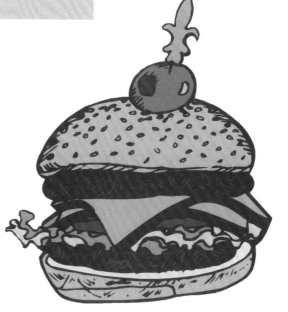

How to Size Up Your Portions

- If you eat all the right foods, but eat too much, you will gain weight.
- Control portions to control weight. Portions count just like calories.

Meat, Poultry, Fish (Cooked)

3 oz. = the palm of a lady's hand (don't count fingers!)
  = a deck of cards
  = amount in a typical homemade sandwich
  = amount in a "quarter pounder" (cooked)
  = half chicken breast (3 inches across)
6 oz. = restaurant split chicken breasts (6 inches across)
  = typical luncheon or cafeteria portion
8 oz. = typical evening restaurant portion
6-8 oz. = typical restaurant burger

Cheese

1 oz. = 1 slice on sandwich or hamburger
  = 1 inch cube
  = 3 Tbsp. (1/4 c.) grated
1/2 c. = 1 small scoop cottage cheese

Salads

1 c. = dinner salad
2-4 c. = salad bar or salad entree

Vegetables

1/2 c. = cafeteria or restaurant portion
  = coleslaw or beans at a barbecue restaurant

Potato

1 small (3 oz., red new potato) = 80 calories = 1/2 c.
1 medium small (4 oz.) = 100 calories = 3" long
1 medium (6 oz.) = 160 calories = 4" long
1 medium large (8 oz.) = 200 calories = 5" long
1 large (10 oz.) = 250 calories = restaurant size
1 huge (16 oz.) = 400 calories = meal-in-one larger
  potato

Fruit

| 1 small (3" across) fruit | = 60 calories |
| 1 large fruit (apple, banana, pear) | = 120 calories |

Ice Cream

1/2 c. = 4 oz. = 1 small scoop
1 c. = 8 oz. = 1 large scoop

Beverages

6 oz. (3/4 c.)	= 100 calories	= typical juice portion
8 oz. (1 c.)	= 100 calories	= common fat-free milk carton
4 oz.	= 100 calories	= small glass of wine
6 oz.	= 150 calories	= usual glass of wine
12 oz.	= 150 calories	= a can of beer or soft drink
1 1/2 oz.	= 100 calories	= 1 jigger per alcoholic drink
16-20 oz.	= 200-250 cal.	= bottled teas; sodas
32 oz.	= 320 calories	= sodas
44 oz.	= 440 calories	= sodas

Theater Popcorn

Popped in oil	without butter	w/butter
Small (4 c.)	= 300 calories	475 calories
Medium (10 c.)	= 650 calories	900 calories
Large (15-20 c.)	=1000 calories	1500 calories

MEASURE UP!

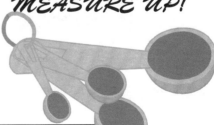

➢ *See more on portions in Step 9.*

Fats

1 tsp. margarine/butter	=	50 calories	=	1 pat
1 Tbsp. mayonnaise	=	100 calories	=	typical amount on sandwiches
2 Tbsp. dressing	=	150 calories	=	typical amount on a dinner salad
4 Tbsp. (1/4 c.) dressing	=	300 calories	=	1 large ladle!!

It's Time to Act

As you read about the various eating plans, which one will you put into action? Try several, then select your favorite approach and become better acquainted with it by reading the pages recommended. Don't waste time! **START NOW!** As you read other book sections, you'll discover new facts, behaviors and "tricks of the trade" that will help you along the way.

Oops! . . . What If You Blow It?

Don't let one meal over a one-week period (that's 21 meals!) destroy your frame of mind and enthusiasm. Even three meals "off" shouldn't cause you to throw in the towel. Make up the extra calories and fat by eating two to four extra "all-vegetable" or "fat-free" meals that week. It will all balance out. (All-vegetable plates cut 250-500 calories per meal.) Get back on track and keep moving! Don't look back.

> **Success Tip**
>
> It's the week's balance of meals that counts - not necessarily a single meal!

Beyond Diet

Habits

Along with any of these healthy eating approaches, eating habits are key to lifelong weight success. Learning to plan and eat three meals daily, choosing low-fat snacks, eating slowly and establishing other healthy habits requires repeated practice. Repeated patterns become habits. Once new habits are established, they reinforce the eating styles that enable healthy weight control without as much conscious effort. The sooner you get started, the better.

Exercise

Along with healthy eating habits, you must move more or exercise! Remember, burn 200-300 calories aerobically, four to five times a week to burn sufficient fat calories and body fat. Add two or three 20-30 minute sessions of resistance or strength training weekly to build muscle (lean body mass), which speeds metabolism. Five days a week of exercise will increase fitness; three days a week will maintain fitness. Make exercise time count! Walk a little farther or faster, or uphill (inclined on a treadmill) to burn more calories per exercise session.

> **Success Tip**
>
> # Move, Move!
>
> - Park further away
> - Climb every stair case (not elevators or escalators)
> - Walk long corridors
> - Avoid trams at airports

If your busy schedule prevents exercise now and then, look for ways to increase daily activity by taking stairs; longer walking routes to meetings, offices, your car, etc.; and walking long hotel and airport corridors. Keep moving!

Lifelong Weight Maintenance

The above behaviors will help you lose weight and keep it off. In addition, become familiar with the meal sizes and food portions that will enable you to enjoy your desired weight for life!

Choose Your Own Eating Plan

Now that you've learned the basic components of healthy eating, it's time to design your own eating plan! Select one of the following approaches, based on your personality, lifestyle and preferences...and READ ON!

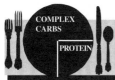

PLAN A: "HEALTHY CHOICES" APPROACH

This is for people who say, "I don't want a plan!" Based on the United States Department of Agriculture's Food Guide Pyramid for healthy eating, you simply **emphasize high-fiber** plant foods (fruit, vegetables, whole grains, peas, beans, starches) and **limit fats** (such as margarine and oils) and keep protein-rich foods moderate. The concept is to make healthy choices as consistently as possible and follow the **"3/4th Plate Rule"** for portions. I also call this the "Look at your Plate" approach.

This approach is the most flexible and least structured. Here are the basic guidelines:

High-Fiber
You will eat **10+ complex carbohydrates** (plant foods) a day (fruit, vegetables, whole grains, beans), giving you 20+ grams of needed fiber daily. Fiber-rich foods are filling and fat-free. Take advantage of large vegetable servings to consume the most food for the fewest calories and least fat. *As a reminder: 1 serving = 1/2 c. vegetable or grain or bean; 1 fruit; 1 slice bread.*

Low-Fat
You will eat daily: • 5-6 oz. of lean protein (meat/fish/ poultry) • 3-6 tsp. (1-2 Tbsp.) of added oils/fats

Your plate should look like this: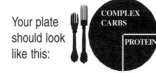

> ➤ *Select 6-7 fruit and vegetable servings per day if you consume 1300-1600 calories.*
> ➤ *Select 8-10 fruits and veggies/day if you consume 1800 calories or more.*

Sample Healthy Choices Plan			
Choose	**Calories**	**Fat (g)**	**Fiber (g)**
2 c. fat-free milk/yogurt	200	0	0
5-6 oz. lean meat/fish/poultry	250-300	5-18	0
3-4 small fruit (2 small = 1 large fruit)	180-250	0	6-8
3 vegetables (1/2 c. each) and a salad	100	0	6-8
5-7 starches (1 slice bread; 1/2 c. pasta, rice, potato, cereal, etc.)	400-700	0-10	5-10
3-6 tsp. fat = "1 tsp." means: *1 tsp. margarine, oil, mayonnaise; or* *2 tsp. salad dressing; or* *3 tsp. (1 Tbsp.) light dressings and margarine)*	150-300	15-30	0
Total	**1250-1850**	**20-60**	**20+**

Continued

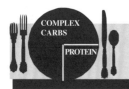

PLAN A: "HEALTHY CHOICES" APPROACH

"Look At Your Plate" Menus

These plates illustrate the "Healthy Choices" or "Look at Your Plate" simple approach to balance as well as portion and calorie-controlled meals. These dinner menus are from this book's 1600 Calorie Menus, p. 76-80, and range from 400 to 700 calories, depending on the calories and fat consumed from other foods that day.

1600 CALORIE MENUS

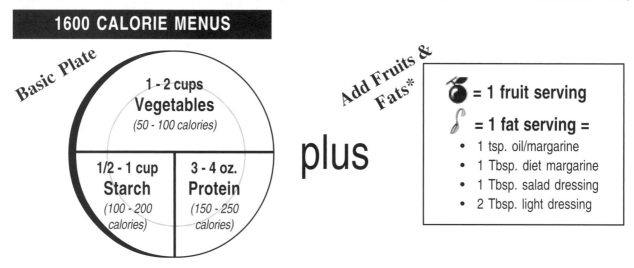

Basic Plate

- 1 - 2 cups **Vegetables** (50 - 100 calories)
- 1/2 - 1 cup **Starch** (100 - 200 calories)
- 3 - 4 oz. **Protein** (150 - 250 calories)

plus

Add Fruits & Fats*

🍎 = 1 fruit serving

🥄 = 1 fat serving =
- 1 tsp. oil/margarine
- 1 Tbsp. diet margarine
- 1 Tbsp. salad dressing
- 2 Tbsp. light dressing

* A Note about fats in these menus: You may use "light" margarine and "light" salad dressings to decrease total calories. If your other meals daily contained 3 or more tsp. of fats, adjust the fat indicated on these **dinner** menus to fit the 6 fat tsp. total for the day.

To make into 1300 CALORIE MENUS:

Reduce starches to 1/2 cup servings, protein (entrees) to 3 oz. servings, and use half the fat servings.

DAY 1   Chicken Dinner

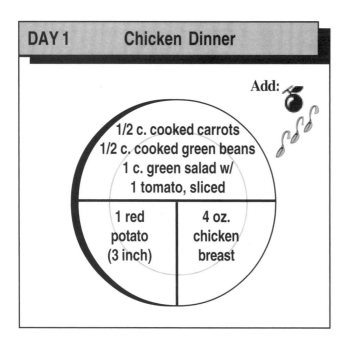

Add:

- 1/2 c. cooked carrots
- 1/2 c. cooked green beans
- 1 c. green salad w/ 1 tomato, sliced
- 1 red potato (3 inch)
- 4 oz. chicken breast

DAY 2   Seafood Dinner

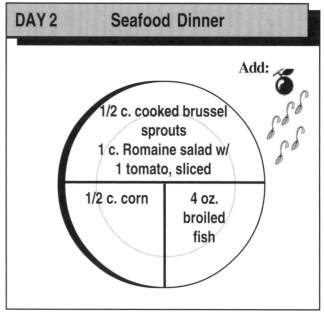

Add:

- 1/2 c. cooked brussel sprouts
- 1 c. Romaine salad w/ 1 tomato, sliced
- 1/2 c. corn
- 4 oz. broiled fish

DAY 3 — Steak Dinner

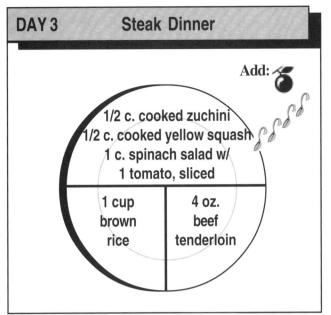

Add:

1/2 c. cooked zuchini
1/2 c. cooked yellow squash
1 c. spinach salad w/
1 tomato, sliced

| 1 cup brown rice | 4 oz. beef tenderloin |

DAY 4 — Spaghetti Dinner

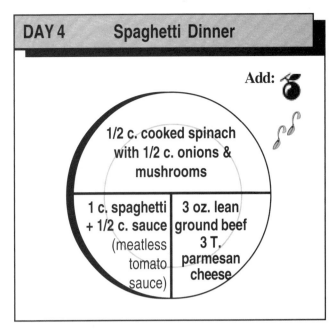

Add:

1/2 c. cooked spinach
with 1/2 c. onions &
mushrooms

| 1 c. spaghetti + 1/2 c. sauce (meatless tomato sauce) | 3 oz. lean ground beef 3 T. parmesan cheese |

DAY 5 — Seafood Dinner

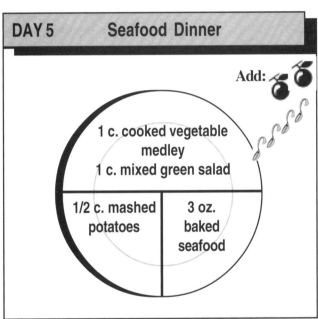

Add:

1 c. cooked vegetable medley
1 c. mixed green salad

| 1/2 c. mashed potatoes | 3 oz. baked seafood |

DAY 6 — Take-out Pizza

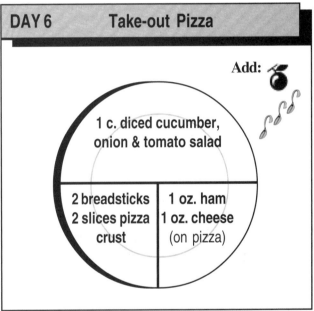

Add:

1 c. diced cucumber,
onion & tomato salad

| 2 breadsticks 2 slices pizza crust | 1 oz. ham 1 oz. cheese (on pizza) |

DAY 7 — Taco Salad

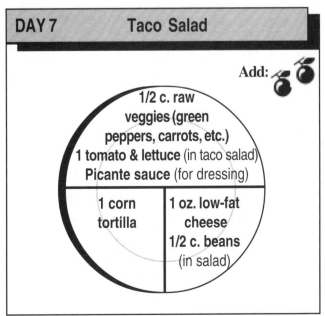

Add:

1/2 c. raw veggies (green peppers, carrots, etc.)
1 tomato & lettuce (in taco salad)
Picante sauce (for dressing)

| 1 corn tortilla | 1 oz. low-fat cheese 1/2 c. beans (in salad) |

DAY 8 — Vegetarian Stir-fry

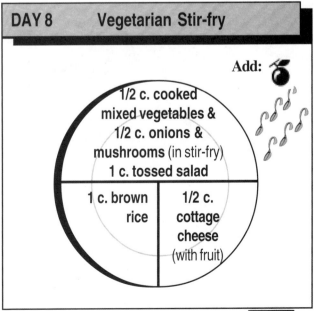

Add:

1/2 c. cooked mixed vegetables &
1/2 c. onions & mushrooms (in stir-fry)
1 c. tossed salad

| 1 c. brown rice | 1/2 c. cottage cheese (with fruit) |

DAY 9 — Chicken Dinner

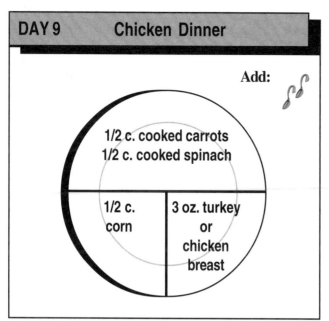

Add: 🎵🎵

- 1/2 c. cooked carrots
- 1/2 c. cooked spinach
- 1/2 c. corn
- 3 oz. turkey or chicken breast

DAY 10 — Seafood Dinner

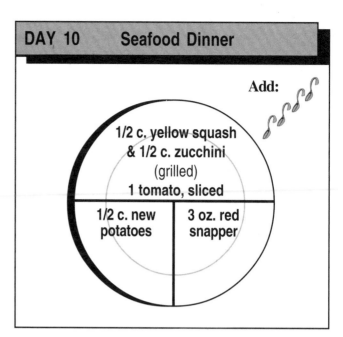

Add: 🎵🎵🎵🎵🎵

- 1/2 c. yellow squash & 1/2 c. zucchini (grilled)
- 1 tomato, sliced
- 1/2 c. new potatoes
- 3 oz. red snapper

DAY 11 — Frozen Dinner

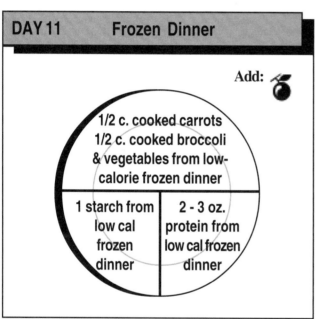

Add: 🍊

- 1/2 c. cooked carrots
- 1/2 c. cooked broccoli & vegetables from low-calorie frozen dinner
- 1 starch from low cal frozen dinner
- 2 - 3 oz. protein from low cal frozen dinner

DAY 12 — Shrimp Creole

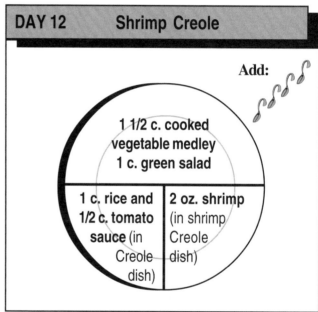

Add: 🎵🎵🎵🎵

- 1 1/2 c. cooked vegetable medley
- 1 c. green salad
- 1 c. rice and 1/2 c. tomato sauce (in Creole dish)
- 2 oz. shrimp (in shrimp Creole dish)

DAY 13 — Fajitas

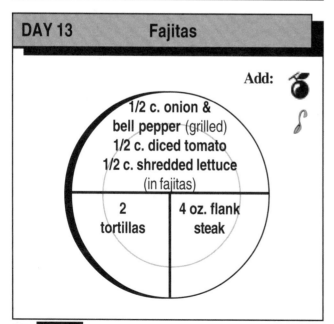

Add: 🍊 🎵

- 1/2 c. onion & bell pepper (grilled)
- 1/2 c. diced tomato
- 1/2 c. shredded lettuce (in fajitas)
- 2 tortillas
- 4 oz. flank steak

DAY 14 — Mini Pizzas

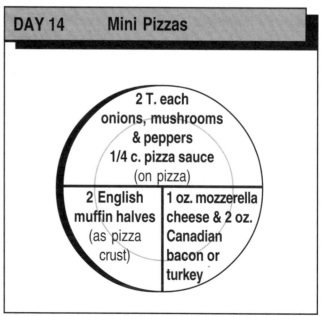

- 2 T. each onions, mushrooms & peppers
- 1/4 c. pizza sauce (on pizza)
- 2 English muffin halves (as pizza crust)
- 1 oz. mozzarella cheese & 2 oz. Canadian bacon or turkey

If the "Healthy Choices" option seems too vague for starters, begin with one of the four "Select-A-Plan" approaches for specific meal plans; later advance to "Healthy Choices" as a lifelong approach, being mindful of portions. Below are four options. Try all four and then decide which single or combined approach works best for your lifestyle and personality.

4 Select-A-Plan Options:

1 **SELECT BY FOOD GROUPS**

Simply eat a set number of servings daily from each of six food groups to plan your own meals. You'll lose weight while enjoying the maximum *flexibility* plus *structure* in meal planning—and no calorie counting!

2 **SELECT BY MENU**

To jump start your program, follow two weeks of **Sample Menus** at 1300 or 1600 calories. These low-fat, high-fiber menus utilize food groups for meal planning. Think of them as a start-up guide. Take note of portions and the mix of food choices per meal, the emphasis on plant foods, and smaller protein and fat servings. After two to four weeks, "spice up your life" with more food variety by creating your own menus (Approach 1).

3 **SELECT BY MEAL**

Using **Mix-and-Match Meals**, combine any of the quick-fix, preplanned P-C-F breakfast, lunch and dinner meals. The result? You'll automatically eat healthy, nutritionally balanced meals and 1300 or 1600 calories daily with 30-50 grams of fat. This plan works well for busy people who eat on the run, and need *flexibility* and *convenience*. Think of the meals as "calorie clusters."

4 **SELECT BY CALORIE-COUNT**

Sometimes it's more convenient and appropriate to choose snacks or meals based on calories. Restaurant meals, fast foods, snack foods and frozen dinners particularly fit this system. Choose specific "Meals Out" (p. 174-183) and Fast Foods (Appendix C), as well as labeled snacks and purchased meals, that fit this calorie-based method. Make use of a simplified calorie-counting system (p. 97).

Choose 1 , 2 , 3 , 4 or any combination!

Here's an Example of How You Can Combine 1, 2, 3, 4!

| 1 | 3 | 2 | 4 |

Breakfast
FOOD GROUP

1 dairy = 1 c. milk
2 grains = 1 c. oatmeal
2 fruit = 1/2 c.
orange juice
&
1 c. straw-
berries

Lunch
**MIX & MATCH
MEAL**

sandwich + fruit

(= 450 calories,
10 g fat)

Dinner
SAMPLE MENU

3 oz. baked chicken
1 small potato
1/2 c. broccoli
1/2 c. carrots
salad w/ 1 Tbsp.
dressing
1/2 c. fresh pineapple

Snack
CALORIE COUNT

100-calorie frozen
yogurt (small)

Remember

- All plans are interchangeable.
- *Calories* are the bottom line.
- *Quality calories* are the goal.

Bottom Line

Women: Select daily:
1300 - 1400 calories,
30 - 40 grams fat,
20 - 30 grams fiber.

Men: Select daily:
1500 - 1800 calories,
50 - 60 grams fat,
20 - 30 grams fiber.

For more details, read on!

SELECT-A-PLAN $\boxed{1}$, $\boxed{2}$, $\boxed{3}$, $\boxed{4}$ APPROACHES

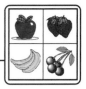

No matter which meal-planning approach pleases you most, you will want to consume daily the following foods and quantities to assure optimal nutrition and appropriate calories. All Select-A-Plan approaches are based on these eating plans.

WOMEN: 1300-1400 Calories

Choose	Calories	Fat (g)
2 c. fat-free milk/yogurt	200	0
5 oz. lean meat/fish/poultry	250	5-15
3 small fruit (or 1 large + 1 small fruit)	180	0
3 vegetables (1/2 c. each) and a green salad; or 2 veggies (1/2 c. each) and a big tossed salad	75	0
5 starches (1 slice bread; 1/2 c. pasta, rice, potato, cereal, etc.)	400-500	0-5
4 tsp. fat ("1 tsp." means 1 tsp. margarine, oil, mayonnaise; or 2 tsp. salad dressing; or 3 tsp. (1 Tbsp.) light dressing, margarine, mayonnaise)	200	15-20
Total	**1300-1400**	**20-40**

MEN: 1600-1800 Calories

Choose	Calories	Fat (g)
2 c. fat-free milk/yogurt	200	0
6 oz. lean meat/fish/poultry	300	6-18
4 small (or 2 large) fruit	200	0
3 vegetables (1/2 c. each) and a salad = 4 total	100	0
6-7 starches (1 slice bread; or ½ c. pasta, rice, potato, corn, cereal, etc.)	500-700	0-10
6 tsp. fat ("1 tsp." means 1 tsp. margarine, oil, mayonnaise; or 2 tsp. salad dressing; or 3 tsp. (1 Tbsp.) light dressing, margarine, mayonnaise)	300	30
Total	**1600-1800**	**35-60**

① SELECT-A-PLAN: BY FOOD GROUPS

Never count calories or fat grams! Use "Food Groups" to create your meals if you want structure, flexibility and simplicity. All foods fit into six groups according to their nutrient and calorie content. Simply select a specific number of servings from each group daily based on your weight loss category, and you automatically consume the right amount of fiber, fat and calories, and optimal nutrition.

Weight Loss Categories: Sample Daily Eating Plans				
Weight Loss Categories	**Protein Sources**	**Fat Sources**	**Carbohydrate Sources**	**This Results in**
Most Women	5 oz. meat/sub 2 c. fat-free milk	4 tsp. fat	3 fruit (small) 5 starches 3 vegetables	1300 calories 30 g fat
Very Active Women	6 oz. meat/sub 2 c. fat-free milk	5 tsp. fat	3 fruit (small) 6 starches 3 vegetables	1500 calories 40 g fat
Less Active Men*	6 oz. meat/sub 2 c. fat-free milk	6 tsp. fat	4 fruit (small) or 2 large 6 starches 4 vegetables	1600 calories 50 g fat
Most Men	7 oz. meat/sub 2 c. fat-free milk	6 tsp. fat	4 fruit (small) or 2 large 7 starches 4 vegetables	1800 calories 55 g fat
Very Active Men	7 oz. meat/sub 2 c. fat-free milk	7 tsp. fat	6 fruit (small) or 3 large 7 starches 4 vegetables	2000 calories 60 g fat

also weight maintenance for most women

Design your own eating plan using this chart. Follow these steps:

Step 1. Choose your appropriate category for weight loss.

Step 2. Note the number of servings you can eat daily from each food group.

Step 3. Record the "totals" of servings from each group in the far right column of your Eating Plan chart (p. 61).

Step 4. Distribute the servings into three meals and snacks, recording them on your chart so that now you have a meal plan for each meal. See example next page.

Step 5. Familiarize yourself with the food groups and serving sizes (p. 62, 64-67).

Sample Daily Eating Plan

Category: _Weight Loss for Most Women_   Calories: _1300-1400_   Fat Grams: _30 - 40_

	Breakfast	Snack	Lunch	Snack	Dinner	Snack	TOTALS
Milk	1			1			2
Meat			2 oz.		3 oz.		5 oz.
Starches	1		2		1-2	1	5-6
Fruit	1		1	1			3
Vegetables			1		2		3
Fats			1		2	1	4
Extras							
Calories	240		400	150	400-500	130	1300-1400
Fat Grams	0		10-15	0	15-20	5	30-40

Notes:

Sample Daily Eating Plan

Category:	*Weight Loss for Men & Weight Maintenance for Women (Weight Maint. for Men by adding 250-500 Calories)* Calories: **1500-2000** Fat Grams: **50 - 60**

	Breakfast	Snack	Lunch	Snack	Dinner	Snack	TOTALS
Milk	1					1	2 cups
Meat			3 oz.		3 oz.		6 oz.
Starches	2		2		1 - 2	1	6 - 7+
Fruit	1		1	1			3+
Vegetables			1+		2+		3+
Fats	1 - 2		1 - 3		1 - 3		3 - 8
Extras							
Calories	350 - 400		500 - 600	50 - 100	450 - 600	150-200	1500-1900
Fat Grams	5 - 10		10-25	0	10-25	0	25-60

Notes:

© 2009, *The Cooper Clinic Solution to the Diet Revolution* by Georgia G. Kostas, M.P.H., R.D., L.D., Dallas, Texas

My Daily Eating Plan

Category: _____   Calories: _____   Fat Grams: _____

	Breakfast	Snack	Lunch	Snack	Dinner	Snack	TOTALS
Milk							
Meat							
Starches							
Fruit							
Vegetables							
Fats							
Extras							
Calories							
Fat Grams							

Notes:

Food Group Quick List

Here is an easy, at-a-glance look at the foods and serving sizes that make up the six food categories.

Milk (100 calories)

1c. milk: fat-free, low-fat, 1%
1 c. yogurt: nonfat, low-fat, sugar-free
2 c. light hot cocoa: fat-free, sugar-free
1/2 c. cottage cheese: nonfat, low-fat
2 oz. (1-2 slices) fat-free or veggie/soy cheese
   (30-50 calories/1 oz. slice)
1 oz. (1 slice) low-fat, reduced fat, light cheese
   (3-7 g. fat/oz.; 50-70 calories/oz.)

Meat/Protein (50 calories/oz.)

1 oz. poultry, fish, lean beef,* pork,* lamb, venison,
   shellfish, soyburger, tofu, etc.
1/4 c. tuna, salmon, cottage cheese, chicken, beef
1/4 c. dried beans/peas, tofu, soy crumbles
1 egg or 2 egg whites or 1/4 c. egg substitute
2 Tbsp. mozzarella, Parmesan, feta cheeses
1 oz. (3 Tbsp.) low-fat or fat-free cheese **
1-2 oz. lean cold cuts (read labels)

lean cuts listed on p. 64
**cheeses with no more than 3 g fat per oz. see p. 64,*
   124-125

Fruit (60 calories)

1 small fruit = 1/2 large = 60 calories

1 small fresh fruit (orange, peach, pear, apple)
1/2 large fruit (apple, pear, banana)
1 c. grapes, cherries, melon, strawberries
1/2 c. sliced fresh fruit or frozen, or canned without
   sugar; most berries
1/2 banana, grapefruit, mango, papaya
1/4 cantaloupe
3 dates, prunes, apricots (6 halves)
2 plums, kiwi
1/2 c. fruit juice
1/4 c. dried fruit
1/8 c. (2 Tbsp.) raisins

Note: Count 1 large fruit as 2 servings = 120 calories
   (1 banana, 1 large apple, grapefruit, etc.)

Starches/Bread/Grains/ Starchy Vegetables (80-100 calories)

1 slice bread, roll, tortilla
2 slices light bread
1/2 English muffin, small bagel (1 oz.), hamburger or
   hot dog bun, pita pocket
4-6 crackers, mini-rice cakes
1/2 c. cooked cereal (oatmeal, grits, etc.)
1 oz. ready-to-eat cereals:
       1 c. puffed
       3/4 c. flakes
       1/2 c. bran type
       1/4 c. dense (Grape-Nuts, low-fat
          granola, Muselix)
3 Tbsp. wheat germ, flour, bread crumbs
1 pancake (4"), waffle (4 1/2" square)
1/2 c. rice, pasta, grains
1/2 c. potato, corn, peas, lima beans, dried beans,
   sweet potatoes, acorn or butternut squash (starchy
   vegetables)
1 small potato or red new potato (4 oz.)
1/2 medium potato (8 oz.)

Vegetables (25 calories)

1/2 c. cooked vegetables
1 c. raw vegetables
1 dinner salad
1/2 c. tomato or vegetable juice

Fat (50 calories)

1 tsp. oil, soft or liquid margarine, mayonnaise,
   butter*
1 Tbsp. light margarine, light mayonnaise
2 tsp. salad dressing, peanutbutter, soy butter
1 Tbsp. seeds, nuts; cream,* cream cheese,* gravy*
2 Tbsp. light salad dressing; sour cream,* soynuts, dips*
5 large olives, 1 strip bacon*
1/8 avocado

high in saturated fat; limit these foods

Why the System Works

The chart below shows the average nutrient content in each Food Group serving.

Food Groups						
Food Group	Serving Size	Calories	Fat (g)	Carbo-hydrate (g)	Protein (g)	Fiber (g)
Milk (fat-free)^P	1 cup	100	0-3	15	8	0
Meat/Protein^P	1 ounce (cooked)	50	1-3	0	8	0
Starch/Bread^C	1/2 cup; 1 slice	80-100	0-2	15	3	1-2
Fruit^C	1 small; 1/2 cup	60	0	15	0	2
Vegetable^C	1/2 cup, 1 cup raw or 1 salad	25	0	5	2	2
Fat^F	1 teaspoon	50	5	0	0	0

P = Lean protein sources   C = Complex carbohydrate sources (plant foods)   F = Fat sources

Here is how these food servings can be translated into calories:

1300- to 1400-Calorie Eating Plan (Women)					
You select:			You automatically consume:		
Amount	Food Group & Calories Per Group		Calories	Fat (g)	Fiber (g)
3	Fruit	x 60 =	180	0	6+
3	Vegetables	x 25 =	75	0	6+
5	Starches	x 80-100 =	400-500	0-5	10+
2 c.	Milk (fat-free)	x 100 =	200	0	0
5 oz.	Lean meat	x 50 =	250	5-15	0
4 tsp.	Fats/oils	x 50 =	200	15-20	0
Totals			**1300-1400**	**20-40 (Average)**	**22+**

Serving Size Tools

- food weighing scale - for meat and cheese
- standard measuring cups and spoons (teaspoons and tablespoons) for other foods/liquids.

  Know how much you eat!

Measuring and Weight Equivalents

1 oz. = 28 g	4 Tbsp. = 1/4 c. (except cheese)
1 lb. = 16 oz.	1 pt. = 2 c. = 16 oz.
1 c. = 8 oz. = 16 Tbsp.	2 pt. = 4 c. = 1 qt. = 32 oz.
1 Tbsp. = 3 tsp.	4 qt. = 1 gal. = 64 oz.
2 Tbsp. = 1 fluid oz. (i.e., dressings)	1 oz. cheese = 3 Tbsp. = ¼ c.

A Closer Look at Each Food Group

See p. 62 for foods in each group.

See p. 62 for foods in each group.

MILK

1. **Choose 2-3 c. fat-free milk and other dairy foods daily** for strong bones, nails, teeth; proper growth and healing; the prevention of colon cancer, high blood pressure and osteoporosis.

2. Drink up! **Calcium-fortified orange juice** contains as much calcium as milk.

MEAT/PROTEIN

1. **Select fish 2-5 times weekly,** especially cold water fish such as salmon, mackeral, sardines, tuna.

2. **Choose chicken, turkey, poultry, bison, game, beans** 4-5 times a week.

3. **Choose lean meat cuts** (3-4 oz. portions, three to four times a week).

Per 3 oz. portion, these cuts contain less than 200 calories and less than 10 g fat:

- **Beef cuts:** tenderloin (filet), top sirloin, sirloin tips, London broil, kabobs, club, strip steaks, skirt steak, eye of round, top round, rinsed ground round or sirloin (10% fat), fajita meat
- **Lamb:** leg, loin, chops, shoulder
- **Pork/ham:** loin, chops, tenderloin

Note: The words *"loin"* and *"round"* guarantee lean cuts. See *www.beef.org* for 29 lean beef cuts.

---

3 oz. Servings

- 1 pork or veal chop, 3/4" thick
- 2 rib lamb chops or 1 shoulder chop
- 1/2 breast or 1 leg and thigh of 3 lb. chicken
- 1 meat patty, 3" x 3/4"
- 2 thin slices roast meat, each 3" x 3" x 1/4"
- 3 medium-size pieces of stew meat
- 1 small beef filet or 1/2 small sirloin tip
- 1 fish filet, 3" x 3" x 1/2"
- 3/4 c. tuna, salmon, crab, cottage cheese
- 15 large shrimp
- 3 boiled crabs or 18 oysters
- 1/2 Rock Cornish hen

---

4. **Select nonfat or low-fat cheeses** (0-5 g fat per oz.): cottage cheese, Laughing Cow, parmesan, mozzarella, Kraft 2% milk cheese, skim ricotta, Cabot 50% & 70% reduced fat cheese.

Calories & Fat per 1 oz. Meat

	Calories	Fat (g)
Fish	40	0-1
Poultry (no skin)	50	1
Poultry (with skin)	60	2
Lean meat	60	3
Low-fat cheese or tofu	35-50	2-3
Reduced-fat cheese	50-80	3-5
1/4 c. beans	50	0
Average	50	0-3

Note: 4 oz. (1/4 lb.) lean meat = 3 oz. cooked.

5. **Limit cholesterol-rich, fatty cuts:** brisket, corned beef, ground beef, rib steaks, rib roasts, spare ribs, sausage, hot dogs, cold cuts, deviled ham, meatloaf, fried meats, casseroles, meats with gravies, chicken fried steak, etc.

6. **Cook "lean":** Trim all visible fat off meat before cooking; remove poultry skin before or after cooking. Rinse cooked ground beef in a sieve under hot water to wash away fat. Then add beef to skillet, add tomato sauce, etc.

7. **Remove fat from meat drippings.** Refrigerate drippings; fat will rise to the top and harden; skim off. Or use a "gravy skimmer" to separate fat from hot drippings.

FATS

1. **Choose primarily monounsaturated and polyunsaturated fats** for your best health: *monounsaturated* = olive, canola, peanut *polyunsaturated* = safflower, sunflower, corn, soybean, cottonseed oils; flax seeds; seafood; nuts and seeds.

2. **Choose margarine with "liquid oil"** as the first listed ingredient on the label and "hydrogenated" near the end of the list. "Trans-free" new soft tub and liquid forms are best.

3. **Avoid saturated fats**—meat fat, milk/cheese fat, butter, lard, cream, gravy, dips, bacon, coconut oil, palm oil, cocoa butter and "hydrogenated" (hardened) fats.

4. **Avoid trans fats** in fried foods, commercially baked goods and some margarines.

5. **Know how to estimate hidden fats** when eating away from home, such as in restaurants or at parties. When you tally food groups consumed daily, don't forget to include these easily forgotten fats!

6. **See p. 113 for ways to reduce fats** in cooking.

7. **See Appendix C and Step 4 for more details on fat grams** in foods.

8. **Choose foods with Omega-3's** which promote heart, eye, brain and bone health. (See more on p. 164.)

Hidden Fat: Seek and Find It!

1/2 tsp. fat per …	• 1 oz. meat, fish, poultry (sauteed, stir-fried, pan-fried, basted, marinated)
1 tsp. fat per …	• 1/2 c. restaurant vegetables seasoned with oil or margarine or stir-fried • 1 oz. breaded/fried meat, cheese, starch, vegetable • 1 egg, fried or scrambled
3 tsp. fat (=1 Tbsp.) per …	• 20 French fries ("small" order) or 15 potato chips • 1/2 c. of meat or tuna salad, potato or pasta salad, slaw
2 Tbsp. dressing on …	• 1 c. tossed salad
4 Tbsp. dressing on…	• small Caesar salad or 2 c. tossed salad

STARCHES / BREADS / GRAINS / STARCHY VEGETABLES

1. **Choose wholegrains** whenever possible for fiber and nutrients. Examples: 100% wholewheat bread/pita bread, popcorn, wholegrain cereals, corn tortillas, oatmeal, corn, grits, barley, brown rice, rye crackers, Triscuit crackers. **Three wholegrain servings daily** reduce your risk of cancer, heart disease and diabetes, and help reduce weight and belly fat. (See more on wholegrains on pgs. 67 and 108.)

2. **Choose 1/2 to 1 cup portions** of starches for weight management.

3. **Eat only 2 cups of pasta** when having a meatless meal.

4. **Mix cooked grains with vegetables** for additional nutrient variety: rice/carrots/onion; pasta/broccoli/carrots/onions/tomato/corn/black beans/pico de gallo; etc.

5. **Choose wholegrained cereals** with little, if any, sugar. (See cereal list pg. 225.)

6. **Eat dried beans** several times a week - they are packed with nutrients, antioxidants and phyto-nutrients.

7. Wholegrains retain all grain parts including the nutrient-rich, bio-active bran and germ, important to health. **Remember:** *what keeps the plant alive, keeps the eater alive!*

A Whole Grain Kernel

Endosperm:
• Carbohydrate
• Protein
• Some B Vitamins

Bran: (outer shell)
• Fiber
• B Vitamins
• Trace Minerals
• Phytochemicals

Germ:
• B Vitamins
• Vitamin E
• Trace Minerals
• Phytochemicals
• Antioxidants
• Healthy Fats

Diagram courtesy of Bob's Red Mill.

VEGETABLES

1. For variety, **stock your refrigerator and freezer** with some of the following veggies: beets, broccoli, tomatoes, cabbage, carrots, cucumbers, greens (collards, kale, mustard, spinach, turnip), green beans, mixed vegetables, mushrooms, onions, pea pods, radishes, turnips, zucchini. (See list for a smorgasbord from which to choose.)

2. **Cook vegetables** slightly to preserve their nutritive value.

3. **Eat greens daily**—they contain nutrients such as vitamins A and C, folic acid, lutein, fiber, B vitamins and many minerals (iron, calcium, magnesium, copper, zinc, manganese, selenium, potassium). Greens boost the immune system as well as your energy and build red blood cells. They are heart-healthy. Choose darker greens (romaine, etc.) for more nutrients.

4. **Limit** vegetables that are canned, fried, buttered, creamed, served with sauces or cheese (as in casseroles), and cooked with bacon or sausage.

5. **Eat more red bell peppers** than green to gain benefits from the higher vitamin C content and polyphenols/bioflavonoids.

6. **Be creative:** Eat veggies raw or cooked.

7. **Eat baby carrots daily.** They can be added to many foods: rice, spaghetti sauce, beans, etc.

8. **Add a veggie to lunch daily.**

9. **Eat nutrient-rich beans often** to consume great veggie nutrients when you cannot eat veggies.

Remember Your Veggies

Don't get stuck eating the same vegetables day after day. Look at the list below and choose some new ones to add to your meals.

Artichoke (1/2 medium)	Onions
Asparagus	Rhubarb
Bean sprouts	Rutabaga
Beets	Sauerkraut
Broccoli	Snow peas
Brussels sprouts	Spinach, cooked
Cabbage, cooked	String beans, green
Carrots	or yellow
Cauliflower	Sugar snap peas
Eggplant	Summer squash
Green beans	Tomatoes
Green pepper	Tomato juice
Greens, all types	Turnips
Kohlrabi	Vegetable juice
Mushrooms, cooked	Water chestnuts
Okra	Zucchini, cooked

Eat the following raw vegetables in any quantity:

Cabbage	Lettuce, all types
Celery	Mushrooms
Chicory	Parsley
Chinese Cabbage	Pickles, dill or sour
Cucumbers	Radishes
Endive	Spinach
Escarole	Watercress
Green onions	Zucchini

More Ideas

"20 Easy Ways to Eat More Veggies," see Step 3
"Great Cooking Tips for Veggies," see Step 10
"Nutrient All-Stars", see pg 102-103

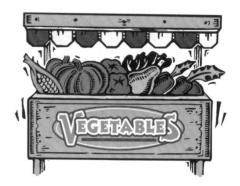

FRUIT

1. **Get the most food for your calories:**

60 Calories:

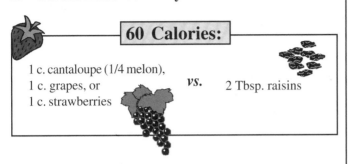

1 c. cantaloupe (1/4 melon),
1 c. grapes, or
1 c. strawberries

vs.

2 Tbsp. raisins

2. **Choose color: fruit with red, yellow and orange pigments contain more vitamins A and C, antioxidants and polyphenols.** Cantaloupe, strawberries, blueberries, all berries, cherries, orange, mango, papaya, peaches, apricots, nectarines, red grapefruit, red grapes, watermelon and tomatoes protect against heart disease and cancer.

3. **Eat citrus daily** for vitamin C and limonene—cancer and heart-disease fighters, and immune-boosters.

4. **A fruit contains about 2 g of fiber** per serving.

5. **Drink calcium-fortified juices** to boost calcium intake. Orange, orange/tangerine, ruby red grapefruit and tomato juice varieties are available with 300 to 400 mg calcium per 8 oz. drink.

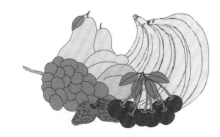

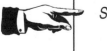 *See "12 Easy Ways to Eat More Fruit" in Step 3*

Wholegrains (WG)

Continued from p. 65

1. **Wholegrains are wholesome.** Do not settle for less! Buy "100% wholegrained" foods!

   "Wholegrained" does not mean:
   " wheat flour"   "cracked wheat"
   "enriched flour"   "stoneground wheat"
   "multi-grain"   "high fiber"
   "natural" grain   brown in color

2. **Read labels!** A true wholegrain (WG) lists as its first ingredient the words "100% wholegrain (*wheat*) flour". Look for the new wholegrain stamp (from the Whole Grains Council) on product packages, showing how much wholegrain they contain.

   Foods with this stamp contain 8 gm WG (= 1/2 "WG serving") GOAL: 6 servings daily (= 48 gms WG)
   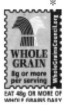
   Foods with this stamp contain 100% wholegrains & 16 gm WG (= 1 "WG serving") GOAL: 3 servings daily (= 48 gms WG)

3. **We need 3 servings** (48 gms) of 100% wholegrains daily. (1 WG serving = 1 grain/starch serving = 80-100 cal)

Sample foods with 100% WG & 16 gm WG/serving
• 4 Triscuit® crackers
• 2/3 c of Cheerios®
• 1/3 c of Wheat Chex®
• 2/5 c of cooked oatmeal
• 1 slice of 100% WG bread
• 1/2 100% WG English muffin or hamburger bun
• 1/3 c cooked wholewheat pasta or brown rice
• 1/3 c cooked bulgur, barley or other cooked WG

Easy ways to include more WG daily:
• Start your day with a WG cereal - ie. Kashi, oat flakes, oatmeal, 100% wholewheat Chex cereals, etc.
• Use wholewheat bread for sandwiches
• Eat brown rice instead of white rice
• Snack on popcorn, WG dry cereals or an ear of corn
• Choose WG crackers - ie. Triscuits.
• Cook wholewheat pasta
• Make a sandwich wrap with a corn or 100% wholewheat tortilla
• Top yogurt, cottage cheese or salad with crunchy WG cereals

* *Stamps: © Whole Grains Council and Oldways preservation Trust .*

A Few Extras

- An occasional treat or "extra" three times a week is fine. Just keep portions reasonable.
- Try to choose foods up to 150 calories and 5 g fat per serving. Some ideas:

Cookies	Cal.	Fat (g)
Snackwell's Cinnamon Graham Cookies (9), Devil's Food Cake (1)	60	0
Snackwell's Chocolate Chip Cookies (6), Oatmeal Raisin Cookies (1)	60	1
Nabisco Devil's Food Cake (1)	70	1
Health Valley fat-free cookies: oatmeal raisin (3), apricot (3), etc.	75	0
Entenmann's fat-free cookies: oatmeal raisin, etc. (1)	80	0
Animal crackers (10), vanilla wafers (5), chocolate snaps (4), ginger snaps (3)	80	3
Homemade cookies: oatmeal (1), sugar (1), chocolate chip (1), etc.	80	3
Chocolate creme-filled (2) or Lovin' Lite brownie (1/24 of mix)	100	3
Fig newtons (2)	120	2
Health Valley fat-free granola bar (1) or fat-free muffin (1)	140	0
Desserts/Sweets		
Angel food cake (1/24 of cake); Entenmann's fat-free cakes (1 oz.)	80	0
Regular gelatin (1/2 c.) or sugar-free pudding (1/2 c.)	80	0
Fat-free pudding snacks (1/2 c.)	100	0
Popsicle twin pop (1 bar), frozen fruit bar, frozen pudding bar	80	0
Fruit ice (1/2 c.), nonfat frozen yogurt (1/2 c.)	80	0
Ice milk (1/2 c.) or low-fat frozen yogurt (1/2 c.)	100	3
Sorbet (1/2 c.)	120	0
Sherbet (1/2 c.)	135	2
Condiments		
Apple butter (1 Tbsp.)	15	0
Sugar, jelly, marmalade, honey, molasses, maple syrup (1 Tbsp.)	55	0
Low-calorie jelly or maple syrup (1 Tbsp.)	8-35	0
Chocolate syrup (1 Tbsp.)	50	0
Low-calorie fudge topping (1 Tbsp.)	35	0
Beverages		
Water, club soda, sugar-free tonic water	0	0
Tonic water (6 oz.)	7	0
Wine, dry (3 oz.)	70	0
Liquor (1 oz., 80 Proof)	70	0
Lite beer (12 oz.)	70-100	0
Regular beer (12 oz.)	150	0
Dessert wine, sherry (3 oz.)	120	0
Port wine (3 oz.)	140	0
Soft drinks, punch (12 oz.)	150	0

A Few Extras for Free!

You can eat a few "extras" for free! These items have only a few calories (less than 20 per serving), are fat-free and may contain a little sugar. A few of these foods have specified portions listed because large amounts will add too many calories. Enjoy without guilt...

water, regular or bottled
baking powder, baking soda
carbonated water
bouillon, consommé without fat*
sugar-free soft drinks
broth*
sugar-free tonic water
chives
club soda
cranberries, unsweetened
sugar-free drink mixes (lemonade, Kool-Aid)
rhubarb, unsweetened
coffee, tea, Postum
lemon, lime
cocoa powder, unsweetened (1 Tbsp.)
gelatin, sugar-free (1/2 c.)
barbecue sauce* (1 Tbsp.)
jam, jelly, regular or sugar-free (1 tsp.)
catsup* (1 Tbsp.)
apple butter (1 Tbsp.)
chili sauce* (1 Tbsp.)

pancake syrup, sugar-free (1 Tbsp.)
pizza sauce (2 Tbsp.)
sugar substitutes
picante sauce, salsa, pico de gallo
whipped toppings (2 Tbsp.)
hot pepper sauce, Tabasco sauce
herbs and spices, all types
taco (hot) sauce*
mustard, prepared* (1 Tbsp.)
tomato paste/puree (1 Tbsp.)
mustard powder
Worcestershire sauce*
pickles, dill/sour*
soy sauce*
pimento (1 Tbsp.)
steak sauce (A-1, etc.)
pepper; most seasonings
vinegar, all flavors
lettuce, parsley, radishes, watercress, celery
butter-flavored sprays
sprinkles

Note: The following foods are included as "free" if 1 Tbsp. of fat-free is used: cream cheese, mayonnaise, salad dressing, sour cream . . . and calories per Tbsp. are 20 or less.

*High in sodium. Buy low-sodium brands.

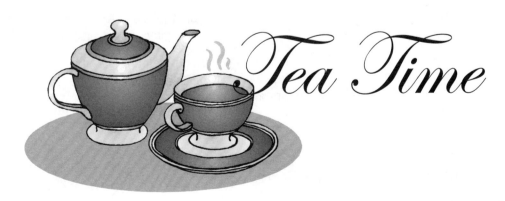

The following 14 days of menus give you meal ideas at 3 different calorie levels. Please note the use of the Food Group System, which enables you to eat well-balanced, healthy, low-fat meals with the P-C-F (protein-carbo-hydrate-fat) mix per meal . . . and you don't need to count fat or calories . . . just food groups!

Helpful Hints Before You Begin:

1. It helps to have a particular pattern of eating at meals, (i.e., a fruit at breakfast, lunch and snack, or 2-3 vegetables at supper). Patterns build consistency.

2. You may save something from a meal for a snack later.

3. Substitute favorite vegetables or fruit for those in menus.

4. You may add garlic, seasonings or butter flavorings (i.e., I Can't Believe It's Not Butter Spray) to any menu items. You may use nonstick vegetable oil cooking sprays whenever desired. If you prefer to use less fat than the menu suggests, go ahead! You'll save 50 calories per fat serving.

5. Drink an 8-16 oz. glass of water at every meal, and 32 oz. additional water throughout the day.

6. You may add 3 "extra" foods a week (up to 100-150 calories each) and still lose weight. Ideas:
    - 1/2 cup (4 oz.) frozen fat-free, sugar-free yogurt or ice milk (80-110 calories)
    - 1/2 cup (4 oz.) fat-free chocolate pudding snack (Jello, Hunt's, etc.) (100 calories)
    - 1 frozen "ice cream" bar treat (80-100 calories)
    - 5 vanilla wafers (80 calories)
    - 2 Fig Newtons (120 calories)
    - 2 Tbsp "lite" syrup (60 calories)
    - See p. 68 for "Extra's" listed

7. Soy yogurt, soy cheese and soy milk may replace milk products. Choose fat-free, fortified with calcium.

8. **Vegetarians:** Trade a 2 oz. meat portion for 1/2 cup beans or tofu, or 1 oz. cheese; and trade a 3 oz. meat portion for 3/4 cup beans or tofu, or 1 1/2 oz. cheese.

9. **About breads/grains:**
    - Note these bread substitutes: 2 toasts = 1 English muffin = 1 small bagel (i.e., Lender's) = 1/2 deli bagel.
    - You can substitute grits, oatmeal, hot cereal/grains for cold cereals; or let cereal replace bread (2 toasts = 1 cup cereal).
    - Choose 100% wholegrains!

10. Add "free" (calorie-free) foods as desired. See p. 69.

11. **Calcium:** add calcium-fortified foods or a calcium supplement daily to add 300 mg calcium per day.

12. **About fats:**
    - Feel free to add "lower-fat" versions of cheese, dressings, mayonnaise, etc., in the menus.
    - "Light" dressings refer to those averaging 25 calories per tablespoon. Read labels. They can range from 15 to 50 calories per tablespoon.

13. **About vegetables:**
    - If you can eat more vegetables per menu, add them! Never skimp on veggies! Eat as many as you can!
    - If you don't like a listed vegetable, substitute one you enjoy. Baby carrots, fresh tomatoes, salads, frozen veggies are convenient options. Other ideas: grilled or roasted veggies (eggplant, cabbage, red bell pepper, etc.), steamed fresh celery and carrots, or blend frozen vegetables, such as 1 package broccoli with 1 package broccoli with cheese sauce, or 1 package spinach with 1 package creamed or buttered spinach. And don't forget to try sugar-snap beans (fresh or frozen)—everyone's favorite!
    - Ever try edamame beans (in the pods)? Delicious and fun food to eat! Just steam a frozen bag for 5 minutes and eat as finger food! Count 1/2 c. (with pods) as 3 vegetables! (Just don't eat the pods!)These are soybeans . . . sweet and delicious!

14. **About seasonings:** Add salsa, cilantro, pico de gallo, onion, garlic, bell pepper, jalapenos, spices and herbs to add "pizzazz" to any menu items.

15. **About juices:** Always choose calcium-fortified citrus juices (orange, grapefruit, tangerine, etc.).

16. **About color:** Note the "red" and "green" in most lunch and dinner menus . . . signs of super-nutrition!

17. **With a little prior thought,** you can plan delicious, healthy meals!

Bon Appetit!

14-Day Weight Loss Menus for Women

1300 Calories, 30-40 grams fat

2 Milk *(Mk)*	5 Meat *(Mt)*	5 Starches *(St)*	3 Fruits *(Fr)*	3+ Vegetables *(Vg)*	4 Fat *(Ft)*

- To make 1200 calories: omit 2 fat servings.
- To make 1400 calories: add 100 calories of choice as a snack, extra starch or a large fruit (see Calorie Counter p. 97).
- Today we recommend 1300 calories plus 30 minutes brisk physical activity daily rather than 1200 calories/day.

> *For a complete shopping list, see p. 85-87.*

DAY 1

BREAKFAST
1/2 c. calcium-fortified orange juice or
   1 fresh orange *(1Fr)*
1 wholewheat toast *(1 St)* with
   1 tsp. sugar-free jam/jelly *(free)*
   & 1/2 Tbsp. peanutbutter or
   1 tsp. tub margarine *(1 Ft)*
1 c. fat-free milk *(1 Mk)*

LUNCH
Tuna Sandwich:
   2 slices wholewheat bread *(2 St)*
   1/2 c. water-packed tuna *(2 Mt)*
   1 Tbsp. light mayonnaise *(1 Ft)*
   1/4 c. apple, celery, pickle *(free)*
   lettuce and tomato slices *(free)*
1/2 c. grape tomatoes *(1 Vg)*
1 small apple *(1 Fr)*
1 c. fat-free milk or yogurt *(1 Mk)*

DINNER
3 oz. skinless chicken breast, grilled *(3 Mt)*
1 small red (new) potato *(1 St)*
   with butter-flavored pump spray *(free)*
1/2 c. carrots, steamed *(1 Vg)*
1/2 c. green beans, steamed *(1 Vg)*
   with butter-flavored pump spray *(free)*
1 c. green salad *(free)* with
   1 sliced tomato *(1 Vg)* and
   2 Tbsp. light dressing *(1 Ft)*
1/2 c. fresh pineapple chunks *(1 Fr)*

SNACK
3 c. microwave light popcorn *(1 St, 1 Ft)*

DAY 2

BREAKFAST
1 c. cubed or 1/4 of a cantaloupe *(1Fr)*
1/2 wholewheat English muffin *(1 St)*
   with 1 tsp. apple butter *(free)* &
   1/2 Tbsp. peanutbutter or 1 tsp.
   tub margarine *(1 Ft)*
1 c. fat-free milk *(1 Mk)*

LUNCH
1 small wholewheat bagel or 2 bread *(2 St)*
2 oz. low-fat cheese *(2 Mt)*
1 raw carrot, in sticks *(1 Vg)*
1 small pear *(1 Fr)*
1 c. nonfat, sugar-free yogurt *(1 Mk)*

DINNER
3 oz. broiled fish with lemon *(3 Mt)*
   & 1 tsp. olive oil *(1 Ft)*
1/2 c. corn, steamed *(1 St)*
1/2 c. Brussels sprouts, steamed *(1 Vg)*
1 tsp. (or 1 Tbsp. light) margarine for
   vegetables *(1 Ft)*
1 c. Romaine salad *(free)* with
   1 tomato, slices *(1 Vg)* and
   2 Tbsp. light dressing or 1 Tbsp.
   French dressing *(1 Ft)*
1/2 c. fresh fruit salad *(1 Fr)*

SNACK
5 wholewheat low-fat Triscuit crackers *(1 St)*

DAY 3

BREAKFAST
1/2 banana *(1 Fr)*
1/2 c. bran flakes or Kashi cereal *(1 St)*
1 Tbsp. almonds *(1 Ft)*
1 c. fat-free milk *(1 Mk)*

LUNCH
Sandwich:
   2 slices wholewheat bread *(2 St)*
   2 oz. turkey *(2 Mt)*
   1 Tbsp. light mayonnaise *(1 Ft)*
   Lettuce, tomato slices *(free)*
1/2 c. raw baby carrots *(1 Vg)*
1 small apple *(1 Fr)*
1 c. fat-free milk *(1 Mk)*

DINNER
3 oz. lean beef tenderloin *(3 Mt)*
1/2 c. brown rice *(1 St)*
   cooked in broth *(free)*
1/2 c. zucchini *(1 Vg)* and
1/2 c. yellow squash *(1 Vg)*
   stir-fried in 1 tsp. oil *(1 Ft)*
1 spinach salad *(free)* with
   1 small tomato *(1 Vg)* and
   2 Tbsp. light dressing *(1 Ft)*
1 orange, in sections *(1 Fr)*

SNACK
3 graham cracker squares *(1 St)*

> *Legend*
> Tbsp. = tablespoon
> tsp. = teaspoon
> c. = cup
> oz. = ounce

DAY 4

BREAKFAST
1/2 grapefruit *(1 Fr)*
1 small wholewheat bagel *(2 St)* with
   1 1/2 Tbsp. light cream cheese *(1 Ft)*
1 c. fat-free milk or yogurt *(1 Mk)*

LUNCH
1 small red (new) potato *(1 St)* topped w/
   1/2 c. low-fat cottage cheese *(2 Mt)*
1 large Romaine salad w/sliced
   cucumbers, onions, celery,
   cherry tomatoes *(free)*
   2 Tbsp. light dressing *(1 Ft)*
1/2 c. asparagus *(1 Vg)*
   sautéed in 1 tsp. oil *(1 Ft)*
1 c. strawberries *(1 Fr)*

DINNER
Spaghetti:
   3 oz. extra lean ground beef,
     cooked & drained *(3 Mt)* and
   1/2 c. meatless spaghetti sauce *(1 St)*
     over 1/2 c. spaghetti *(1 St)*
4 c. raw spinach (1/2 c. cooked) *(1 Vg)* &
   1/2 c. mushrooms & onions *(1 Vg)*
     sautéed in 1 tsp. olive oil *(1 Ft)*
     and lemon juice
1 c. melon, cubed *(1 Fr)*

SNACK
8 oz. carton lemon nonfat, sugar-
   free yogurt *(1 Mk)*

DAY 5

BREAKFAST
1 orange or 1/2 c. blueberries *(1 Fr)*
1/2 c. oatmeal cooked *(1 St)*
1 Tbsp. walnuts *(1 Ft)*
1 c. fat-free milk *(1 Mk)*

LUNCH
Pita Sandwich:
   1 wholewheat pita pocket *(2 St)*
   2 oz. turkey *(2 Mt)*
   1 oz. (2 slices) low-fat cheese *(1 Mk)*
   lettuce, tomato slices *(free)*
   1 Tbsp. mustard *(free)*
1 c. grapes *(1 Fr)*
1/2 c. V-8 or tomato juice (w/
   calcium added) *(1 Vg)*

DINNER
3 oz. baked seafood *(3 Mt)*
1/2 c. mashed potatoes *(1 St)*
   with 1 Tbsp. light margarine *(1 Ft)*
1 c. broccoli-carrot-onion-mush-
   room mix *(2 Vg)*, stir-fried
   with 1 tsp. olive oil *(1 Ft)*
Mixed green salad *(free)*
   with 2 Tbsp. light dressing *(1 Ft)*
1/2 cup fruit salad *(1 Fr)*

SNACK
2 large flavored rice cakes or 1 c.
   Cheerios or 1/2 c. dry Chex
   cereal mix *(1 St)*

DAY 6

BREAKFAST
1 c. nonfat plain yogurt *(1 Mk)*
   topped with 1/2 banana *(1 Fr)*
   and 1/3 c. Kashi Go Lean
   Crunch cereal *(1 St)*

LUNCH
Chef Salad:
   2 c. mixed salad greens *(free)* w/
   1/2 c. raw broccoli & 1/2 c. raw
     cauliflower *(1 Vg)*
   1 tomato, sliced *(1 Vg)*
   2 oz. turkey ham *(2 Mt)*
   1 oz. low-fat cheese *(1 Mt)*
   4 Tbsp. light dressing *(2 Ft)*
1 fresh peach *(1 Fr)*
1 c. vegetable soup or 4 Rye Krisps
   (1 St)

DINNER
2 slices of a medium cheese pizza,
   thin crust *(2 Mt, 2 St, 2 Ft)*
1 c. cucumber, onion and tomato *(1 Vg)*
1 1/4 c. watermelon *(1 Fr)*

SNACK
16 oz. (2 c.) sugar-free, fat-free hot
   cocoa *(1 Mk)*
3 graham cracker squares or
   5 low-fat Triscuit crackers *(1 St)*

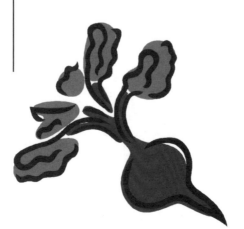

   © 2009, *The Cooper Clinic Solution to the Diet Revolution* by Georgia G. Kostas, M.P.H., R.D., L.D., Dallas, Texas

DAY 7

BREAKFAST
1/2 c. calcium-fortified orange juice or 1/2 c. blueberries *(1 Fr)*
1 wholewheat 4" pancake *(1 St)*
   with 1 Tbsp. "lite" syrup *(1 Ft)*
   and 1 Tbsp. light margarine *(1 Ft):*
   (or replace syrup & fat w/1/2 c. fresh or frozen berries + Splenda, heated in microwave)
1 c. fat-free milk *(1 Mk)*

LUNCH
3 oz. skinless chicken breast *(3 Mt)*
1/2 c. rice, cooked in chicken broth *(1 St)*
1/2 c. green peas, steamed *(1 St)*
1/2 c. carrots, steamed *(1 Vg)*
   with 1 tsp. margarine *(1 Ft)*
1/2 c. cabbage, shredded (slaw) *(free)*
   with 2 Tbsp. light dressing *(1 Ft)*
1 c. cubed or 1/4 of a cantaloupe *(1 Fr)*

DINNER
Taco Salad:
   1/2 c. pinto or kidney beans
      (1 St, 1 Mt)
   1 oz. (1/4 c.) low-fat cheese *(1 Mt)*
   1 tomato, sliced *(1 Vg)*
   1 c. raw vegetables (bell pepper, carrots, red onions, etc.) *(1 Vg)*
   1 c. lettuce *(free)*
   1 corn tortilla, toasted and broken into chips *(1 St)*
   4 Tbsp. Picante sauce *(free)*
1/2 c. fresh pineapple chunks *(1 Fr)*

SNACK
1 c. nonfat, sugar-free strawberry yogurt *(1 Mk)*

DAY 8

BREAKFAST
1 fresh orange *(1 Fr)*
1 wholewheat English muffin *(2 St)*
   topped with 1/4 c. 2% cheese (calcium-added) *(1 Mt)*
1 c. fat-free milk *(1 Mk)*

LUNCH
Fast food grilled chicken breast sandwich (no mayonnaise) *(2 St, 3 Mt)*
1 small apple *(1 Fr)*
1 c. fat-free milk *(1 Mk)*
   (or occasional 4 oz. fat-free, sugar-free frozen yogurt)

DINNER
Vegetarian Stir-fry:
   Heat in skillet in 3 tsp. oil: *(3 Ft)*
   1 1/2 c. mixed vegetables *(3 Vg)*
   1/2 c. onions and mushrooms
      (1 Vg)
1/2 c. steamed brown rice *(1 St)*
1/2 c. fresh pineapple chunks *(1 Fr)* with 1/4 c. low-fat cottage cheese *(1 Mt)*
1 fortune cookie *(free)*

SNACK
1 wedge/slice of low-fat cheese *(1 Mt)*

DAY 9

BREAKFAST
1/4 cantaloupe *(1 Fr)*
1 cinnamon-raisin bagel *(2 St)* with 1 1/2 Tbsp. light cream cheese *(1 Ft)*
8 oz. carton nonfat, sugar-free peach yogurt *(1 Mk)*

LUNCH
1 c. lentil or bean soup *(1 St, 1 Vg, 1 Mt)*
1 c. tossed salad *(free)* with 1 Tbsp. walnuts *(1 Ft)* & 3 Tbsp. Parmesan cheese *(1 Mt)* & 1 Tbsp. (or 2 Tbsp. light) Ranch dressing *(1 Ft)*
1 wholewheat roll or 5 crackers *(1 St)*
1/2 c. fresh fruit salad *(1 Fr)*

DINNER
3 oz. turkey or skinless chicken breast, roasted *(3 Mt)*
1/2 c. corn, steamed *(1 St)*
1/2 c. carrots, steamed *(1 Vg)*
4 c. raw spinach (1/2 c. cooked) *(1 Vg)* sautéed in 1 tsp. olive oil *(1 Ft)*
15-calorie sugar-free popsicle *(free)*

SNACK
1 c. fat-free milk *(1 Mk)*
1 c. grapes *(1 Fr)*

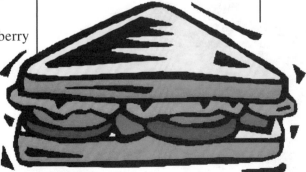

1300 Calorie Menus

© 2009, *The Cooper Clinic Solution to the Diet Revolution* by Georgia G. Kostas, M.P.H., R.D., L.D., Dallas, Texas

DAY 10

BREAKFAST

1 banana *(2 Fr)*
1 c. shredded wheat *(2 St)*
1 Tbsp. chopped nuts *(1 Ft)*
1 c. fat-free milk *(1 Mk)*

LUNCH

Soft Tacos:
    2 corn tortillas *(2 St)*
    2 oz. skinless chicken *(2 Mt)*
    1/4 c. low-fat cheese, grated *(1 Mk)*
    1/4 tomato, diced *(free)*
    lettuce, shredded *(free)*
    3 Tbsp. picante sauce *(free)*
1 fresh peach *(1 Fr)*

DINNER

3 oz. red snapper *(3 Mt)*
    sautéed in 2 tsp. oil *(2 Ft)*
1/2 c. red new potatoes, grilled *(1 St)*
1/2 c. yellow squash, grilled *(1 Vg)*
1/2 c. zucchini, grilled *(1 Vg)*
1/2 c. red bell pepper *(free)*
1 tsp. olive oil (to grill vegetables) *(1 Ft)*
    + 2 Tbsp. Balsamic vinegar *(free)*
1 fresh tomato, in wedges *(1 Vg)*

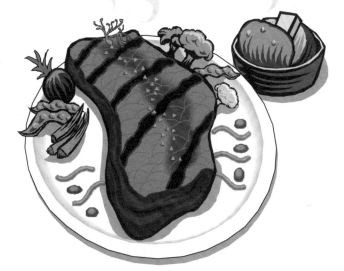

DAY 11

BREAKFAST

1 c. fresh strawberries *(1 Fr)*
1/3 c. Kashi Go Lean Crunch *(1 St)* &
1 Tbsp. nuts *(1 Ft)* on top of
8 oz. plain, nonfat yogurt *(1 Mk)*

LUNCH

Tuna Sandwich:
    2 slices light wholewheat bread
      (1 St)
    1/2 c. water-packed tuna *(2 Mt)*
    1 Tbsp. light mayonnaise *(1 Ft)*
    3 Tbsp. chopped celery, apple,
      pickle *(free)*
    lettuce and tomato slices *(free)*
1 fresh small pear or apple *(1 Fr)*

DINNER

Low-calorie frozen dinner (up to 300
    cal., 10 g fat) *(3 Mt, 1 St, 1 Vg)*
1/2 c. broccoli, steamed *(1 Vg)*
    w/1 Tbsp. slivered almonds *(1 Ft)*
    & 1 tsp. margarine *(1 Ft)*
1/2 c. carrots, steamed *(1 Vg)*
1 wholewheat roll or bread slice *(1 St)*
    w/butter-flavored pump spray *(free)*

SNACK

1 c. fat-free milk *(1 Mk)*
1 c. grapes *(1 Fr)*
3 graham cracker squares *(1 St)*

DAY 12

BREAKFAST

1/2 grapefruit *(1 Fr)*
1 fat-free Eggo or Kashi waffle *(1 St)*
    with 1 Tbsp. "lite" syrup *(1 Ft)*
    and 1 Tbsp. light margarine *(1 Ft)*
    (or replace syrup & fat w/1/2 c. fresh or
    frozen berries + Splenda, heated in micro-
    wave)
8 oz. nonfat, sugar-free strawberry
    yogurt or 1 c. fat-free milk *(1 Mk)*

LUNCH

Hamburger:
    1 wholewheat bun *(2 St)*
    3 oz. extra-lean (90% lean)
      ground beef patty or veggie
      burger *(3 Mt)*
    1 slice low-fat cheddar cheese
      (50 cal./oz.) *(1 Mt)*
    lettuce, tomato, mustard *(free)*
1 c. watermelon slices *(1 Fr)*
1 c. fat-free milk *(1 Mk)*
    (or occasional 4 oz. fat-free,
    sugar-free pudding snack)

DINNER

Shrimp Creole:
    1 oz. (5 large) boiled shrimp *(1 Mt)*
    heated in 1/2 c. spaghetti sauce *(1 St)*
    served over 1/2 c. brown rice *(1 St)*
1 1/2 c. vegetable mix (broccoli,
    cauliflower, carrots, etc.) *(3 Vg)*
    stir-fried in 2 tsp. oil *(2 Ft)*
1 c. cantaloupe slices (1/4 melon) *(1 Fr)*

SNACK

1 c. fat-free milk *(1 Mk)*
1 c. grapes *(1 Fr)*

DAY 13

BREAKFAST

1/2 c. calcium-fortified orange juice or
  1 fresh orange *(1 Fr)*
1 wholewheat toast *(1 St)*
  with 1 tsp. sugar-free jam *(free)*
1 poached egg *(1 Mt)*
1 c. fat-free milk *(1 Mk)*

LUNCH

Pasta Salad:
  1 c. pasta, cooked *(2 St)*
  1/2 c. vegetables (broccoli,
    carrots, onions, red bell
    pepper) *(1 Vg)*
  3-4 Tbsp. light Italian dressing *(2 Ft)*
  3 Tbsp. Parmesan, grated *(1 Mt)*
Spinach Salad *(free)* with
  2 Tbsp. light Catalina dressing *(1 Ft)*
1/2 c. fresh fruit salad *(1 Fr)*
1 c. fat-free milk *(1 Mk)*

DINNER

Fajitas:
  2 soft wholewheat tortillas *(2 St)*
  3 oz. grilled flank steak *(3 Mt)*
  marinated in 2 Tbsp. lime juice *(free)*
  and 1/2 tsp. fajita seasoning *(free)*
  1/2 c. onion and bell peppers *(1 Vg)*
    grilled in 1 tsp. oil *(1 Ft)*
  1/2 c. tomato, diced *(1 Vg)*
  1/2 c. lettuce, shredded *(free)*
1/2 c. fresh pineapple chunks *(1 Fr)*

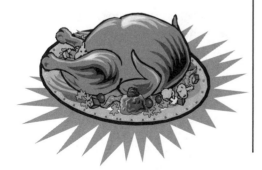

DAY 14

BREAKFAST

1 c. strawberries or 1/2 c. blueberries
  (1 Fr)
2 wholewheat pancakes (4") *(2 St)*
  with 2 Tbsp. "lite" syrup *(1 Ft)*
1 c. fat-free milk or yogurt *(1 Mk)*

LUNCH

3 oz. skinless chicken breast *(3 Mt)*
  marinated in 3 Tbsp. fat-free
  Italian dressing *(free)*
  and baked, grilled or broiled
1/2 c. mashed potatoes *(1 St)* with
  1 tsp. (1 Tbsp. light) margarine *(1 Ft)*
1/2 c. cabbage, shredded *(free)*
  with 1 Tbsp. coleslaw dressing *(1 Ft)*
1/2 c. yellow squash, steamed *(1 Vg)*
1/2 c. green beans, steamed *(1 Vg)*
1 Tbsp. light margarine *(1 Ft)*
1 c. watermelon slices *(1 Fr)*
1 c. fat-free milk *(1 Mk)*

DINNER

Mini-pizzas:
  1 wholewheat English muffin *(2
    St)* topped w/
  1 oz. (3 Tbsp.) grated part-skim
    mozzarella cheese *(3 Mt)*
  1 oz. (2 slices) Canadian bacon
    or smoked turkey *(1 Mt)*
  2 Tbsp. mushrooms, sliced *(free)*
  2 Tbsp. onion, diced *(free)*
  2 Tbsp. green pepper, diced *(free)*
  1/4 c. pizza sauce *(free)*
1 c. raw vegetables *(1 Vg)*
  (carrot sticks, celery, broccoli,
  tomato, cucumber, etc.)
1 fresh orange, in slices *(1 Fr)*

SNACK

1 c. fat-free yogurt or
  2 c. fat-free, sugar-free hot
  cocoa *(1 Mk)*

1300 Calorie Menus

14-Day Weight Loss Menus for Men or Weight Maintenance for Women

1600 Calories, 40-50 grams fat

2 Milk *(Mk)*	6 Meat *(Mt)*	6 Starches *(St)*	4 Fruits *(Fr)**	4+ Vegetables *(Vg)*	6 Fat *(Ft)*

* 4 small = 2 large

◆ To make 1500 calories: omit 2 fat servings (i.e., use "light" rather than regular margarine, dressings, etc.)

➢ *For a complete shopping list, see p. 85-87.*

DAY 1

BREAKFAST
1/2 c. calcium-fortified orange juice or
    1 fresh orange *(1 Fr)*
2 wholewheat toast or 1 bagel *(2 St)*
    with 2 tsp. sugar-free jam/jelly *(free)*
    & 1/2 Tbsp. peanutbutter or
    1 tsp. tub margarine *(1 Ft)*
1 c. fat-free milk or yogurt *(1 Mk)*

LUNCH
Tuna Sandwich:
    2 slices wholewheat bread *(2 St)*
    with 1/2 c. water-packed tuna *(2 Mt)*
    1 Tbsp. light mayonnaise *(1 Ft)*
    and 1/4 c. apple, celery, pickle *(free)*
    Lettuce and tomato slices *(free)*
1/2 c. grape tomatoes *(1 Vg)*
1 large apple *(2 Fr)*
1 c. fat-free milk *(1 Mk)*

DINNER
4 oz. skinless chicken breast *(4 Mt)*
1 small red (new) potato *(1 St)* with
    butter-flavored pump spray *(free)*
1/2 c. carrots, steamed *(1 Vg)*
1/2 c. green beans, steamed *(1 Vg)*
2 tsp. margarine for vegetables *(2 Ft)*
1 c. green salad *(free)* w/1 sliced
    tomato *(1 Vg)* & 2 Tbsp. light
    dressing *(1 Ft)*
1/2 c. fresh pineapple chunks *(1 Fr)*

SNACK
3 c. microwave "light" popcorn *(1 St, 1 Ft)*

DAY 2

BREAKFAST
1 c. cubed or 1/4 of a cantaloupe *(1 Fr)*
1 wholewheat English muffin *(2 St)* with
    2 tsp. apple butter *(free)*
    & 1/2 Tbsp. peanutbutter or
    1 tsp. tub margarine *(1 Ft)*
1 c. fat-free milk *(1 Mk)*

LUNCH
1 small wholewheat bagel or 2 bread *(2 St)*
    with 2 oz. low-fat cheese *(2 Mt)*
1 raw carrot, in sticks *(1 Vg)*
1 large pear *(2 Fr)*
1 c. nonfat, sugar-free yogurt *(1 Mk)*

DINNER
4 oz. broiled fish with lemon *(4 Mt)*
    & 2 tsp. oil *(2 Ft)*
1/2 c. corn, steamed *(1 St)*
1 c. Brussel sprouts, steamed *(2 Vg)*
2 tsp. (2 Tbsp. light) margarine *(2 Ft)*
1 c. Romaine salad *(free)* with
    1 tomato, sliced *(1 Vg)* and
    1 Tbsp. French dressing or
    2 Tbsp. light dressing *(1 Ft)*
1/2 c. fresh fruit salad *(1 Fr)*

SNACK
5 wholewheat low-fat Triscuit
    crackers *(1 St)*

> ### Legend
> *Tbsp. = tablespoon*
> *tsp. = teaspoon*
> *c. = cup*
> *oz. = ounce*

DAY 3

BREAKFAST
1/2 banana *(1 Fr)*
1/2 c. bran flakes or Kashi cereal *(1 St)*
1 Tbsp. chopped almonds *(1 Ft)*
1 c. fat-free milk *(1 Mk)*

LUNCH
Sandwich:
    2 slices wholewheat bread *(2 St)*
    2 oz. turkey *(2 Mt)*
    1 Tbsp. light mayonnaise *(1 Ft)*
    Lettuce, tomato slices *(free)*
1/2 c. raw baby carrots *(1 Vg)*
1 large apple *(2 Fr)*
1 c. fat-free milk *(1 Mk)*

DINNER
4 oz. lean beef tenderloin *(4 Mt)*
1 c. brown rice *(2 St)*
    cooked in broth *(free)*
1/2 c. zucchini *(1 Vg)* and
1/2 c. yellow squash *(1 Vg)*
    stir-fried in 2 tsp. olive oil *(2 Ft)*
1 spinach salad *(free)* with
    1 small tomato *(1 Vg)*,
    1 Tbsp. walnuts *(1 Ft)* and
    2 Tbsp. light dressing *(1 Ft)*
1 orange, in sections *(1 Fr)*

SNACK
3 graham cracker squares *(1 St)*

© 2009, *The Cooper Clinic Solution to the Diet Revolution* by Georgia G. Kostas, M.P.H., R.D., L.D., Dallas, Texas

DAY 4

BREAKFAST

2 grapefruit halves *(2 Fr)*
1 small wholewheat bagel *(2 St)* with
    1 1/2 Tbsp. light cream cheese *(1 Ft)*
1 c. fat-free milk or yogurt *(1 Mk)*

LUNCH

1 small red (new) potato *(1 St)* topped with
    1/2 c. low-fat cottage cheese *(2 Mt)*
1 large Romaine salad w/sliced
    cucumbers, onions, celery &
    grape tomatoes *(free)*
    2 Tbsp. dressing *(2 Ft)*
1/2 c. asparagus, sautéed *(1 Vg)* in
    1 tsp. olive oil *(1 Ft)* and lemon juice
1 c. strawberries *(1 Fr)*

DINNER

Spaghetti:
    3 oz. 90% lean ground beef,
        cooked and drained *(3 Mt)*
    1/2 c. meatless spaghetti sauce *(1 St)*
        over 1 c. spaghetti *(2 St)*
    3 Tbsp. Parmesan cheese *(1 Mt)*
4 c. raw spinach (1/2 c. cooked) *(1 Vg)*
    & 1/2 c. mushrooms & onions *(1 Vg)*
    sautéed in 2 tsp. olive oil *(2 Ft)*
1/2 c. carrots, steamed *(1 Vg)*
1 c. melon, cubed *(1 Fr)*

SNACK

8 oz. carton lemon nonfat, sugar-free
    yogurt *(1 Mk)*

DAY 5

BREAKFAST

1 orange or 1/2 c. blueberries *(1 Fr)*
1 c. oatmeal, cooked *(2 St)*
1 Tbsp. chopped nuts *(1 Ft)*
1 c. fat-free milk *(1 Mk)*

LUNCH

Pita Sandwich:
    1 wholewheat pita pocket *(2 St)*
    3 oz. turkey *(2 Mt)*
    1 oz. (2 slices) low-fat cheese *(1 Mk)*
    lettuce, tomato slices *(free)*
    1 Tbsp. light mayonnaise *(1 Ft)*
1 c. grapes *(1 Fr)*
1 c. V-8 or tomato juice (w/calcium
    added) *(2 Vg)*

DINNER

3 oz. baked seafood *(3 Mt)*
1/2 c. mashed potatoes *(1 St)*
    with 1 Tbsp. light margarine *(1 Ft)*
1 c. vegetable mix *(2 Vg)*
    stir-fried with 1 tsp. olive oil *(1 Ft)*
Mixed green salad *(free)* with
    1 1/2 Tbsp. Italian dressing *(2 Ft)*
1 c. fruit salad *(2 Fr)*

SNACK

2 large flavored rice cakes or
    1 c. Cheerios or
    1/2 c. dry Chex cereal mix *(1 St)*

DAY 6

BREAKFAST

1 c. nonfat plain yogurt *(1 Mk)*
    topped with 1 banana *(2 Fr)*
    & 2/3 c. Kashi Go Lean Crunch
    (2 St) and
    1 Tbsp. chopped walnuts *(1 Ft)*

LUNCH

Chef Salad:
    2 c. mixed salad greens *(free)* with
    1/2 c. raw broccoli & 1/2 cup raw
        cauliflower *(1 Vg)*
    1 tomato, sliced *(1 Vg)*
    3 oz. turkey ham *(3 Mt)*
    1 oz. low-fat cheese *(1 Mt)*
    3-4 Tbsp. light dressing *(2 Ft)*
1 c. vegetable soup or
    4 Rye Krisps *(1 St)*
1 fresh peach *(1 Fr)*

DINNER

2 slices of a medium cheese pizza,
    thin crust *(2 Mt, 2 St, 2 Ft)*
1 c. cucumber, onion and tomato *(1 Vg)*
    w/1 Tbsp. French dressing *(1 Ft)*
1 c. watermelon *(1 Fr)*

SNACK

16 oz. (2 c.) sugar-free, fat-free hot
    cocoa *(1 Mk)*
3 graham cracker squares or
    5 low-fat Triscuits *(1 St)*

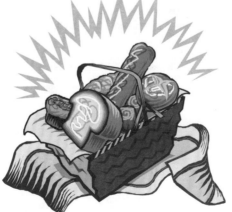

1600 Calorie Menus

© 2009, *The Cooper Clinic Solution to the Diet Revolution* by Georgia G. Kostas, M.P.H., R.D., L.D., Dallas, Texas

DAY 7

BREAKFAST

1/2 c. calcium-fortified orange juice or 1/2 c. blueberries *(1 Fr)*

2 wholewheat 4" pancakes *(2 St)* topped with 2 Tbsp. "lite" syrup *(1 Ft)* and 2 Tbsp. light margarine *(2 Ft)* (or replace syrup & fat w/1/2 c. fresh or frozen berries + Splenda, heated in microwave)

1 c. fat-free milk *(1 Mk)*

LUNCH

4 oz. roasted skinless chicken breast *(4 Mt)*

1 c. rice *(2 St)* cooked in chicken broth

1/2 c. green peas, steamed *(1 St)*

1 c. carrots, steamed *(2 Vg)* with 1 tsp. margarine *(1 Ft)*

1/2 c. cabbage, shredded (slaw) *(free)* with 2 Tbsp. light dressing *(1 Ft)*

1 c. cubed or 1/4 of a cantaloupe *(1 Fr)*

DINNER

Taco Salad:

1/2 c. pinto or kidney beans *(1 St, 1 Mt)*

1 oz. (3 Tbsp.) grated low-fat cheese *(1 Mt)*

1 tomato, sliced *(1 Vg)*

1 c. raw vegetables (green pepper, carrots, red onions, etc.) *(1 Vg)*

1 c. lettuce *(free)*

1 corn tortilla, toasted and broken into chips *(1 St)*

1/4 c. Picante sauce *(free)*

1 c. fresh pineapple chunks *(2 Fr)*

SNACK

1 c. nonfat, sugar-free strawberry yogurt *(1 Mk)*

DAY 8

BREAKFAST

1 fresh orange *(1 Fr)*

1 wholewheat English muffin *(2 St)* topped with 1/4 c. 2% cheese (calcium added) *(1 Mt)*, melted

LUNCH

Fast food grilled chicken breast sandwich (no mayonnaise) *(2 St, 3 Mt)*

1 large apple or fruit cup *(2 Fr)*

1 c. fat-free milk *(1 Mk)* (or occasional 4 oz. fat-free, sugar-free frozen yogurt)

DINNER

Vegetarian Stir-fry:

Heat in skillet in 3 tsp. oil *(3 Ft)*:

1 1/2 c. mixed frozen Japanese vegetables *(3 Vg)*

1/2 c. diced onions and mushrooms *(1 Vg)*

1 c. steamed brown rice *(2 St)*

Tossed salad *(free)* with 2 Tbsp. Italian dressing *(3 Ft)*

1/2 c. fresh pineapple chunks *(1 Fr)* with 1/2 c. low-fat cottage cheese *(2 Mt)*

1 fortune cookie *(free)*

SNACK

1 wedge/slice low-fat cheese *(1 Mt)*

DAY 9

BREAKFAST

1/4 cantaloupe *(1 Fr)*

1 small cinnamon-raisin bagel *(2 St)* with 1 1/2 Tbsp. light cream cheese *(1 Ft)*

8 oz. carton nonfat, sugar-free vanilla yogurt *(1 Mk)*

LUNCH

1 c. lentil or bean soup *(1 St, 1 Vg, 1 Mt)*

1 c. tossed salad *(free)* with 3 Tbsp. Parmesan cheese *(1 Mt)* & 1 Tbsp. walnuts *(1 Ft)* & 2 Tbsp. Ranch dressing *(2 Ft)*

1 wholewheat roll *(1 St)* with 1 tsp. margarine *(1 Ft)*

1 c. fresh fruit salad *(2 Fr)*

DINNER

3 oz. turkey or skinless chicken breast, roasted *(3 Mt)*

1/2 c. corn, steamed *(1 St)*

1 c. carrots, steamed *(2 Vg)*

4 c. raw spinach (1/2 c. cooked) *(1 Vg)*, sautéed in 1 tsp. olive oil *(1 Ft)*

15-calorie sugar-free popsicle *(free)*

SNACK

Half Sandwich:

1 slice wholewheat bread *(1 St)*

1 oz. turkey ham *(1 Mt)*

mustard, lettuce, tomato *(free)*

1 c. grapes *(1 Fr)*

1 c. fat-free milk *(1 Mk)*

1600 Calorie Menus

DAY 10

BREAKFAST

1 banana (2 Fr)
1 c. shredded wheat (2 St)
1 Tbsp. chopped nuts (1 Ft)
1 c. fat-free milk (1 Mk)

LUNCH

Soft Tacos:
  3 corn tortillas (3 St)
  3 oz. skinless, cooked chicken, (or
    1/2 c. fat-free refried beans) (3 Mt)
    browned in 1 tsp. oil (1 Ft)
  1/4 tomato, diced (free)
  lettuce, shredded (free)
  3 Tbsp. picante sauce (free)
1 fresh peach (1 Fr)

DINNER

3 oz. red snapper (3 Mt)
  sautéed in 2 tsp. oil (2 Ft)
1/2 c. red new potatoes, grilled (1 St)
1/2 c. yellow squash, grilled (1 Vg)
1/2 c. zucchini, grilled (1 Vg)
1 c. red bell pepper, grilled (1 Vg)
2 tsp. olive oil for vegetables (2 Ft) +
  2 Tbsp. Balsamic vinegar (free)
1 small fresh tomato, in wedges (1 Vg)

SNACK

2 c. (16 oz.) fat-free, sugar-free hot
  cocoa or 8 oz. nonfat, sugar-free
  lemon yogurt (1 Mk)
1 c. grapes (1 Fr)

DAY 11

BREAKFAST

1 c. fresh strawberries (1 Fr) and
  1/3 c. Kashi Go Lean Crunch (1 St)
  on top of 8 oz. plain, nonfat
  yogurt (1 Mk)
1 slice wholewheat toast (1 St)
  with 1 tsp. margarine (1 Ft) or
  1/2 Tbsp. peanutbutter (1 Ft)

LUNCH

Tuna Sandwich:
  2 slices wholewheat bread (2 St)
  1/2 c. water-packed tuna (2 Mt)
  1 Tbsp. light mayonnaise (1 Ft)
  3 Tbsp. celery, apple, pickle (free)
  lettuce and tomato slices (free)
1/2 c. grape tomatoes (1 Vg)
1 fresh large pear or apple (2 Fr)

DINNER

Low-calorie frozen dinner (up to 300
  cal., 10 g fat) (3 Mt, 1 St, 1 Vg)
1/2 c. broccoli, steamed (1 Vg) with
  1 Tbsp. slivered almonds (1 Ft)
  with 1 tsp. margarine (1 Ft)
1/2 c. carrots, steamed (1 Vg)
1 c. grapes (1 Fr)

SNACK

1 c. fat-free milk (1 Mk)
1/2 small (1 oz.) bagel (1 St)
1 oz. low-calorie cheese (1 Mt)

DAY 12

BREAKFAST

1 whole grapefruit (2 Fr)
2 fat-free Eggo or Kashi waffles (2 St)
  with 2 Tbsp. "lite" reduced-calorie
  syrup (1 Ft) and
  1 Tbsp. light margarine (1 Ft)
  (or replace syrup & fat w/1/2 c. fresh or
  frozen berries + Splenda, heated in microwave)
8 oz. nonfat, sugar-free yogurt
  or 1 c. fat-free milk (1 Mk)

LUNCH

Hamburger:
  1 wholewheat bun (2 St)
  3 oz. extra lean (90% lean)
    ground beef patty or veggie
    burger (3 Mt)
  1 slice low-fat cheddar cheese
    (50 cal./slice) (1 Mt)
  lettuce, tomato, mustard (free)
1 c. watermelon slices (1 Fr)
1 c. fat-free milk (1 Mk)
  (or occasional 4 oz. fat-free,
  sugar-free pudding snack)

DINNER

Shrimp Creole:
  1 oz. (5 large) boiled shrimp (1 Mt)
  in 1/2 c. spaghetti sauce, (1 St)
  served over 1 c. brown rice (2 St)
2 c. vegetable mix (broccoli, cauliflower, carrots, onions, etc.) (4 Vg)
  stir-fried in 2 tsp. oil (2 Ft)
Tossed salad (free)
  with 2 tsp. olive oil (2 Ft) and
  2 tsp. balsamic vinegar (free)

SNACK

1 c. cantaloupe (1/3 melon) (1 Fr) with
  1/4 c. low-fat cottage cheese (1 Mt)

1600 Calorie Menus

© 2009, The Cooper Clinic Solution to the Diet Revolution by Georgia G. Kostas, M.P.H., R.D., L.D., Dallas, Texas

BREAKFAST

1/2 c. calcium-fortified orange juice or
    1 fresh orange *(1 Fr)*
1 wholewheat toast *(1 St)*
    with 1 Tbsp. light margarine *(1 Ft)*
1 poached egg *(1 Mt)*
1 c. fat-free milk *(1 Mk)*

LUNCH

Pasta Salad:
    1 c. pasta, cooked *(2 St)*
    1 c. steamed vegetables (broccoli,
        carrots, red bell pepper) *(2 Vg)*
    3-4 Tbsp. light Italian dressing *(2 Ft)*
    3 Tbsp. Parmesan, grated *(1 Mt)*
Spinach Salad *(free)* with
    1/2 c. mandarin or orange slices *(1 Fr)*
    w/ 2 Tbsp. light Catalina dress-
    ing *(1 Ft)*
1 c. fat-free milk *(1 Mk)*

DINNER

Fajitas:
    2 soft wholewheat tortillas *(2 St)*
    4 oz. grilled flank steak *(4 Mt)*
        marinated in 2 Tbsp. lime
        juice *(free)* and
        1/2 tsp. fajita seasoning *(free)*
    1/2 c. onion and bell pepper *(1 Vg)*
        grilled in 1 tsp. oil *(1 Ft)*
    1/2 c. tomato, diced *(1 Vg)*
    1/2 c. lettuce, shredded *(free)*
1 c. fresh pineapple chunks *(2 Fr)*

SNACK

3 c. microwave "light" popcorn *(1 St, 1 Ft)*

BREAKFAST

1/2 c. calcium-fortified grapefruit juice *(1 Fr)*
1 c. strawberries or 1/2 c. blueberries *(1 Fr)*
2 wholewheat pancakes (4") *(2 St)*
    with 2 Tbsp. "lite" syrup *(1 Ft)*
1 c. fat-free milk or yogurt *(1 Mk)*

LUNCH

3 oz. skinless chicken breast *(3 Mt)*
    marinated in 3 Tbsp. fat-free
        Italian dressing *(free)*
    and baked, grilled or broiled
1/2 c. mashed potatoes *(1 St)*
    with 1 tsp. (or 1 Tbsp. light)
    margarine *(1 Ft)*
1/2 c. cabbage, shredded *(free)*
    with 1 Tbsp. coleslaw dressing *(1 Ft)*
1 c. yellow squash, steamed *(2 Vg)*
1 c. green beans, steamed *(2 Vg)*
1 Tbsp. light margarine for vegetables *(1 Ft)*
1 c. watermelon slices *(1 Fr)*

DINNER

Mini-pizzas:
    1 wholewheat English muffin
        (2 St) topped with
    1 oz. (3 Tbsp.) part-skim
        mozzarella cheese *(1 Mt)*
    2 oz. Canadian bacon or
        smoked turkey *(2 Mt)*
    2 Tbsp. mushrooms, sliced *(free)*
    2 Tbsp. onion, diced *(free)*
    2 Tbsp. green pepper, diced *(free)*
    1/4 c. pizza or spaghetti sauce *(free)*
1/2 c. mixed fresh fruit *(1 Fr)*

SNACK

1 c. Cheerios *(1 St)*
1 c. fat-free milk *(1 Mk)*

1600 Calorie Menus

14-Day Weight Maintenance Menus for Men

2000 Calories, 50-70 grams fat

2 Milk *(Mk)*	7 Meat *(Mt)*	7 Starches *(St)*	6 Fruits *(Fr)**	4+ Vegetables *(Vg)*	7 Fat *(Ft)*

*6 small fruit = 3 large

- ◆ Women may need to adjust to smaller portions to make 1700 - 1800 calories.
- ◆ More active or taller men may need to add more food to make 2200 - 2500 calories.

➢ *For a complete shopping list, see p. 85-87.*

DAY 1

BREAKFAST
1 c. calcium-fortified orange juice *(2 Fr)*
2 wholewheat toast or 1 small bagel *(2 St)*
   w/2 tsp sugar-free jam/jelly *(free)*
   & 1/2 Tbsp. peanutbutter *(1 Ft)*
1 wedge Laughing Cow cheese *(1 Mt)*
1 c. fat-free milk or yogurt *(1 Mk)*

LUNCH
Tuna Sandwich:
   2 slices wholewheat bread *(2 St)*
   1/2 c. water-packed tuna *(2 Mt)*
   1 Tbsp. light mayonnaise *(1 Ft)*
   1/4 c. chopped apple, celery,
      pickle *(free)*
   Lettuce and tomato slices *(free)*
1/2 c. grape tomatoes *(1 Vg)*
1 large apple *(2 Fr)*
1 c. fat-free milk *(1 Mk)*

DINNER
4 oz. skinless chicken breast, grilled *(4 Mt)*
1 medium red potato *(2 St)* with
   1 Tbsp. light margarine *(1 Ft)*
1 c. carrots, steamed *(2 Vg)*
1 c. green beans, steamed *(2 Vg)*
2 tsp. margarine for vegetables *(2 Ft)*
1 c. green salad *(free)* with
   1 sliced tomato *(1 Vg)* and
   2 Tbsp. light dressing *(1 Ft)*
1 c. fresh pineapple chunks *(2 Fr)*

SNACK
3 c. light microwave popcorn *(1 St, 1 Ft)*

DAY 2

BREAKFAST
2 c. cubed or 1/2 of a cantaloupe *(2 Fr)*
1 wholewheat English muffin *(2 St)*
   with 2 tsp. apple butter *(free)*
   & 1/2 Tbsp. peanutbutter or
   1 tsp. tub margarine *(1 Ft)*
1 c. fat-free milk *(1 Mk)*

LUNCH
1 small wholewheat bagel or
   2 bread slices *(2 St)* with
   2 oz. low-fat cheese *(2 Mt)*
1 raw carrot, in sticks *(1 Vg)*
1 large pear *(2 Fr)*
1 c. nonfat, sugar-free yogurt *(1 Mk)*

DINNER
5 oz. broiled fish w/ lemon *(5 Mt)* and
   2 tsp. oil *(2 Ft)*
1 c. corn, steamed *(2 St)*
1 c. Brussel sprouts, steamed *(2 Vg)*
2 tsp. (2 Tbsp. light) margarine for
   vegetables *(2 Ft)*
1 c. Romaine salad *(free)* with
   1 tomato, sliced *(1 Vg)* and
   2 Tbsp. French dressing *(2 Ft)*
1 c. fresh fruit salad *(2 Fr)*

SNACK
5 wholewheat low-fat Triscuits *(1 St)*

Legend
Tbsp. = tablespoon	*c.= cup*
tsp. = teaspoon	*oz. = ounce*

DAY 3

BREAKFAST
1/2 c. calcium-fortified orange juice
   (1 Fr)
1 banana *(2 Fr)*
1 c. bran flakes or Kashi cereal *(2 St)*
1 Tbsp. chopped almonds *(1 Ft)*
1 c. fat-free milk *(1 Mk)*

LUNCH
Sandwich:
   2 slices wholewheat bread *(2 St)*
   3 oz. turkey *(3 Mt)*
   2 tsp. mayonnaise *(2 Ft)*
   Lettuce, tomato slices *(free)*
1 large apple *(2 Fr)*
1 c. raw baby carrots *(1 Vg)*
1 c. fat-free milk *(1 Mk)*

DINNER
4 oz. lean beef tenderloin *(4 Mt)*
1 c. brown rice *(2 St)*
   cooked in broth *(free)*
1/2 c. zucchini *(1 Vg)* and
1/2 c. yellow squash, steamed *(1 Vg)*
   stir-fried in 2 tsp. olive oil *(2 Ft)*
1 spinach salad *(free)* with
   1 small tomato *(1 Vg)* and
   1 Tbsp. walnuts *(1 Ft)* and
   2 Tbsp. light dressing *(1 Ft)*
1 orange, in sections *(1 Fr)*

SNACK
3 graham cracker squares *(1 St)*

DAY 4

BREAKFAST

2 grapefruit halves *(2 Fr)*
1 small wholewheat bagel *(2 St)*
    with 1-1/2 Tbsp. light cream
    cheese *(1 Ft)*
1 c. fat-free milk or yogurt *(1 Mk)*

LUNCH

1 medium red (new) potato *(2 St)* with
    1/2 c. low-fat cottage cheese *(2 Mt)*
    and salsa *(free)*
1 large Romaine salad *(free)* w/sliced
    cucumber, onion, celery, grape
    tomatoes *(free)* and
    2 Tbsp. ranch dressing *(2 Ft)*
1 c. asparagus, sautéed *(2 Vg)* in
    2 tsp. olive oil *(2 Ft)* and lemon juice
2 c. strawberries *(2 Fr)*

DINNER

Spaghetti:
    3 oz. 90% lean ground beef,
      cooked and drained *(3 Mt)*
    1/2 c. meatless spaghetti sauce *(1 St)*
    over 1 c. spaghetti *(2 St)*
    4 Tbsp. Parmesan cheese *(2 Mt)*
4 c. raw spinach, (1/2 c. cooked) *(1 Vg)* &
    1/2 c. mushrooms & onions *(1 Vg)*
    sautéed in 2 tsp. olive oil *(2 Ft)*
1 c. melon, cubed *(1 Fr)*

SNACK

8 oz. carton lemon nonfat, sugar-free
    yogurt *(1 Mk)*
1/2 c. pineapple *(1 Ft)*

DAY 5

BREAKFAST

1 orange or 1/2 c. blueberries *(1 Fr)*
1 c. cooked oatmeal *(2 St)* topped
    with 2 Tbsp. raisins *(1 Fr)*
    & 1 tsp. brown sugar *(free)*
    & 1 Tbsp. chopped nuts *(1 Ft)*
1 c. fat-free milk *(1 Mk)*

LUNCH

Pita Sandwich:
    1 wholewheat pita pocket *(2 St)*
    3 oz. turkey *(2 Mt)*
    1 oz. (2 slices) low-fat cheese *(1 Mk)*
    lettuce, tomato slices *(free)*
    1 Tbsp. light mayonnaise *(1 Ft)*
2 c. grapes *(2 Fr)*
1/2 c. V-8 or tomato juice (calcium
    added) *(1 Vg)*

DINNER

4 oz. baked seafood *(4 Mt)*
1 c. mashed potatoes *(2 St)*
    with 1 Tbsp. light margarine *(1 Ft)*
2 c. broccoli-carrot-onion-mix *(4 Vg)*
    stir-fried with 2 tsp. olive oil *(2 Ft)*
Mixed green salad *(free)* with
    1 1/2 Tbsp. Italian dressing *(2 Ft)*
1 c. fruit salad *(2 Fr)*

SNACK

2 large flavored rice cakes or
    1 c. Cheerios or
    1/2 c. dry Chex cereal blend *(1 St)*

DAY 6

BREAKFAST

1 c. calcium-fortified orange juice *(2 Fr)*
1 c. nonfat plain yogurt *(1 Mk)*
    topped with 1 banana *(2 Fr)* &
    2/3 c. Kashi Go Lean Crunch
    cereal *(2 St)* & 1 Tbsp. chopped
    walnuts *(1 Ft)*

LUNCH

Chef Salad:
    2 c. mixed salad greens *(free)* with
    1/2 c. raw broccoli & 1/2 c. raw
      cauliflower *(1 Vg)*
    1 tomato, sliced *(1 Vg)*
    3 oz. turkey ham *(3 Mt)*
    1 oz. low-fat cheese *(1 Mt)*
    3-4 Tbsp. light dressing *(2 Ft)*
1 c. vegetable soup or 4 Rye Krisps *(1 St)*
1 fresh peach *(1 Fr)*

DINNER

3 slices of a medium cheese pizza
    (3 Mt, 3 St, 3 Ft)
1 c. cucumber, onion and tomato
    (1 Vg) with 1 Tbsp French
    dressing *(1 Ft)*
1 c. watermelon *(1 Fr)*

SNACK

16 oz. (2 c.) sugar-free, fat-free hot
    cocoa *(1 Mk)*
5 wholewheat low-fat Triscuits or
    1 biscotti *(1 St)*

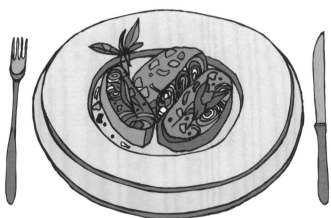

DAY 7

BREAKFAST

1 c. calcium-fortified orange juice *(2 Fr)* or 1/2 c. blueberries

4 wholewheat 4" pancakes *(4 St)* with 4 Tbsp. "lite" syrup *(2 Ft)* and 2 Tbsp. light margarine *(2 Ft)* (or replace syrup & fat w/1 c. fresh or frozen berries + Splenda, heated in microwave)

1 c. fat-free milk *(1 Mk)*

LUNCH

4 oz. roasted skinless chicken breast *(4 Mt)*

1 c. rice *(2 St)* cooked in chicken broth

1/2 c. green peas, steamed *(1 St)*

1 c. carrots, steamed *(2 Vg)* with 1 tsp. margarine *(1 Ft)*

1/2 c. cabbage, shredded (slaw) *(free)* with 2 Tbsp. light dressing *(1 Ft)*

2 c. cubed or 1/2 of a cantaloupe *(2 Fr)*

DINNER

Taco Salad:

    3/4 c. pinto or kidney beans *(1 St, 2 Mt)*

    3 Tbsp. grated low-fat cheese *(1 Mt)*

    1 tomato, sliced *(1 Vg)*

    1 c. raw vegetables (green pepper, carrots, red onions) *(1 Vg)*

    1 c. lettuce *(free)*

    1 corn tortilla, toasted and broken into chips *(1 St)*

    Picante sauce *(free)*

1 c. fresh pineapple chunks *(2 Fr)*

SNACK

1 c. nonfat, sugar-free strawberry yogurt *(1 Mk)* topped with 1 Tbsp. almonds *(1 Ft)*

DAY 8

BREAKFAST

1 fresh orange *(1 Fr)*

1 wholewheat English muffin, in halves *(2 St)*

1/4 c. 2% cheese (calcium added), melted *(1 Mk)*

LUNCH

Fast food grilled chicken breast sandwich (no mayonnaise) *(2 St, 3 Mt)*

1/2 order small fries *(1 St, 1 Ft)*

1 large apple or fruit cup *(2 Fr)*

1 c. fat-free milk *(Mk)* (or occasional 4 oz. fat-free, sugar-free frozen yogurt)

DINNER

Vegetarian Stir-fry:

Heat in skillet in 3 tsp. oil *(3 Ft)*:

    2 c. mixed frozen Japanese vegetables *(4 Vg)*

    1/2 c. onions and mushrooms *(1 Vg)*

1 c. steamed brown rice *(2 St)*

Tossed salad *(free)* with 2 Tbsp. Parmesan cheese *(1 Mt)* & 2 Tbsp. Italian dressing *(3 Ft)*

1 c. fresh pineapple chunks *(2 Fr)* with 1/2 c. low-fat cottage cheese *(2 Mt)*

1 fortune cookie *(free)*

DAY 9

BREAKFAST

1/2 cantaloupe *(2 Fr)*

1 small cinnamon-raisin bagel *(2 St)* w/ 1 1/2 Tbsp. light cream cheese *(1 Ft)*

8 oz. carton nonfat, sugar-free vanilla yogurt *(1 Mk)*

LUNCH

1 c. lentil or bean soup *(1 St, 1 Vg, 1 Mt)*

1 c. tossed salad *(free)* w/1 Tbsp. walnuts *(1 Ft)* & 3 Tbsp. Parmesan cheese *(1 Mt)* & 2 Tbsp. Ranch dressing *(2 Ft)*

1 wholewheat roll *(1 St)* with 1 tsp. margarine *(1 Ft)*

1 c. fresh fruit salad *(2 Fr)*

DINNER

3 oz. turkey or skinless chicken breast *(3 Mt)*

1 c. corn, steamed *(2 St)*

1 c. carrots, steamed *(2 Vg)*

8 c. raw spinach (1 c. cooked) *(2 Vg)*, sautéed in 1 tsp. olive oil *(1 Ft)*

15-calorie sugar-free popsicle *(free)*

SNACK

Half sandwich:

    1 slice wholewheat bread *(1 St)*

    2 oz. turkey ham *(2 Mt)*

    mustard, lettuce, tomato *(free)*

2 c. grapes *(2 Fr)*

1 c. fat-free milk *(1 Mk)*

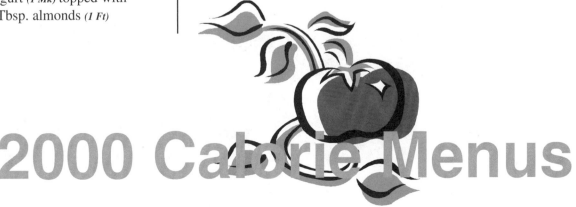

2000 Calorie Menus

DAY 10

BREAKFAST

1/2 c. calcium-fortified orange juice *(1 Fr)*
1 banana *(2 Fr)*
1 1/2 c. shredded wheat *(3 St)*
1 Tbsp. chopped nuts *(1 Ft)*
1 c. fat-free milk *(1 Mk)*

LUNCH

Soft Tacos:
    3 corn tortillas *(3 St)*
    3 oz. skinless, cooked chicken, *(3 Mt)*
        (or 1/2 c. fat-free refried beans)
        browned in 1 tsp. oil *(1 Ft)*
    1/4 tomato, diced *(free)*
    lettuce, shredded *(free)*
    3 Tbsp. picante sauce *(free)*
1 fresh peach *(1 Fr)*

DINNER

4 oz. red snapper *(4 Mt)*
    sautéed in 2 tsp. oil *(2 Ft)*
1/2 c. red new potatoes, grilled *(1 St)*
1/2 c. yellow squash, grilled *(1 Vg)*
1/2 c. zucchini, grilled *(1 Vg)*
1 c. red bell pepper, grilled *(1 Vg)*
2 tsp. olive oil (to grill veggies) *(2 Ft)* &
    2 Tbsp. Balsamic vinegar *(free)*
1 small fresh tomato, in wedges *(1 Vg)*
1 c. strawberries *(1 Fr)*

SNACK

2 c. fat-free, sugar-free hot cocoa or
    8 oz. nonfat, sugar-free lemon
    yogurt *(1 Mk)*
1 c. grapes *(1 Fr)*

DAY 11

BREAKFAST

1 c. fresh strawberries *(1 Fr)* on top of
    8 oz. plain, nonfat yogurt *(1 Mk)*
1 slice wholewheat toast *(1 St)*
    with 1 tsp. margarine *(1 Ft)*

LUNCH

1 c. tomato soup *(1 St)*
Tuna Sandwich:
    2 slices wholewheat bread *(2 St)*
    1/2 c. water-packed tuna *(2 Mt)*
    1 Tbsp. light mayonnaise *(1 Ft)*
    3 Tbsp. chopped celery, apple,
        pickle *(free)*
    lettuce and tomato slices *(free)*
1 fresh large pear or apple *(2 Fr)*
1 c. raw baby carrots *(1 Vg)*

DINNER

Low-calorie frozen dinner (up to 300
    cal., 10 g fat) *(3 Mt, 1 St, 1 Vg)*
1/2 c. broccoli *(1 Vg)*, steamed with
    1 Tbsp. slivered almonds *(1 Ft)*
    and 1 tsp. margarine *(1 Ft)*
1/2 c. carrots, steamed *(1 Vg)* with
    1 tsp. margarine *(1 Ft)*
1 c. grapes *(1 Fr)*

SNACK

1 c. fat-free milk *(1 Mk)*
1 small bagel *(2 St)*
2 oz. low-calorie cheese *(2 Mt)*
1 banana *(2 Fr)*

DAY 12

BREAKFAST

1 whole grapefruit *(2 Fr)*
2 fat-free Eggo or Kashi waffles *(2 St)*
    with 2 Tbsp. "lite" reduced-
    calorie syrup *(1 Ft)*
    and 1 Tbsp. light margarine *(1 Ft)*
    (or replace syrup & fat w/1 c. fresh or
    frozen berries + Splenda, heated in micro-
    wave)
8 oz. nonfat, sugar-free strawberry
    yogurt or 1 c. fat-free milk *(1 Mk)*

LUNCH

Hamburger:
    1 wholewheat bun *(2 St)*
    3 oz. extra lean (90% lean)
        ground beef patty or veggie
        burger *(3 Mt)*
    1 slice (50 cal. per slice) low-fat
        cheese *(1 Mt)*
    lettuce, tomato, mustard *(free)*
1/2 c. baked beans *(1 St, 1 Mt, 1 Ft)*
2 c. watermelon slices *(2 Fr)*
1 c. fat-free milk *(1 Mk)*
    (or 1/2 c. nonfat frozen yogurt)

DINNER

Shrimp Creole:
    2 oz. (10 large) boiled shrimp *(2 Mt)*
    in 1/2 c. spaghetti sauce, *(1 St)*
    served over 1 c. brown rice *(2 St)*
2 c. vegetable mix (broccoli, cauli-
    flower, carrots, onions, etc.) *(4 Vg)*
    stir-fried in 2 tsp. oil *(2 Ft)*
Tossed salad *(free)* with
    2 tsp. olive oil *(2 Ft)* and
    2 tsp. balsamic vinegar *(free)*

SNACK

2 c. cantaloupe slices (1/2 melon) *(2 Fr)*

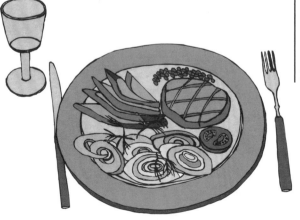

BREAKFAST

1 c. calcium-fortified orange juice or
   1 banana *(2 Fr)*
2 slices wholewheat toast *(2 St)*
   with 1 Tbsp. light margarine *(1 Ft)*
1 poached egg *(1 Mt)*
1 c. fat-free milk *(1 Mk)*

LUNCH

Pasta Salad:
   1 c. pasta, cooked *(2 St)*
   1 c. steamed vegetables, sliced
      (broccoli, carrots, onions, red
      bell pepper)* *(2 Vg)*
   4-5 Tbsp. fat-free Italian dress-
      ing *(3 Ft)*
   4 Tbsp. Parmesan, grated *(2 Mt)*
Spinach Salad (free) with
   1/2 c. mandarin or orange slices *(1 Fr)*
   w/ 2 Tbsp. light Catalina dress-
      ing *(1 Ft)*
1 c. fat-free milk *(1 Mk)*

DINNER

Fajitas:
   3 soft wholewheat tortillas *(3 St)*
   4 oz. grilled flank steak, sliced *(4 Mt)*
      in 2 Tbsp. lime juice *(free)* and
      1/2 tsp. fajita seasoning *(free)*
   1/2 c. onion and bell pepper, *(1 Vg)*
      grilled in 1 tsp. oil *(1 Ft)*
   1/2 c. tomato, diced *(1 Vg)*
   1/2 c. lettuce, shredded *(free)*
1 c. fresh pineapple chunks *(2 Fr)*
   + 1 c. red grapes *(1 Fr)*

SNACK

3 c. microwave "light" popcorn *(1 St, 1 Ft)*

* may use leftovers from dinner – day 12

BREAKFAST

1 c. calcium-fortified grapefruit juice *(2 Fr)*
1 c. strawberries or
   1/2 c. blueberries *(1 Fr)*
3 wholewheat pancakes (4") *(3 St)*
   with 2 Tbsp. "lite" syrup *(1 Ft)*
1 c. fat-free milk or yogurt *(1 Mk)*

LUNCH

3 oz. skinless chicken breast, *(3 Mt)*
   marinate in 3 Tbsp. fat-free Italian
   dressing *(free)* & bake, grill or broil
1/2 c. mashed potatoes *(1 St)* with
   1 tsp. (or 1 Tbsp. light) margarine *(1 Ft)*
1/2 c. cabbage, shredded *(free)*
   w/ 1 Tbsp. coleslaw dressing *(1 Ft)*
1/2 c. yellow squash, steamed *(1 Vg)*
1/2 c. green beans, steamed *(1 Vg)*
1 Tbsp. light margarine on veggies *(1 Ft)*
1 c. melon slices *(1 Fr)*

DINNER

Mini-pizzas:
   1 wholewheat English muffin (2
      halves) *(2 St)* w/4 Tbsp. grated
      part-skim mozzarella cheese
      (2 Mt)
   2 oz. Canadian bacon or smoked
      turkey *(2 Mt)*
   2 Tbsp. mushrooms, sliced *(free)*
   2 Tbsp. onion, diced *(free)*
   2 Tbsp. green pepper, diced *(free)*
   1/4 c. pizza or spaghetti sauce *(free)*
   1 c. raw vegetables (carrots,
      celery, broccoli, tomato, etc.)
      (1 Vg) w/ 2 Tbsp. light Ranch
      dressing *(1 Ft)*
1 c. fresh pineapple slices or mixed
   fresh fruit *(2 Fr)*

SNACK

76 pretzel sticks or 24 3-ring twists
   (1 1/2 oz.), or 2 c. Cheerios *(2 St)*
1 c. fat-free milk *(1 Mk)*

Shopping   List

Shopping   tips

Buy pantry items in the smallest
available package.

Shop at stores with salad bars or
pre-cut fruits & vegetables for your
convenience.

Keep extra bread products,
cheese, deli and butcher meats in
the freezer until needed.

Take advantage of the deli, butcher
and bakery areas to buy individual
portions.

Condiments

(keep on hand):

Light cream cheese
Soft tub margarine
Light tub margarine
   (1 Tbsp.= 35-50 calories)
Light or fat-free salad dressings
   (Ranch, Italian, vinaigrette,
   coleslaw, Catalina)
Balsamic vinegar
Picante sauce
Sugar free jam/jelly
Apple butter
"Lite" maple syrup
Light or fat-free mayonnaise
Mustard
Olive oil
Dill pickles
Knorr bouillon cubes (chicken)

2000 Calorie Menus

	1300 Calorie Week #1	Week #2	1600 Calorie Week #1	Week #2	2000 Calorie Week #1	Week #2
REFRIGERATED SECTION:						
Calcium-fortified orange juice, 1 qt. (4 c.) or buy frozen can (makes 1 qt.)	1 c.	1/2 c.	1 c.	1/2 c.	3 c.	2 c.
Fat-free milk, 1/2 gallon (8 c.) + 1 qt. (4 c.)	10 c.	10 c.	10 c.	10 c.	10 c.	11 c.
Nonfat, sugar free yogurt, 8 oz. (1 c.) cartons	4	4	4	4	4	4
Low-fat cheese (1 oz. serving=approx. 50 calories) - i.e. 2% milk American cheese slices (Kraft), mini-Bonbel rounds or wedges (Laughing Cow), or string cheese (Mozzarella)	4 oz.	4 oz.	4 oz.	6 oz.	5 oz.	6 oz.
Parmesan cheese, grated, 1 small can/container	0	4 Tbsp.	3 Tbsp.	1/2 c.	1/2 c.	1/2 c.
Mozzarella cheese, grated, 4 oz. package (1 c.)	0	1 oz.	1 oz.	2 oz.	2 oz.	2 oz.
Low-fat cottage cheese, 4 oz. carton (1 c.)	1/2 c.	1/4 c.	1/2 c.	3/4 c.	1/2 c.	3/4 c.
Eggs or egg substitute (i.e., Eggbeaters)	0	1	0	1	0	1
BAKERY: (Freeze unused portions)						
100% wholewheat bread	3 slices	3 slices	5 slices	5 slices	5 slices	5 slices
100% wholewheat English muffin	1 whole	2 whole	2 whole	2 whole	2 whole	2 whole
100% wholewheat bagel	2	1	3	3	3	3
100% wholewheat Pita pocket	1	0	1	0	1	0
Bread sticks, 4"	2	0	2	0	2	0
Wholewheat roll	2	0	2	2	2	2
Hamburger bun	0	1	0	1	0	1
Corn tortilla (can substitute wholewheat), 6"	1	2	1	3	1	3
Wholewheat tortilla (can substitute corn), 6"	2	0	2	2	2	2
DELI/BUTCHER:						
Boneless, skinless chicken breasts, 3-4 oz. each	2	3	3	3	3	3
Fresh fish, 4-5 oz. filets, (some butchers poach fish for you)	2	1	2	1	2	1
Sliced turkey (1/2 lb. = 8 sandwich slices, 1 oz. each)	6 oz.	1 oz.	8 oz.	3 oz.	8 oz.	3 oz.
Sliced turkey ham	2 oz.	0 oz.	3 oz.	2 oz.	3 oz.	2 oz.
Canadian bacon (1 oz. = 2 slices)	0	1 oz.	0	1 oz.	0	1 oz.
Extra lean ground beef- 1/4 lb. (4 oz.) raw, cooks to 3 oz.	3 oz.	3 oz.	4 oz.	3 oz.	4 oz.	3 oz.
Beef tenderloin/Flank steak- 1/4 lb. (4 oz.) raw, cooks to 3 oz.	3 oz.	3 oz.	3 oz.	4 oz.	3 oz.	4 oz.
Shrimp	0	10 large	0	10 oz.	0	10 large
FRESH FRUIT:						
Apples	2 small	1 small	2 large	1 large	2 large	1 large
Pear	1 small	0	1 large	0	1 large	0
Banana	1	1	1	1	1	2
Fresh peach or seasoned fruit	1	1	1	1	1	1
Oranges	2	2	2	2	2	2
Grapefruit	1	1	1	1	1	1
Cantaloupe	1/2	1/2	1	1	1 1/4	1 1/4
Watermelon, (1/4th = 4 c.)	1 1/4	2 1/2 c.	1 1/4 c.	2 1/2 c.	1 1/4 c.	3 1/2 c.
Grapes	1 c.	2 c.	1 c.	2 c.	2 c.	4 c.
Strawberries, (1 pint = 2 c.)	1 1/4 c.	2 1/2 c.	1 1/4 c.	2 1/2 c.	2 c.	3 1/2 c.
Fresh pineapple, 1 whole	1	1	1	1	2 c.	3 c.
Fresh fruit salad	1 c.	1 c.	1 1/2 c.	1 c.	2 c.	1 c.
MISCELLANEOUS:						
Grilled chicken fast-food sandwich	0	1	0	1	0	1
Small order fast-food french fries	0	0	0	0	0	1/2
Fortune cookie	0	1	0	1	0	1

	1300 Calorie		1600 Calorie		2000 Calorie	
	Week #1	Week #2	Week #1	Week #2	Week #1	Week#2

FRESH VEGETABLES: (Add extra vegetables to salads, any dish or snack)

	1300 W#1	1300 W#2	1600 W#1	1600 W#2	2000 W#1	2000 W#2
1 Lettuce (1 head = 8 salads)	8 salads	4 salads	8 salads	4 salads	8 salads	6 salads
Small tomato	9	5	9	6	9	7
Regular carrot (10 baby carrots = 1 regular carrot = 1 c.)	4 reg.	3 reg.	4 reg.	4 reg.	6 reg	6 reg.
Cucumber	1	1	1	1	1	1
Mushrooms (1/2 c.= 3 large mushrooms)	1/2 c.	1/2 c.	1/2 c.	1/2 c.	1/2 c.	1/2 c.
Onion, large (1 onion = 1 c.)	1	1	2	2	2	2
Broccoli, flowerets	1/2 c.	1 c.	1 c.	1 1/2 c.	1 c.	1 1/2 c.
Cauliflower, flowerets	1/2 c.	0	1 c.	1 c.	1 c.	1 c.
Zucchini	1	1	1	1	1	1
Yellow squash	1	1	1	1	1	1
Shredded cabbage, bagged (add extra to salads/sandwiches)	1/2 c.	1/2 c.	1 c.	1 c.	1 c.	1 c.
Fresh spinach	1 c.	1 c.	1/2 c.	1 c.	1 c.	1 c.
Asparagus (5 spears = 1/2 c.)	0	1/2 c.	1/2 c.	1/2 c.	1 c.	1/2 c.
New potatoes (1 small = 1/2 c.)	2 small	1 small	2 small	1 small	2 lg., 1 sm.	1 small
Red or green bell peppers	1	1	1	1	1	1
Celery stalks	0	0	3	3	3	3

FROZEN SECTION:

	1300 W#1	1300 W#2	1600 W#1	1600 W#2	2000 W#1	2000 W#2
Cheese Pizza, 1 medium	2 slices	0	2 slices	0	3 slices	0
Low-calorie frozen dinners (<300 calories, <10 g fat)	0	1	0	1	0	1
Eggo or Special K low-fat waffles	0	1	0	2	0	2
Wholewheat pancakes	2	2	0	2	0	3
Sugar-free popsicles	1	1	0	1	4	2
Green beans	1/2 c.	1/2 c.	1/2 c.	0	1 c.	0
Brussel sprouts	1/2 c.	0	1/2 c.	0	1 c.	1 c.
Spinach	1/2 c.	1/2 c.	1/2 c.	1/2 c.	1 c.	1/2 c.
Peas	1/2 c.	0	1/2 c.	1/2 c.	1/2 c.	1 c.
Corn	1/2 c.	1/2 c.	1/2 c.	1/2 c.	1 c.	1/2 c.
Japanese vegetable blend, 16 oz. bag (= 3 c.)	0	1 1/2 c.	0	1 c.	0	2 c.
California or any vegetable blend, 16 oz. bag (= 3 c.)	0 c.	2 c.	1 c.	1/2 c.	2 c.	1 c.

PANTRY ITEMS:

	1300 W#1	1300 W#2	1600 W#1	1600 W#2	2000 W#1	2000 W#2
Oatmeal (amounts shown are cooked)	1/2 c.	0	1 c.	0	1 c.	0
Spaghetti, small package (amounts shown are cooked)	1/2 c.	1 c.	1 c.	1 c.	1 c.	1 c.
Rice, small box (amounts shown are cooked)	1/2 c.	1 c.	2 c.	1 c.	2 c.	1 c.
Pizza sauce, small jar	0	1/4 c.	0	1/4 c.	0	1/4 c.
Spaghetti Sauce, small jar	1/2 c.	0	1/2 c.	0	1/2 c.	0
Tuna packed in water (3 oz. can)	1	1	1	1	1	1
Tomato soup, 1 can	1	1	0	0	0	1
Lentil or Bean Soup, 1 can (1/2 can = 1 c.)	0	0	0	1	0	1 c.
Vegetable Soup, 1 can (1/2 can = 1 c.)	1 c.	1 c.	1 c.	0	1 c.	1 c.
Pinto or Kidney Beans (16 oz. can = 2 c.)	3/4 c.	3/4 c.	3/4 c.	3/4 c.	3/4 c.	0
Baked beans	0	0	0	0	0	1/2 c.
Cereals: Bran Flakes, single serving box	1/2 c.	0	1/2 c.	0	1/2 c.	0
Shredded Wheat, single serving box	0	1 c.	0	1 c.	0	1 c.
Grapenuts or low-fat granola, small box	1/3 c.	1/3 c.	1/2 c.	1/3 c.	1/2 c.	1/3 c.
Large Rice Cakes, small bag	2	0	2	0	4	0
Light microwave popcorn (i.e., Orville Redenbacher Smartpop)	1/2 c.	1/2 bag	1/2 bag	0	1 bag	0
Pretzels, tiny twists, 1 oz. snack bag (= 1 c.)	1/2 c.	0	3/4 c.	1/4 c.	1 1/2 c.	1 1/2 c.
Low-fat Triscuit crackers	0	0	0	0	6	6
Graham crackers, 1 package	3	3	3	2	6	0
Sugar-free, fat-free hot cocoa mix, individual packets	2	2	2	2	2	2
V-8 tomato juice (6 oz. cans)	1	0	1	0	1	0
Chicken broth, 14.5 oz. can, = 2 c.	1 can	1 can	2 cans	1 can	2 cans	1 can
Raisins, 1.5 oz. box = 4 Tbsp.	0	0	0	0	2 Tbsp.	0

This approach allows you to choose well-balanced, low-fat, high-fiber P-C-F meals very easily.

◇ Combine any of the following breakfast, lunch or dinner meals on the following pages.

◇ You'll consume your desired 1300-1600 calories/day, and 20-30 grams fiber per 1,000 calories.

◇ Most meals are conveniently "assembled," with little or no cooking.

◇ "Miscellaneous" refers to snacks or extras you can eat at mealtimes.

For Weight Loss, I Recommend:

WOMEN: Eat 1300-1400 calories a day and 30-40 g fat as:

	Calories	Fat
Breakfast:	250-300	0-5 g
Lunch:	400-500	10-15 g
Supper:	450-500	15-25 g
Misc./Snack:	100-200	0-5 g

MEN: Eat 1600-1800 calories a day and 50-60 g fat as:

	Calories	Fat
Breakfast:	300-400	0-10 g
Lunch:	600-700	10-25 g
Supper:	600-700	10-25 g
Misc./Snack:	100-200	0-5 g

Results

With moderate daily activity, a woman will lose 2-4 pounds a month, and a man will lose 4-6 pounds a month.

For Weight Maintenance, I Recommend:

WOMEN: Eat 1500-1800 calories a day and 30-60 g fat as:

	Calories	Fat
Breakfast:	300	0-5 g
Lunch:	500-600	10-15 g
Supper:	600-700	15-25 g
Misc./Snack:	100-200	0-5 g

MEN: Eat 2000-2500 calories a day and 50-75 g fat as:

	Calories	Fat
Breakfast:	400-500	0-10 g
Lunch:	700-900	15-30 g
Supper:	700-900	15-30 g
Misc./Snack:	200	0-10 g

Quick and Easy Breakfast Ideas

200 - 300 Calories, < 10 Grams Fat

- ✧ Healthy breakfast meals include fruit, wholegrains and protein (milk or meat) for the P-C-F balance.
- ✧ Note: Meals with the same food groups, (as below), tend to have the same number of calories and fat.
- ✧ 🛍 Means brown-bag "grab-'n-go" meal . . . pack the night before.

C = Complex Carbohydrate	P = Protein	F = Fat (in grams)	Cal. = Calories
c. = cup *Tbsp. = tablespoon*	*tsp. = teaspoon*	*red. = reduced*	

FOOD GROUP		Cal.	Fat		Cal.	Fat		Cal.	Fat
Fruit (C)	2 Tbsp. raisins	60		1/2 banana	60		1/2 c. blueberries	60	
Starch (C)	3/4 c. bran flakes	100		3/4 c. Kashi Crunch			1/2 c. shredded wheat	100	
Milk (P,C)	1 c. fat-free milk	100		cereal	100	1	1/2 c. whole milk	75	4
Fat (F)	1 Tbsp. almonds	50	5	3/4 c. 2% milk	100	4			
TOTALS		**310**	**5**		**260**	**5**		**235**	**4**
Fruit (C)	1/2 c. applesauce	60		1/4 cantaloupe	60		1 c. strawberries	60	
Starch (C)	1/2 wholewheat tortilla	80	1	1/2 wholewheat pita			3 Tbsp. Grapenuts	80	
	topped with			pocket	80				
Milk (P,C) or	1/4 c. part-skim ricotta			1/2 c. low-fat			1 c. nonfat yogurt	100	
Meat (P,F)	cheese	100	5	cottage cheese	100	2			
Fat (F)	*(Put fruit and cinnamon*			3 tsp. light marga-			1 Tbsp. chopped		
	* over cheese; broil)*			rine	50	5	walnuts or almonds	50	5
				(Top fruit w/cheese)					
TOTALS		**240**	**6**		**290**	**7**		**290**	**5**
2 Fruit (C)	1 c. fruit salad	120		1/2 banana	60		1 banana, sliced	120	
				1 c. strawberries	60				
Starch (C)	1/2 c. grits topped with	80		4 rye crackers	80	1	2 slices light		
Milk (P,C) or	1 oz. (3 Tbsp.) mozza-						wholewheat bread	80	
Meat (P,F)	rella cheese, grated or			1 c. fat-free milk	90		1 Tbsp. peanutbutter	100	8
	2 Tbsp. cheddar	80	5	*(Blend fruit & milk*					
				* into a smoothie)*					
TOTALS		**280**	**5**		**290**	**1**		**300**	**8**
Fruit (C)	1/2 c. orange juice	60		1 large apple	120		1 orange	60	
Starch (C)	1 wholewheat toast	80	1	5 wholewheat			1/2 c. oatmeal	80	
				crackers	100	1			
Milk (P,C) or	1 egg, poached/boiled	80	5	1 oz. string cheese			1 c. fat-free milk	100	
Meat (P,F)				or 2 2% milk					
Fat (F)	1 tsp. margarine or	45	5	cheese slices	80	5	1 Tbsp. walnuts on		
	1 Tbsp. jam on toast						oatmeal	50	5
TOTALS		**265**	**11**		**300**	**6**		**290**	**5**

Continued

© 2009, *The Cooper Clinic Solution to the Diet Revolution* by Georgia G. Kostas, M.P.H., R.D., L.D., Dallas, Texas

200-300 Calorie Breakfast Ideas

FOOD GROUP		Cal.	Fat		Cal.	Fat		Cal.	Fat
Fruit (C)	1/2 grapefruit	60		6 oz. tomato juice	35		1 small pear	60	
2 Starch C)	1 small bagel (1 oz.)	160		1 English muffin	160		2 corn tortillas	160	1
Meat (P,F) or	1 oz. turkey ham	50	1	1 oz. lean ham	50	2	1 oz. (3 Tbsp.) 2% milk		
Milk (P,C)							cheese,* grated,		
Fat (F)	1 Tbsp. light cream			1 tsp. margarine (or 1			melted on tortillas	80	5
	cheese on bagel	40	3	oz. low-fat cheese)	45	5			
TOTALS		**310**	**4**		**290**	**7**		**300**	**6**
Fruit (C)	1 small pear	60		1 medium peach	60		1 small apple	60	
2 Starch C)	1 c. dry Chex cereal mix			1 c. canned vegetable			1 wholewheat		
	(Rice, Wheat, Corn,			soup	80	2	English muffin or		
	Bran Chex, shredded			5 melba toast crackers	80	2	1 small bagel	160	1
	wheat)	160	1						
Milk (P,C) or	1 oz. fat-free string			1 c. fat-free milk	100		1 wedge Laughing		
Meat (P,F)	cheese	50	2				Cow light cheese	50	3
TOTALS		**270**	**3**		**320**	**4**		**270**	**4**
Fruit (C)	1/8 honeydew	60		1 orange	60		1 c. pineapple	60	
Starch (C)	1/2 English muffin	80		1 wholewheat toast	80	1	2 light wholewheat toast	80	1
2 Meat (P,F)	1 egg, poached	80	5	1 egg (or egg substitute)	80	5	1 oz. 2% milk Kraft		
	1 oz. low-fat cheese*			blended with 1/4 c.			cheddar cheese slice*	80	5
	(3 Tbsp.) grated	80	5	low-fat cottage cheese	50	1	1 oz. (2 slices)		
				(Omelet, cooked with			Canadian Bacon	40	2
	(Open-faced sandwich)			nonstick spray)					
TOTALS		**300**	**10**		**270**	**7**		**260**	**8**
Fruit (C)	1 c. grapes	60		1/2 grapefruit	60		1/2 c. orange juice+	60	
Starch (C)	2 slices light whole-			1/2 wholewheat English			2 light wholewheat		
	wheat bread	80		muffin	80		bread	80	
2 Meat (P,F)	1 low-fat "single" cheese			2 oz. Canadian Bacon	80	4	2 oz. hamburger		
1/2 Fat (F)	slice*	50	2	1/2 tsp. margarine	15	2	patty, broiled (or		
	1 oz. lean ham	50	1				soy burger)	160	10
							tomato, lettuce,		
	(Grill or broil)						mustard	0	
							+ Calcium fortified		
TOTALS		**240**	**3**		**235**	**6**		**300**	**10**

*NOTE: **Nonfat cheeses** (fat-free) refer to Kraft Free slices, etc.

      Low-fat cheeses (< 3 g fat per oz.) refer to Weight Watchers slices, Laughing Cow light wedges, etc.

      Reduced-fat cheeses (≤ 6 g fat per 1 oz.) refer to part-skim mozzarella, Parmesan, Kraft reduced-fat 2% milk Cheddar or Swiss, etc.

      Light cheeses may be low-fat or reduced-fat, and contain 50% less fat than original product.

      Light refers to 35-40 calories per slice bread and 50 calories per tablespoon margarine or mayonnaise.

© 2009, *The Cooper Clinic Solution to the Diet Revolution* by Georgia G. Kostas, M.P.H., R.D., L.D., Dallas, Texas

Quick and Easy Brown-Bag Lunches

300 - 500 Calories, < 20 Grams Fat

C = Complex Carbohydrate   **P = Protein**   **F = Fat (in grams)**   **Cal. = Calories**

c. = cup   *Tbsp. = tablespoon*   *tsp. = teaspoon*   *red. = reduced*

SANDWICHES	Cal.	Fat		Cal.	Fat
Tuna Sandwich			**Turkey/Beef Sandwich**		
2 slices wholewheat bread (C)	160		2 slices light wholewheat bread (C)	80	
1/2 c. tuna-in-water (P,F)	80	2	2 oz. chicken, turkey or lean beef (P,F)	100	2
3 tsp. light mayonnaise (F)	50	5	1 tsp. mayonnaise or light cheese (F)	50	5
lettuce, pickle	0		lettuce, tomato slices	0	
1 large apple or			1 small orange (C)	60	
8 oz. apple juice (C)	120		25 stick pretzels (C)	80	
1/2 c. baby carrots (C)	25				
TOTALS	**435**	**7**	**TOTALS**	**370**	**7**
Peanutbutter Sandwich			**Veggie Sandwich**		
2 slices light wholewheat bread (C)	80		1 wholewheat pita pocket (C)	160	1
1 Tbsp. peanutbutter (P,F)	100	8	1 c. vegetables, cooked or grilled (C)	50	
1 banana (C)	120		1 oz. grated mozzarella cheese (P,F)	80	5
1 c. skim fat-free milk (P,C)	100		1 peach (C)	60	
TOTALS	**400**	**8**	**TOTALS**	**350**	**6**
Lean Ham Sandwich			**Burger**		
2 slices wholewheat bread (C)	160	2	fast-food hamburger* (P,C,F)	350	10
2 oz. lean ham (P,F)	100	4	(1/4 lb. meat, no mayonnaise)		
1 Tbsp. fat-free mayonnaise (F)	15		1 large apple (from home) (C)	120	
lettuce	0		water	0	
1/2 c. carrot sticks (C)	25				
1 large pear (C)	120		*or grilled chicken sandwich (no sauce)*		
TOTALS	**420**	**6**	**TOTALS**	**470**	**10**

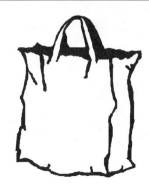

300-500 Cal. Brown-Bag Lunches

COLD SALADS	Cal.	Fat		Cal.	Fat
Pasta Salad			***Fruit Salad***		
1/2 c. spaghetti (C)	100		1 c. low-fat cottage cheese (P,F)	100	2
1 c. raw vegetables (C)	25		1 c. pineapple chunks (C)	60	
1 oz. (3 Tbsp.) grated mozzarella cheese (P,F)	80	5	1 c. strawberries (C)	60	
			1/2 banana, sliced (C)	60	
3 Tbsp. nonfat Italian dressing (F)	75		topping: 3 Tbsp. Grapenuts (C)	80	
1 fresh fruit or 2 small ones (plums, kiwi) (C)	60		1 Tbsp. almonds (F)	50	
TOTALS	**340**	**5**	**TOTALS**	**410**	**2**
Caesar Salad			***Fajita or Taco Salad***		
2 c. lettuce (C)	25		2 c. lettuce (C)	25	
1/2 c. croutons (C,F)	80	3	1/2 c. pinto or kidney beans (P,C)	100	
1/4 c. (1 oz.) Parmesan cheese	80	5	3 Tbsp. light cheddar, grated (P,F)	80	5
4 Tbsp. nonfat Caesar dressing (on side)	100	8	1/4 c. salsa	0	
3 oz. chicken breast, steamed	150	3	1/2 medium tomato	25	
			4 Tbsp. nonfat Ranch dressing	100	8
TOTALS	**435**	**19**	**TOTALS**	**330**	**13**
Rice-Vegetables Salad			***Chef Salad***		
1 c. cooked rice (C)	200		2 c. mixed salad greens (C)	25	
1 c. raw vegetables (C)	25		1/2 medium tomato	25	
2 oz. cooked chicken (P,F)	100	2	2 oz. turkey ham (P,F)	100	
3 tsp. light mayonnaise	50	5	1/2 c low-fat cottage cheese (P,F)	100	2
1 small fresh fruit (C)	60		2 Tbsp. light dressing (F)	50	5
			5 rye crisp crackers	100	
TOTALS	**435**	**7**	**TOTALS**	**400**	**7**

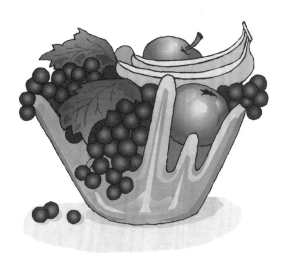

   © 2009, *The Cooper Clinic Solution to the Diet Revolution* by Georgia G. Kostas, M.P.H., R.D., L.D., Dallas, Texas

300-500 Cal. Brown-Bag Lunches

MISCELLANEOUS	Cal.	Fat		Cal.	Fat
Yogurt/Fruit Sundae			**_Baked Potato & Salad_**		
1 c. plain fat-free yogurt (P,C)	100		1 restaurant-size baked potato (C) with	250	
1 c. fresh strawberries (C)	60		1 oz. (3 Tbsp.) mozzarella cheese (P,F)	80	5
4 graham crackers or			Tossed salad	25	
8 wholewheat crackers (C)	160	1	1 Tbsp. salad dressing (F)	80	5
TOTALS	**320**	**1**	**TOTALS**	**435**	**11**
Soups, Etc.			**_Frozen Meal_**		
1 c. minestrone soup (C,F)	80	2	Low-calorie frozen meal (< 300 cal,	300	9
6 wholewheat crackers (C,F)	120	1	< 10 g fat, such as Lean Cuisine,		
1 oz. low-fat cheese (i.e.,	50	3	Weight Watchers, etc.) (P,C,F)		
Laughing Cow light cheese) (P,F)			1/2 c. sugar snap peas or cherry		
1 c. grapes or cherries (C)	60		tomatoes (C)	25	
			1 large fruit (C)	120	
TOTALS	**310**	**6**	**TOTALS**	**445**	**9**
Grab-n-Go			**_Grab-n-Go_**		
1 1/2 oz. box raisins (4 Tbsp.) (C)	120		1 large bagel	300	
5 graham crackers			1 nonfat yogurt	100	
or 1 c. dry cereal mix (C)	160	4	1 large apple	120	
1 c. fat-free milk or nonfat yogurt (P,C)	100				
TOTALS	**380**	**4**	**TOTALS**	**520**	**0**

Other Ideas

1. Pick up sandwich at local deli at lunch or before work (some delis are in grocery stores). Add fresh fruit from home.
2. Pack leftovers. If at a restaurant the night before, add "extra vegetables to go" with half of your entrée for tomorrow.
3. Keep supply of soup, frozen meals, cheese and crackers, peanutbutter, fruit, and popcorn at work.
4. See breakfast and dinner ideas to use at lunch.
5. Choose fresh fruit, green salads, non-creamy soups and potatoes from your local grocery store delis.

Quick and Easy Dinner Ideas

250 - 500 Calories, < 15 Grams Fat

C = Complex Carbohydrate	P = Protein	F = Fat (in grams)	Cal. = Calories
c. = cup *Tbsp.* = tablespoon	*tsp.* = teaspoon		*red.* = reduced

	Cal.	Fat		Cal.	Fat
Mini Pizza and Fruit			**Stuffed Vegetables**		
2 oz. Canadian Bacon (P,F)	80	4	Fill and bake tomato, green pepper,		
1 oz. (3 Tbsp.) mozzarella (P,F)	80	5	squash or eggplant (C) with:	25	
1/2 c. raw mushrooms (C)	15		2 oz. lean ground turkey, cooked	100	2
1/2 c. tomato sauce (C) on	35		1/2 c. cooked rice (C) and	100	
2 pita pocket halves or 2 tortillas or			1/2 c. chopped onions and green	25	
2 English muffin halves (C)	160		peppers in 1/2 c. tomato sauce (C)	35	
1 large fruit (i.e., pear) (C)	120		1 fruit (i.e. 1 c. melon slices) (C)	60	
			1 wholewheat dinner roll (C)	80	1
TOTAL	**490**	**9**	**TOTAL**	**425**	**3**
Chalupa or Taco			**Baked Potato, Salad and Fruit**		
1 corn tortilla (C)	80	1	1 medium potato (C) with	250	
2 oz. lean ground beef, drained (P,F)	160	10	1 oz. (3 Tbsp.) 2% milk cheddar		
1 oz. (3 Tbsp.) low-fat cheddar* (P,F)	40	3	cheese (P,F)	80	5
1/2 c. diced tomato and onion (C)	25		Tossed salad with raw vegetables (C)	25	
lettuce, pepper, picante sauce	0		with 1 Tbsp. French dressing (F)	60	6
			1 c. watermelon	60	
1 c. fat-free milk (P,C)	100				
1 c. strawberries (C)	60				
TOTAL	**465**	**14**	**TOTAL**	**475**	**11**
Soup, Salad and Fruit			**Soup, Sandwich and Fruit**		
1 c. vegetable soup (C)	80	2	1 c. chicken noodle soup (C)	80	2
Tossed salad w/ raw vegetables (C) w/	25		2 slices wholewheat bread (C)	160	2
2 Tbsp. light Italian dressing* (F) and	50	5	3 oz. lean meat (P,F)	160	10
1 oz. grated Parmesan cheese (P,F)	80	5	mustard, lettuce, tomato	0	
1 slice French bread (C)	80	5	1 small pear or apple	60	
1/2 c. fruit salad (C)	60				
TOTAL	**375**	**17**	**TOTAL**	**460**	**4**

refer to p. 96

250-500 Calorie Quick Dinners

	Cal.	Fat		Cal.	Fat
Cheese Toast, Fruit Salad			***Cold Plate***		
1 slice wholewheat toast (C)	80	1	1 c. raw vegetables (C) with	25	
1 oz. light Laughing Cow cheese wedge	50	3	1/2 c. nonfat plain yogurt (dip) (P,C)	50	
1 c. fruit salad (C)	120		mixed with herbs and spices	0	
1 c. V-8 juice (C)	50		2 oz. 2% milk Swiss cheese* (P,F)	160	10
			8 wholewheat crackers (C)	160	2
			1 c. grapes (C)	60	
TOTAL	**300**	**4**	**TOTAL**	**455**	**12**
Chicken & Rice Dinner			***Taco Salad and Fruit***		
3 oz. chicken breast (no skin) or fish (P,F)	150	3	Lettuce	0	
seasoned with 2 Tbsp. light Italian			1/2 medium tomato, sliced	25	
dressing* (F), grilled or baked	50	5	2 oz. lean ground turkey (P,F)	100	3
1/2 c. steamed spinach, etc. (C)	25		cooked in 1/2 c. picante sauce (C)	0	
1/2 c. steamed carrots, etc. (C)	25		1/2 c. pinto or kidney beans (P,C)	100	
1 c. brown or wild rice (C)	200		with optional chili powder added		
1/4 cantaloupe (C)	60		1 oz. grated low-fat cheese* (P,C)	80	3
			1 c. strawberries (C)	60	
TOTAL	**510**	**8**	**TOTAL**	**365**	**6**
Steamed Vegetables with Rice			***Ham Dinner***		
2 c. mixed steamed vegetables (C)	100		3 oz. lean ham (P,F)	150	7
1 c. brown rice (C)	200		Small baked sweet potato (C)	150	
1 c. plain nonfat yogurt (P,C) and	100		1 c. broccoli/cauliflower, steamed (C)	50	
1 c. pineapple/orange fruit mix (C)	120		2 tsp. light margarine (F)	30	3
TOTAL	**520**	**0**	**TOTAL**	**380**	**10**
Tuna-Noodle Casserole			***Frozen Dinner***		
Mix and heat until cheese melts:			Low-cal. frozen meal (P,C,F)	300	10
3 oz. water-packed tuna (P,F)	100	3	(< 300 calories, < 10 g fat)		
1 c. cooked noodles (C)	200		(Lean Cuisine, Healthy Choice, etc.)		
1 c .steamed carrots (C)	50		1 c. steamed vegetables (fresh or		
1 oz. grated red.-fat cheese* (P,F)	80	5	frozen) (C)	50	
1/4 c. fat-free milk (P, C)	25		1 c. fresh fruit salad (C)	120	
1 small apple (C)	60				
TOTAL	**515**	**8**	**TOTAL**	**470**	**10**

250-500 Calorie Quick Dinners

	Cal.	Fat
Beef Dinner		
3 oz. beef tenderloin (P,F)	170	8
Corn on cob (6" long) (C)	80	
Tossed lettuce with raw vegetables (C)	25	
with 1 Tbsp. fat-free dressing (C)	15	
1/2 c. green beans w/ mushrooms (C)	25	
2 tsp. light margarine (F)	30	3
TOTAL	**345**	**11**

	Cal.	Fat
Tuna Melt Sandwich		
1 wholewheat English muffin (C,F)	160	1
3 oz. water-packed tuna (P, F) mixed	100	3
with 1 Tbsp. light mayonnaise (F)	50	5
2 Tbsp. part-skim grated mozzarella		
cheese (P,F)	50	4
1 c. raw vegetables (C) (carrots,		
celery, tomato slices)	25	
1/2 banana (C)	60	
TOTAL	**445**	**13**

	Cal.	Fat
Spaghetti		
1 c. spaghetti (C), topped with	200	
1/2 c. meatless spaghetti sauce (C,F)	80	2
2 Tbsp. grated parmesan cheese	50	4
Fresh spinach salad (C)	0	
w/ 2 Tbsp. fat-free Italian dressing (C)	30	
1 slice Italian bread (C)	80	
1 c. fat-free milk (P,C)	100	
TOTAL	**540**	**6**

	Cal.	Fat
Shrimp Creole		
Mix & heat: 1 c. white rice (C)	200	
1 c. tomato sauce (C) and	70	
steamed celery, onion, seasonings	0	
Add: 2 oz. (10) frozen cooked		
shrimp (P,F)	100	2
Romaine salad with tomatoes &	25	
2 Tbsp. light dressing* (F)	50	5
1 sliced fresh peach	60	
TOTAL	**505**	**7**

	Cal.	Fat
Stir-Fry		
2 c. frozen vegetables (C) cooked in	100	
1 tsp. canola oil (F) with	50	5
3 oz. skinless chicken breast (P,F)	150	3
1/2 c. linguini (C)	100	
1/2 c. fresh fruit salad (C)	60	
TOTAL	**460**	**8**

	Cal.	Fat
Vegetarian Dinner		
1 c. beans (P,C)	200	
1 c. rice (C)	200	
Tossed salad with raw vegetables (C)	25	
with 2 Tbsp. light dressing* (F)	50	5
1 c. cantaloupe (1/4 melon) (C)	60	
TOTAL	**535**	**5**

*NOTE:

Nonfat cheeses (fat-free) refer to Kraft Free slices, etc.

Light cheeses may be low-fat or reduced-fat cheeses and contain half the fat of the original product or 1/3 fewer calories.

Low-fat cheeses (< 3 g fat per 1 oz.) refer to Weight Watchers slices, Laughing Cow light wedges, etc.

Reduced-fat cheeses (≤ 6 g fat per 1 oz.) refer to part-skim mozzarella, Parmesan, Kraft 2% milk Cheddar, Swiss, etc.

Light or reduced-calorie refers to 35-40 calories per slice bread and 50 calories per tablespoon margarine or mayonnaise.

Nonfat salad dressings ("fat-free") contain 5-25 calories per tablespoon.

Light salad dressings contain 25-50 calories per tablespoon.

A Simplified Counter

Keep it simple . . . count by 50's and 100's. Easy as 50 - 100 - 150!

MILK/DAIRY

	Cal.
Fat-free milk/yogurt (1 c.)	100
1% cottage cheese (1/2 c.)	100
Cheese (1 oz. = 3 Tbsp. = ¼ c.)	100
Parmesan or Mozzarella (2 Tbsp.)	50
Low-fat cheese (1 slice)	50
Frozen nonfat yogurt or ice milk (1/2 c.)	100

STARCHES

Rice/pasta/potatoes (1/2 c.)	100
Rice/pasta/potatoes (3/4 c.)	150
Corn/peas (1/2 c.)	100
Corn (6-inch ear)	100
Beans, most (1/2 c.)	100
Cereal: hot/cold (1 c., avg.)	150
Bread (2 slices)	150-200
Corn tortillas (2)	150
English muffin	150
Bagel, small	150
Bagel, large	300
New potato (4 oz.)	100
Baked potato (medium, 8-10 oz.)	200-250
Baked potato (large, 12 oz.)	300
Baked potato (extra large,16 oz.)	500
Sweet potato	300

FRUITS & VEGETABLES

Fruit Juice (1 c.)	100
Fresh fruit (1 medium or 1 c.)*	100
Frozen fruit (1 c.)	100
Vegetables (1 c.)	50
Soup (1 c.)	100
Cream soup (1 c.)	150
Spaghetti sauce (1/2 c.)	100-150

* *1/2 cantaloupe; 1 banana, apple, pear;*
   1 grapefruit, mango, papaya;
   2 c. melon, strawberries, cherries, grapes;
   1 c. blueberries, pineapple;
   2 peaches, oranges, plums

PROTEIN

	Cal.
Tuna in water (1/2 c.)	100
Fish/poultry/lean meat (1 oz.)	50
Fish/poultry/lean meat (2 oz.)	100
Fish/poultry/lean meat (3 oz.)	150
Fish/poultry/lean meat (4 oz.)	200
Shrimp (10 big)	100

FATS / "EXTRAS"

Butter/margarine/oil (1 Tbsp.)	100
(Olive/canola oils are excellent.)	
Light margarine (1 Tbsp.)	50
Mayonnaise/peanutbutter (1 Tbsp.)	100
Light mayonnaise (1 Tbsp.)	50
Salad dressings (2 Tbsp.)	150
Light dressings (2 Tbsp.)	50-100
Fat-free dressings (2 Tbsp.)	25-50
Nuts/seeds (2 Tbsp. = 1 oz.)	100
Cream, cream cheese (2 Tbsp.)	100
Sour cream (3 Tbsp.)	100
Jam, jelly, sugar, honey, syrup (1 Tbsp.)	50

SNACKS

Crackers, 4 to 6	100
Wheat Thins, 12 to 14	100
Fig Newtons, 2	100
Pretzels, 15 tiny twists or 8 large thins	100
Chips, 10 small or 8 large	100
Popcorn, light or low-fat, 4-6 c.	100
Low-fat granola bar	100
Raisins, 1 oz. or 4 Tbsp.	100
Chex mix, 1/2 c.	100
100-calorie snack packs, any	100
1 Cocovia (chocolate bar)	80
1 chocolate candy bar	300

Select Foods With More Bites for the Calories

Make Every Bite Count!

100-Calorie Food Equivalents

2 cups vegetables (non-starchy)
1 med. fruit (i.e., 1/2 cantaloupe, 2 c. grapes or berries, 1 apple, etc.)
1 small red new potato (4 oz.)
4 cups popcorn (without butter)
1/2 cup starch (potato, rice, pasta, etc.)
1/2 cup beans (lentils, pinto, garbanzo, etc.)
1 1/2 slices bread (or 1 slice bread with 1/2 tsp. margarine)
1 1/2 c. (1 bowl) non-creamy soup at home; 1 c. at restaurants
2 oz. fish or poultry
1 1/2 oz. lean meat (flank, filet, tenderloin)
1 oz. high-fat meat (prime rib, brisket, etc.)
1 oz. cheese or 2 oz. low-fat cheese
1 cup fat-free milk or yogurt
1/2 cup low-fat cottage cheese, tuna, crab, salmon, tofu
1 1/2 Tbsp. salad dressing
1 Tbsp. margarine, mayonnaise, oil, peanut-butter

Go for volume!

100-Calorie "Extras"

Cookies

    5 vanilla wafers
    3 gingersnaps
    1 chocolate chip
    2 fig bars

Candy

    15 jelly beans
    10 malted milk balls
    6 gumdrops
    4 large marshmallows
    1 cubic inch of fudge
    1/2 of a 1.25 oz. Kit Kat candy bar

Frozen Treats

    1 fruit-juice pop
    1 chocolate mini-treat pop
    1/2 c. scoop ice milk or frozen yogurt
    1 frozen pudding on a stick

Healthier 100-Calorie "Extras"

Grains

    1 c. Cheerios
    1 slice raisin toast with 1/2 Tbsp. cream cheese
    1 frozen toaster wholegrain waffle with 1 Tbsp. light maple syrup
    1 slice wholewheat toast, topped with 1 Tbsp. grated cheese or 1/2 Tbsp. jam

Fruit

    1/2 cantaloupe
    2 c. (20) cherries
    2 c. watermelon
    2 c. grapes
    3 kiwis

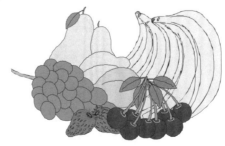

Step 3
Add More Plant Foods -
Natural Wonders

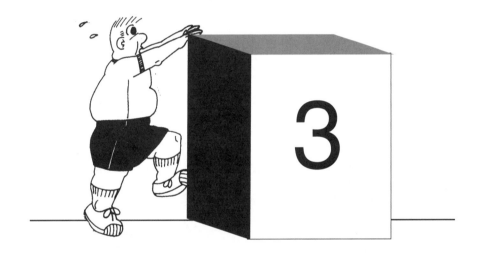

_____

Step 3

Mini-Step 1:
Understand what "5+/day" means . . . and "strive for five" daily.

Mini-Step 2:
Try 3 or more ways to eat more fruit and 3 ways to eat more vegetables.

Every day, scientists discover something new about the food we eat. Findings about new vital food components, as well as new roles and functions for nutrients, keep us ever mindful that "food is medicine", as Hippocrates said 2,500 years ago.

So what do you need to know to make the healthiest food selections?

This chapter focuses on nutrients and other ingredients in plant foods, beginning with phytochemicals in fruits and vegetables. Foods you choose can help prevent heart disease, cancer and eye diseases. So, read on to learn how to select the best.

ACTION STEPS

① Take the "5+/day" challenge!

② Eat red and green foods daily.

③ Add three fruits daily. Make it a habit.

④ Add three vegetables daily. Try new ways to enjoy them.

Select the Best: Eat More Plant Foods

Consuming the recommended **5 to 10 half-cup servings of fruit and vegetables** a day is one of the most important steps you can take to protect and promote your health and to reduce cancer and heart disease risk, according to the National Cancer Institute, the US Dietary Guidelines and USDA Food Guide Pyramid. In addition, this style of eating lowers weight, blood pressure and cholesterol, and helps you feel full! The Dietary Approach to Stop Hypertension (**DASH**) research proved that 8 - 10 servings a day lowers high blood pressure in 6 weeks (just like meds!). The DASH plan includes 2 - 3 Tbsp. of nuts daily and 3 nonfat dairy foods, as well as low-fat, high-fiber foods (see p. 227). When sodium is also limited, DASH lowers blood pressure further.

"Five-to-Ten-a-Day" - How to Do It:

5/day = five **1/2 cup** servings!

10/day = five **1 cup** servings!

How to Eat 5-10 Servings/Day:
(1 serving = 1/2 cup)

5+/day

1 large fruit or 2 small	= 2 servings
1 c. vegetables	= 2 servings
1 salad	= 1 serving

10+/day

3 large fruit or 6 small	= 6 servings
2 c. vegetables	= 4 servings

Sample 10+/Day Options:

1 banana	= 2 servings
1 large apple	= 2 servings
8 oz. orange juice w/ calcium	= 2 servings
(or 1 1/2 oz. box raisins)	
1/2 c. broccoli, cooked	= 1 serving
1/2 c. squash, cooked	= 1 serving
1 c. dinner salad	= 1 serving
1/2 c. raw carrots (snack)	= 1 serving
	10 servings

Foods That Prevent Cancer & Heart Disease

Antioxidants and phytochemicals are plant components that are cancer- and heart-protective.

Top Plant Foods for Top Health

Eat Daily:
- Citrus (1 fruit)
- Tomatoes (1 whole or 1/2 c. fresh; or 3/4 c. cooked)
- Greens: broccoli, spinach, salads, etc. (1 large serving)
- Carrot (1)
- Garlic (1 clove) or onion (1/2)
- Soy with isoflavones: 1 c. soy milk, yogurt or shake; 1/2 c. soy foods (tofu, soy beans); 1 soy burger or soy bar
- Tea, especially green tea (3-5 c.)
- Wholegrains: wholewheat bread, bran cereals, popcorn, oatmeal, etc. (3+ servings)
- Flaxseeds, milled (2 Tbsp.) or flax oil (1 tsp.)

Eat each at least 2 - 4 times weekly:
- Beans, all types
- Red bell pepper
- Red grapes
- Cantaloupe
- Crucifers (broccoli, cauliflower, cabbage, Brussels sprouts)
- Strawberries
- Berries
- Red-blue colored foods
- Sweet potatoes
- Corn, Popcorn

Fruits and Vegetables: Nutrient All-Stars

Nutrition researchers continue to tap into new wonders associated with plants and vegetables. I encourage you to move toward a plant-based diet with:

- at least 3-5 plant foods per meal
- at least 5 fruits/vegetables per day, preferably 10 small (or 5 large) per day
- at least one green salad or green leafy vegetable a day, one citrus fruit a day and one beta-carotene-rich food a day
- more flavonoid-rich foods daily: red grapes, oranges, apples, onion, garlic, tea, etc.

All-Star Benefits

1. **Ten fruits/vegetables a day** will help **lower blood pressure** (from **potassium**) and can **cut a person's risk of heart disease, stroke and cancer by almost half.**

2. **Green leafy vegetables** (rich in **folate**) will **reduce heart disease risk and macular degeneration of the eye**. Research shows that kale, collards, spinach and other greens are rich in the **carotenoids** *lutein* and *zeaxanthin*, which are believed to protect against age-related macular degeneration (ARMD). See table listing great sources for lutein and zeaxanthin.

3. Ten **tomato** servings a week (especially cooked, as in sauces for pizza, chili, spaghetti, soup, etc.) will **cut one's risk of prostate cancer in half** due to **lycopene**.

4. **Vitamin K** and **calcium** in greens will **slow down osteoporosis**.

5. **Vitamins A** (**beta-carotene**) and **C** in red, yellow, orange, and green fruits and vegetables **protect against cancer and heart disease.**

Sources of Lutein and Zeaxanthin	
Fruit or vegetable	Lutein and Zeaxanthin (combined milligrams)
Kale, 1/2 c. cooked	10.3
Spinach, 1 c. raw chopped	6.7
Spinach, 1/2 c. cooked	6.3
Turnip greens, 1/2 c. cooked	6.1
Collard greens, 1/2 c. cooked	5.2
Corn (yellow), 1 fresh ear	2.3
Broccoli, 1/2 c. cooked	1.7
Romaine lettuce, 1 c. fresh	1.5
Zucchini, 1/2 c. raw	1.4
Green peas, 1/2 c. canned	1.1
Brussels sprouts, 1/2 c. cooked	1.0
Corn (yellow), 1/2 c. canned	0.7
Orange, 1 medium	0.2
Papaya, 1 fresh whole	0.2
Tangerine, 1 medium	0.2

Source: USDA-NCC Carotenoid Database (1998)

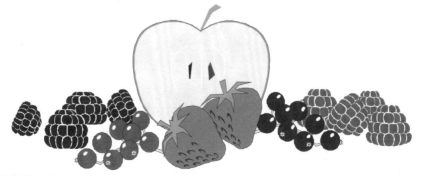

BRIGHTEST ALL-STARS

- **Berries, cherries, red grapes:** go for blueberries, bilberries, strawberries, raspberries, red grapes, cherries. These are rich in antioxidants, polyphenols and anthocyanicides, all of which are cancer-fighters. They are super sources of vitamins A, C and fiber. Red grapes and strawberries also contain ellagic acid, known to fight cancer and heart disease. The flavonoids in all these "red" foods reduce blood clotting, which prevents heart disease and stroke.

- **Citrus fruit family:** oranges, grapefruit, lemons and limes. These contain fiber and vitamin C. Red grapefruit contains lycopene, vitamins A and C, all cancer fighters. Lemons and limes contain limonene, an immune-booster.

- **Crucifers:** Broccoli, cauliflower, Brussels sprouts, cabbage, bok choy and kale are rich in vitamins A (beta-carotene) and C, fiber, indoles and sulfur compounds, all cancer fighters.

- **Dark greens:** Spinach, broccoli, romaine lettuce and collards are rich in vitamins A (beta-carotene) and C, carotenoids, folic acid, vitamin K, fiber, iron, selenium, calcium, magnesium, zinc and B vitamins, all of which boost the immune system. Some ingredients act as antioxidants. The B vitamin folic acid prevents cervical and colon cancer and lowers homocysteine, which reduces heart disease. The lutein and zeaxanthin prevent macular degeneration.

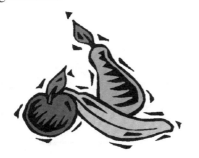

- **Deep yellow-orange-red fruits and veggies** such as carrots, sweet potatoes, red peppers and mangos are super sources of beta-carotene, vitamin C, flavonoids, and fiber. Cooked tomatoes release lycopene, an important carotenoid that reduces one's risk of prostate cancer.

- **Beans/peas:** black beans, navy beans, red beans, pintos, lentils. These contain almost every nutrient known to man, plus fiber. Include these two to five times a week—hot (at breakfast), cold (at lunch), on salads, in soups, part of hot meals or added to pasta, rice, corn dishes or corn tortillas. Beans may lower cholesterol and help regulate blood sugar.

- **Onion, garlic, leeks:** Their flavonoid and sulfur components may boost the immune system, prevent cancer and promote heart health.

- **Soy:** steamed soybeans, soynuts, soy cheeses, soy milk or soy isolate powders, soy shakes, soy crumbles, soy burgers, soy cold cuts, etc. Eat soy daily to reduce cancer and heart disease. Breast and prostate cancer risk may particularly be reduced by soy. (See p. 106 for more details on soy.)

- **Wheat germ, flaxseed, nuts, seeds:** Eat in moderation daily…
  - 1-2 Tbsp. wheat germ for trace minerals, folic acid, magnesium, zinc and copper. Add to oatmeal and dry cereals.
  - 1 Brazil nut for 105 mg. of selenium, a cancer fighter.
  - 1-2 Tbsp. nuts/seeds for alpha linolenic acid and vital trace elements (especially in walnuts & almonds), which lower cholesterol and boost the immune system.
  - 2 Tbsp. flaxseeds (milled) for omega-3 fatty acids and linolenic acid. Add to cereals, salads, yogurt, etc. They may reduce breast cancer and heart disease risk.

12 Easy Ways to Eat More Fruit

Not eating enough fruit? Read on! The ideas are limitless.

1. Eat two fruits in the morning at home; take one or two to go.
Breakfast: banana on cereal, calcium-fortified orange juice
Lunch: apple; eat with sandwich
Snack: grapes

2. Have fruit for dessert each evening: melon, pineapple, cut-up fruit, fruit salads, berries, cherries, apple/ banana/orange salad, etc.

3. Make smoothies: blend banana, frozen peaches or berries, yogurt or juice.

4. Add diced fruit to tuna salad (i.e., apple or grapes).

5. Keep raisins and diced fruit packets at your office for snacks.

6. Add apples, pears, mandarin oranges, raisins, etc., to tossed salads.

7. Puree frozen or canned fruit and pour over frozen yogurt; heat and pour over pancakes (skip the syrup).

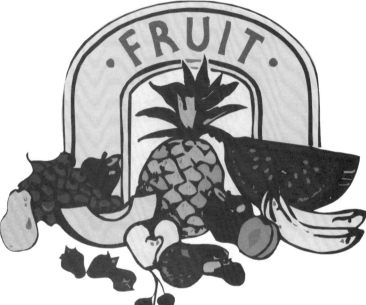

8. Freeze grapes or banana slices for a cool summer treat.

9. Add apple or banana to peanutbutter sandwich.

10. Eat 1/2 cantaloupe or one whole grapefruit to fill up fast and for very few calories (120 calories).

11. Add fruit to sauces, dressings, dips, etc., for festive occasions. Dip berries in chocolate!

12. Add fruit to soy milk or regular milk for healthy smoothies and shakes.

Top 10 Antioxidant Foods	
◆ Blueberries	◆ Kale, collard greens
◆ Plums, prunes, raisins	◆ Spinach
◆ Strawberries	◆ Beets, red bell pepper
◆ Broccoli	◆ Red grapes
◆ Oranges	◆ Brussels sprouts

20 Easy Ways to Eat More Vegetables

1. Eat twice the servings of vegetables as starches per meal—in other words, 2 c. vegetables for 1 c. rice/pasta/potato.

2. Make a colorful, veggie-packed salad once a day. Ideas: dark-green lettuce (romaine, California, etc.), shredded red cabbage, carrots, bell peppers, celery, tomato, cucumber, red onion, leftover cooked veggies (broccoli, cauliflower, etc.).

3. Eat two or more meatless, vegetable-rich meals a week.

4. Drink tomato juice as a snack.

5. Eat at least 2 vegetables and a salad every night.

6. Keep frozen veggies on hand for quick stir-fries.

7. Have fresh sugar snap peas and carrots on hand for snacks.

8. Add veggies to tuna salad (onion, celery, water chestnuts, carrots).

9. Choose fresh or frozen vegetables without sauces rather than canned vegetables.

10. To preserve nutrients and flavor, cook vegetables quickly: steam, stir-fry, microwave, eat raw.

11. Eat broccoli or spinach four times a week; a salad daily. A large serving of broccoli or spinach can replace a salad.

12. Add vegetables to sandwiches—try onion, bell peppers, bean sprouts, broccoli sprouts, cucumber, tomato, lettuce. Veggies fill you up!

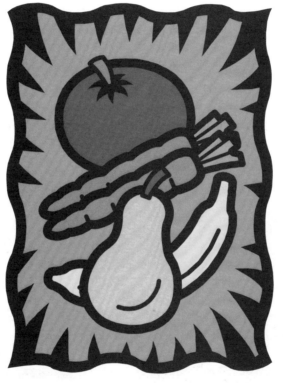

13. Eat onions and garlic daily, added to foods. Keep chopped garlic cloves in olive oil in a jar, refrigerated for quick use. Add to salad dressings, vegetables, meat dishes. Add onion slices to sandwiches, salads, all-cooked vegetable dishes.

14. Add beans to vegetable soup; add vegetables to bean soups.

15. Heat beans with chopped carrots and onion. Add salsa and put on a tortilla.

16. Roast vegetables in a 450-degree oven for great flavors. Spritz yams, carrots, zucchini and bell peppers with olive oil and bake in oven 10 minutes.

17. Eat cabbage twice a week in slaw or added to tossed salads; cooked or added to vegetable soups.

18. Eat crucifers three to four times/week (broccoli, cauliflower, cabbage, bok choy, kale, Brussel sprouts). Oriental stir-fries often contain bok choy and cabbage.

19. Eat tomatoes daily (fresh in salads or as snacks) …or cooked in spaghetti sauces, taco sauces, salsa, pico de gallo, soups, chili, bean dishes, tomato sauces, tomato juice, etc.

20. Combine vegetables together—you will eat more. They are great stir-fried, steamed together, baked as layers, grilled, etc. We eat "with our eyes." Color and variety add appeal.

➢ Note: See p. 210-211 and 228 for ways to make veggies tasty.

Enjoy Soy! Get the Facts on Flax!

Soy: Is it a trend food for the new millennium, or does it really have merit? Studies show that soy is a wonderful food! It may protect against breast cancer, prostate cancer, heart disease and osteoporosis. One serving a day seems worthwhile.

SOY POWER

Soy foods contain healthful soy protein, isoflavones and alpha-linolenic acids. You can find them in stores that specialize in whole foods, or check with your local grocer.

- **Soy protein** and **isoflavones** are phytochemicals found in soy foods. They lower cholesterol and boost the immune system. They also help prevent breast cancer and menopausal "hot flashes" in women.
- **Alpha-linolenic** acids are fatty acids that lower cholesterol and boost the immune system.

Select at least one of the following servings daily:

- 1/2 c. soybeans (1/4 c. soynuts, which are toasted soybeans), tempeh, tofu, silken tofu, textured soy protein or TSP (= 3 oz. cooked)
- 1 c. soy milk or soy yogurt (low-fat and calcium-fortified) (Note: WestSoy Plus contains 130 calories, 300 mg calcium, 4 g fat; WestSoy Non-Fat contains 80 calories, 200 mg calcium, 2 g fat.)
- 1/4 c. soy flour, defatted: add to pancakes, baked goods, breads, etc.
- 2 Tbsp. miso (similar to bouillion powder)

Other soy foods (check labels to be sure foods contain **isoflavones** and not just **soy protein**):

- Soy cheese
- Soy Protein Isolate (powder): add to soups, cereals, shakes, yogurt, pudding, milk, etc.
- Meat alternatives: soy burgers (veggie burgers), soy dogs (veggie dogs), veggie deli meats (chicken, turkey, pastrami, bologna, beef), veggie breakfast links and "bacon" strips, soy crumbles (substitute for ground beef); soy pepperoni
- Soy protein bars and shakes (i.e., Genisoy)

> Recent studies show that 25 gms of soy protein daily (with isoflavones) lowers cholesterol.

INTRODUCING FLAXSEED AND FLAX OIL

What about flax? It, too, is cancer- and heart-protective. Flax contains omega-3 fatty acids, just like seafood.

Flax oil contains omega-3 fatty acids and alpha-linolenic acids... immune boosters and anti-inflammatory agents.

Flaxseeds contain lignins, omega-3 fatty acids and alpha-linolenic acids. Lignins, a type of soluble fiber, have been shown to lower cholesterol and may protect against breast cancer.

Look for both seeds and oil at Whole Foods Markets or other similar grocery stores. Consume 2 Tbsp. ground flaxseed daily or 1 tsp. flax oil:

Seeds:

- Mill seeds with a coffee grinder, then add to batter for quick-breads, cookies, pancakes and other baked goods. Do not use whole seeds.
- Add milled seeds or whole flaxseeds to cereals, oatmeal, yogurt, granola and soup. Put in pepper shaker and shake onto foods for sesame-seed flavor.
- For baking purposes, substitute milled flaxseed for the fat used in baking at a ratio of 3 to 1. For example, 1½ c. of milled flaxseed can replace ½ c. of butter, margarine, shortening or oil in traditional recipes.
- Only grind 1 to 7 days of flaxseeds at one time. Refrigerate in a tightly sealed container.

Oil:

- Combine flax oil with olive oil on salads (1 tsp. flax + 2 tsp. olive oil). Flax oil must be used cold; do not cook with it. Add to pasta salad, potato salad, coleslaw, cooked vegetables, etc. Refrigerate oil.

Take Five or More!

☑ Each day, check a fruit or vegetable icon every time you eat a fruit or vegetable serving. A serving = 1/2 to 1 cup... the bigger, the better. At the end of the week, add up your total number of servings. Your goal is to eat 25 servings (an average of 5 servings per day).

If you achieve this, you are on your way to better health and easier weight management.

Take the "5-A-Day" Challenge!

1 Week	Fruits	Vegetables	Daily Total
Monday			
Tuesday			
Wednesday			
Thursday			
Friday			
Saturday			
Sunday			
Weekly Total			

© 2009, *The Cooper Clinic Solution to the Diet Revolution* by Georgia G. Kostas, M.P.H., R.D., L.D., Dallas, Texas

3 New Simple Strategies
for Weight Loss Success

Good News! Recent research is showing us three new ways to lose weight successfully and keep it off.

1 Wholegrains   **2 Dairy Products**   **3 Breakfast**

☑ Strategy 1: Choose Wholegrains - 3/day

Why? People who eat more wholegrains tend to:

1. weight less
2. have less abdominal fat
3. gain less weight at mid-life (women)
4. feel full longer, which staves off hunger

5. consume more fiber and nutrient variety
6. have less risk of heart disease, diabetes, stroke, digestive problems (constipation, diverticulosis and diverticulitis), certain types of cancer; and have lower cholesterol levels.

☑ Strategy 2: Consume low- or non-fat Dairy Products Daily - 3/day

Why? Recent research reveals you may:

- lose more weight, more body fat and more "middle fat" when including low-fat or non-fat dairy foods daily as part of a reduced-calorie eating plan.
- retain more lean muscle mass as you lose weight.

- gain less weight at mid-life (women) - if comsuming 1000 mg calcium daily.
- increase muscle strength and growth faster when weight training.

How does dairy help with weight loss? Research is underway to discover the mechanism. It appears that calcium and Vitamin D play important roles in signaling the body to burn fat or store it. Vitamin D has also been shown to promote muscle retention in senior adults. Since dairy foods are more effective than calcium and Vitamin D supplements, many believe it is the unique balance and synergy of nutrients within dairy that are the key. So, take advantage of what we DO know: eat dairy daily!

☑ Strategy 3: Start Each Day With Breakfast

Why? Mom was right: breakfast IS the most important meal of the day! Research tells us that people who eat breakfast daily tend to:

- Eat better
- Weight less
- Eat less fat and calories

- Lose weight more easily
- Sustain weight loss
- Prevent weight gain over time

- Miss fewer days from school/work
- perform better academically (students)

Those who skip breakfast tend to over-eat during the day, more than making up for missed morning calories. Breakfast helps "jump-start" your metabolism first thing in the morning and helps stabilize blood sugar, giving you more energy all morning long.

Step 4
Be Food Savvy:
Know Your Best Options

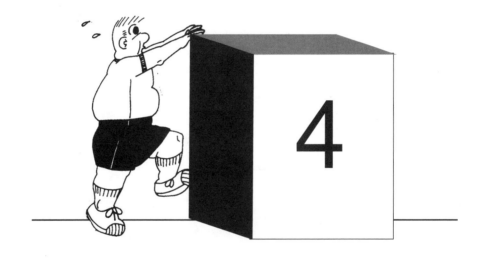

Step 4

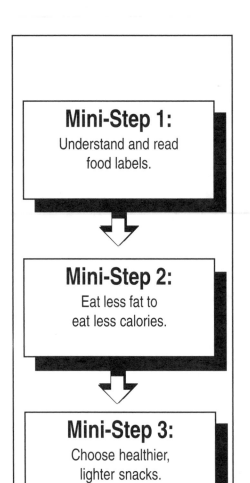

Mini-Step 1:
Understand and read food labels.

Mini-Step 2:
Eat less fat to eat less calories.

Mini-Step 3:
Choose healthier, lighter snacks.

What are you putting in your grocery cart? Do you compare food labels? Whether you're trying to eat more healthfully, lose a few inches or both, food labels can help! Remember, knowledge is power. In the next few pages, I'll explain how to decipher food labels and make them work for your benefit.

You will also learn that the right snack can boost your health, your energy and your weight loss. Note the healthy snack ideas that will keep your appetite down and energy up, all day. If you are tempted by those "Crazy C's" (see p. 123), you'll benefit from some "cures" for your "cravings." Also in this section, I've provided several practical food lists that will serve you as easy-reference guides, helping you trim the fat and save a pound of calories.

Is there much difference between sandwiches, cheeses, dressings, dips and drinks? Take a look at the "Calorie & Fat Comparisons" and find out! Keep this list close to your fridge and on your mind. You control your choices, so gather all the information you can to make wise decisions. Read food labels; then *you* be the judge!

ACTION STEPS

① Begin to look closely at food labels. Select two products... compare, contrast and choose.

② Keep healthy snacks on hand.

③ Trade a higher-fat food for a lower-fat one. Do this again and again.

④ Make food comparison a way of life.

Become a Proficient Label Reader

The more closely you look at labels, the more likely you are to select healthier, nutrient-rich foods. Of all the nutrition principles you glean from this book, learning how to read labels is one of the most important. If you have children at home, teach them while they're young to instill healthy habits—and make grocery shopping a family affair!

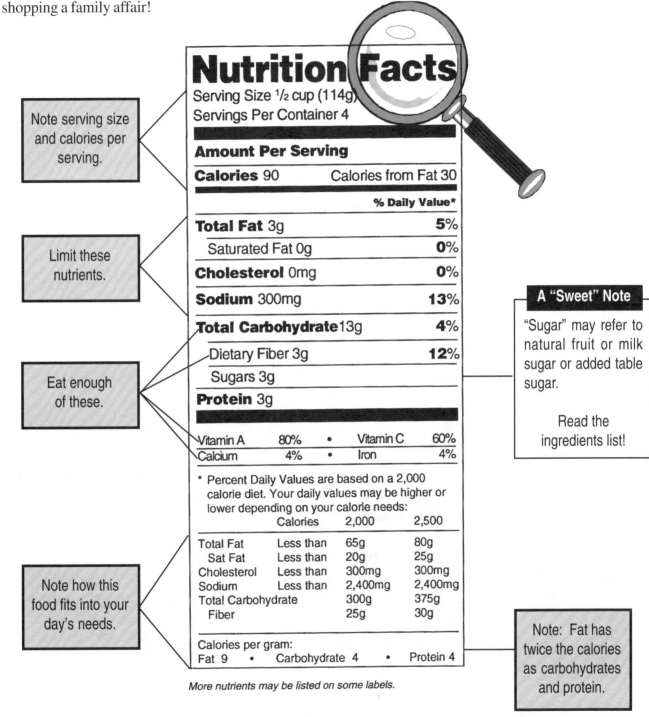

Note serving size and calories per serving.

Limit these nutrients.

Eat enough of these.

Note how this food fits into your day's needs.

Nutrition Facts
Serving Size ½ cup (114g)
Servings Per Container 4

Amount Per Serving

Calories 90   Calories from Fat 30

% Daily Value*

Total Fat 3g	**5%**
Saturated Fat 0g	**0%**
Cholesterol 0mg	**0%**
Sodium 300mg	**13%**
Total Carbohydrate 13g	**4%**
Dietary Fiber 3g	**12%**
Sugars 3g	
Protein 3g	

Vitamin A	80%	Vitamin C	60%
Calcium	4%	Iron	4%

* Percent Daily Values are based on a 2,000 calorie diet. Your daily values may be higher or lower depending on your calorie needs:

		Calories	2,000	2,500
Total Fat	Less than		65g	80g
Sat Fat	Less than		20g	25g
Cholesterol	Less than		300mg	300mg
Sodium	Less than		2,400mg	2,400mg
Total Carbohydrate			300g	375g
Fiber			25g	30g

Calories per gram:
Fat 9   •   Carbohydrate 4   •   Protein 4

More nutrients may be listed on some labels.

A "Sweet" Note

"Sugar" may refer to natural fruit or milk sugar or added table sugar.

Read the ingredients list!

Note: Fat has twice the calories as carbohydrates and protein.

When you know how to read a food label all of the numbers and letters on the sides of boxes become "clues" and you can judge a food by its label. Here's what you need to know to quickly scan the label for the most important information—and comprehend what you read.

List of Ingredients

By law, all ingredients must be listed on the label. The ingredient present in the largest amount, by weight, must be listed first, followed in descending order of weight by the other ingredients. Why does this matter? So you can be sure that first ingredients listed are healthful ones.

Specific names of additives, colors, flavors, preservatives and seasonings also must be included. It has been proposed that all sugars (honey, sugar, corn syrup solids, molasses, etc.) be collectively expressed by weight and individually listed by name.

Nutrition Information on Food Labels

Nutrition information is given on a per-serving basis. The label contains the following details:
- the size of a serving (i.e., one cup, two ounces, one tablespoon)
- the number of servings in the container
- the number of calories per serving
- fat calories per serving
- the amounts (in grams) of protein, carbohydrate and fat per serving

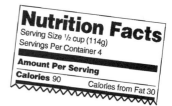

> ➢ Note the size portion you eat. How close does it compare to the box's "serving size"?

Labels must also add the amounts of **cholesterol** (mg), **fiber** (g), **saturated fat** (g), **sodium** (mg), **sugar** or simple carbohydrate (g) and **total carbohydrates** (g); and compare these values to the **Daily Values Recommended**, listed by *percentage* and *grams*. Only two vitamins (A and C) and two minerals (calcium and iron) are required listings, and are compared as *percentages* of the **Daily Value** recommended.

How to Interpret Nutrition Information

Daily Values are the amounts of nutrients that an adult should eat every day to stay healthy. Labels compare the product's nutrients with the **Daily Values Recommended** (average values), based on eating 2,000 or 2,500 calories daily. Daily Values consist of Recommended Daily Intakes (RDI's) for vitamins and minerals, and **Daily Reference Values** (DRV's) for fat, saturated fat, cholesterol, carbohydrates, fiber and sodium. DRV's are 65 grams of fat and 20 grams of saturated fat, based on eating 2,000 calories a day; 80 fat grams and 25 saturated fat grams for those eating 2,500 calories/day. DRV's for people consuming 1,500 calories a day would be 50 grams fat and 15 grams saturated fat. You must adjust these recommended values to your own calorie intake.

New Definitions

All terms on labels ("light," "low-fat," etc.) are defined and consistently used. For example, **"light"** can be used only if the product serving contains 1/3 less calories and 1/2 the fat of the original product equivalent. **"Low-fat"** means the product contains less than 3 grams of fat per serving.

Trim Fat to Trim Calories!

When you start reading food labels, you learn:

1)   As you trim the fat, you trim the calories and . . .
2)   When you trim the calories, you trim your body fat!

One of the easiest, smartest ways to trim calories and fat is to replace a higher-calorie food with a lower-calorie one. Look below at your calorie savings when you make a switch. Small changes…Big results! Even 150 calories less a day adds up to a 15-pound weight loss in a year!

SIMPLE SUBSTITUTES

Instead of:	Cal	Fat(g)	Try This:	Cal	Fat(g)	Save: Cal	Fat(g)
Whole milk, 8 oz.	160	8	Fat-free milk, 8 oz.	90	0	70	8
Sour cream, 4 oz.	240	24	Nonfat yogurt, 4 oz.	60	0	180	24
Rich ice cream, 1 c.	300	20	Nonfat ice milk, 1 c.	200	0	100	20
Ham, 2 oz.	100	5	Turkey breast, 2 oz.	70	2	30	3
Croissant, 1 large	300	15	English muffin	140	1	160	14
Party crackers, 4	80	4	Rye wafers, 2 triple	40	0	40	4
Butter or margarine, 1 Tbsp.	100	12	Parmesan cheese, 1 Tbsp.	25	2	75	10
Chocolate bar, 1 1/2 oz.	240	15	Low fat granola bar, 1	100	2	140	13
Chocolate chip cookie, 1	50	2	Gingersnap, 1	15	0	35	2
Yellow cake w/ icing, 1/12 cake	450	18	Angel food cake, 1/12 cake	120	0	330	18
Danish pastry	275	15	Bran muffin, medium	160	5	115	10
Apple pie, 1/6 of 9-in. pie	400	18	Baked apple w/ 1 Tbsp. nuts, raisins	155	4	245	14
Peanuts, 1 c.	840	72	Popcorn, 1 c. dry	30	0	810	72
Potato chips, 1 oz. (15 chips)	150	10	Pretzels, 8 twists (med.)	100	1	50	9
Peanut butter, 2 Tbsp.	190	16	Low-fat ricotta cheese, 1 Tbsp.	40	3	150	13

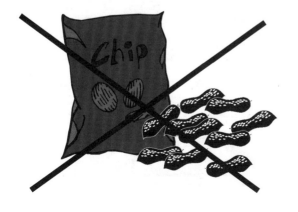

© 2009, *The Cooper Clinic Solution to the Diet Revolution* by Georgia G. Kostas, M.P.H., R.D., L.D., Dallas, Texas

Instead of:	Cal	Fat(g)	Try This:	Cal	Fat(g)
Breakfast					
orange juice, 6 oz.	90	0	orange juice, 6 oz.	90	0
1 egg, fried	110	10	1 egg, poached	80	6
toast, 1 slice	75	0	toast, 1 slice	75	0
butter, 1 pat	35	4	ricotta cheese, 1 Tbsp.	20	1.5
jam, 1 Tbsp.	55	0	jam, 1 Tbsp.	55	0
coffee	0	0	coffee	0	0
half 'n half, 1 Tbsp.	20	2	milk, fat-free, 1 Tbsp.	5	0
TOTAL	385	16	TOTAL	325	7+
Lunch					
Chef salad			Chef salad		
lettuce, 1 c.	10	0	lettuce, 1 c.	10	0
avocado, 1/6	70	7	asparagus, 2 1/2-in. spears	10	0
tomato, 1/2 medium	20	0	tomato, 1/2 medium	20	0
roast beef, 2 oz.	130	6	chicken, 2 oz.	100	5
cheddar cheese, 2 oz.	230	20	cottage cheese, 2 oz. (1/2 c.)	120	5
black olives, 3	30	3			
dressing, 2 Tbsp.	160	18	dressing, 1 Tbsp.	80	9
crackers, 6 rounds	110	6	rye wafers, 2 triple	40	0
chocolate chip cookies, 2	100	4	vanilla wafers, 3	50	2
iced tea with lemon	0	0	iced tea with lemon	0	0
TOTAL	860	64	TOTAL	430	21
Dinner					
Prime Rib, 4 oz.	400	36	flank steak, 4 oz.	220	8
green beans			green beans, 1/2 c.	25	0
with cheese sauce, 2 Tbsp.	60	5	baked potato	200	0
cornbread, 2 1/2" x 2 1/2" square	190	5	margarine, 1 pat	35	4
butter, 1 pat	35	4	(or 1 Tbsp. sour cream)		
cake with icing, 1/12th cake	350	15	pound cake, 1/2-in. slice	110	9
beer, 12 oz.	150	0	wine spritzer, 4 oz.	100	0
TOTAL	1,185	65		690	21
DAILY TOTALS	**2,430**	**145**	**DAILY TOTALS**	**1,445**	**49+**

CALORIES SAVED = 985   FAT GRAMS SAVED = 95+

Instead of:

Try This:

	Cal	Fat(g)		Cal	Fat(g)
Breakfast					
orange juice, 6 oz.	90	0	cantaloupe, 1/4 medium	60	0
cereal, dry, 1 c.	150	0	cereal, cooked, 1 c.	140	0
sugar, 1 Tbsp.	50	0	raisins, 1 Tbsp.	20	0
banana, 1/2 medium	50	0	maple extract, 1/4 tsp.	0	0
milk, whole, 4 oz.	75	5	milk, fat-free, 4 oz.	45	0
coffee	0	0	coffee	0	0
half 'n half, 1 Tbsp.	20	2	milk, fat-free, 1 Tbsp.	5	0
TOTAL	435	7	TOTAL	270	0
Lunch					
Sandwich			Sandwich		
bologna, 2 oz.	200	17	chicken, 2 oz.	100	6
Swiss cheese, 1 oz	100	10	low-calorie cheese, 1 oz.	50	3
bread, 2 slices	150	0	bread, 2 slices	150	0
mayonnaise, 2 tsp.	65	8	mayonnaise, 2 tsp.	65	8
mustard, 2 tsp.	0	0	mustard, 2 tsp.	0	0
lettuce, 1 leaf	0	0	lettuce, 1 leaf	0	0
coleslaw, 1/2 c.	120	10	tomato, 1/2 medium	25	0
			w/wine vinegar, basil	0	0
cola, 12 oz.	150	0	apple juice, 4 oz.	80	0
			with soda water, 6 oz.	0	0
TOTAL	775	46	TOTAL	470	17
Dinner					
Polish pork sausage, 1 link (3 oz.)	275	24	pork tenderloin (lean),	140	4
			applesauce, 2 Tbsp.	15	0
acorn squash, 1 c.	140	0	boiled, roasted potato (small)	100	0
brown sugar, 1 Tbsp.	50	0	with wine-herb baste	0	0
creamed peas and onions, 2/3 c.	100	5	braised peas, onions, mushrooms, 1/2 c.	70	0
			margarine, 1 pat	35	4
apple pie, 1/6 of 9-in. pie	400	18	baked apple with cinnamon	80	0
TOTAL	965	47	TOTAL	440	8
DAILY TOTALS	**2,185**	**99**	**DAILY TOTALS**	**1,180**	**25**

CALORIES SAVED = 1005   FAT GRAMS SAVED = 74

Calorie & Fat Comparisons

A Closer Look at "Add-ons"

Adding fat adds calories…note the following examples. Bottom line:
(1) Keep foods simple, minimizing sauces and fats.
(2) Keep an eye on portions, choosing smaller portions of richer foods and larger portions of lighter foods.

MEAT AND SUBSTITUTES

Chicken, 3 oz.	Cal	Fat (g)
baked, broiled (boneless, skinless)	120	3
+ 2 Tbsp. barbecue sauce	145	3
fried	220	11
Beef Steak, 3 oz.		
sirloin, flank, filet, tenderloin	180	8
T-bone, porterhouse, round steak	180	8
hamburger, medium fat	250	18
prime rib	250	17
brisket	350	27
Fish, 3 oz.		
baked or broiled (cod, trout, snapper, etc.)	90	1
+ 1 Tbsp. butter (or tartar sauce)	190	11
fried (breaded)	260	12

VEGETABLES

Potato (1 small, 1/2 medium, or 1/2 c.)		
baked or broiled	100	0
+ 1 Tbsp. butter (100 cal.), and	200	10
+ 1 Tbsp. sour cream (30 cal.), and	230	13
+ 1 Tbsp. grated cheese (30 cal.)	260	16
hash browns (1/2 c.)	170	9
French fries (20), small order	220	13
potato chips (25)	250	17
Okra, 1/2 c.		
boiled	20	0
fried	200	12
Onions, 1		
boiled	50	0
fried rings, 10	400	26

MIXED DISHES

taco, 1 medium	200-300	13
pizza, 1/8 of 12-in. pizza	200-250	5-10
chili, 1 c.	300-400	22
soups, 1 c.		
broth, bouillon	40	1
broth-based (i.e., chicken noodle)	70	2
creamed	180	7
coleslaw with mayonnaise, 1/2 c.	120	7
pasta salad, 1/2 c.	130	6
tuna salad, 1/2 c.	150	12
potato or macaroni salad, 1/2 c.	175	10
beef stew, 1 c.	220	10
macaroni & cheese, 3/4 c.	325	17
lasagna , 1 c.	700	36
chicken a la king, 1 c.	300	20

SANDWICHES

Meat Only*	Cal	Fat (g)
chicken or turkey (3 oz. baked or smoked)	150	3
bacon (1 oz. or 3 strips)	150	12
hot dog, 1	150	13
chopped ham, 3 oz.	150	8
hamburger patty, 3 oz.	250	18
bologna, 3 oz.	270	24
tuna, 1/2 c.		
in water	100	2
in oil	225	9

*Made with 2 slices bread + 2 Tbsp. mayonnaise adds 340 calories and 22 grams fat. Made with 2 slices bread + no mayonnaise adds 140 calories and no fat.

SNACKS

peanutbutter, 1 Tbsp.	95	8
candy, chocolate, 1 oz.	150	10
nuts, seeds, 1 oz. or 2 Tbsp.	180	10
chips, 1 oz. or 1 small bag	150	10
yogurt, 8 oz.		
plain, nonfat	100	0
plain, low-fat	160	5
fruit flavored	250-300	0
fruit flavored, nonfat, sugar-free	100	0
movie popcorn, popped in oil (no butter)		
"Small," 5 c.	300-400	20-30
"Large," 20 c.	1150	77
microwave popcorn, fat-free, 7 c.	250	10

SWEETS, DESSERTS

cookies		
ginger snaps, 2; vanilla wafers, 4	60	2
chocolate chip, 2 small	100	6
Oreos, 2	100	6
homemade (chocolate chip, oatmeal), 1	100	3
shortbread cookies, 3	100	6
Snackwell's creme-filled, 2	110	3
oatmeal raisin, 1	100	3
chocolate, 1	100	3
glazed donut, 1	180	11
coffee cake, 2.5 oz.	230	7
sweet roll, tart, pastry, 1	270	15
cheesecake, 1 large slice (5 oz.)	430	30
cake with icing (2-layer, 2 1/2 in. wedge)	350-500	15-20
pie (1/8 pie, all types)	300-400	15-20

© 2009, *The Cooper Clinic Solution to the Diet Revolution* by Georgia G. Kostas, M.P.H., R.D., L.D., Dallas, Texas

FROZEN DESSERTS

	Cal	Fat(g)
ice cream, 1/2 c.		
regular	130	7
rich (i.e., Baskin Robbins)	165	9
soft-serve	165	10
very rich (Haagen Daas)	300	20
ice milk, fruit ice, sorbet	100	0
frozen yogurt	110	2
sherbet	130	2
ice cream bar or sandwich (average)	160	11
milkshake, 8 oz.	350	10
hot fudge sundae	650	30

LOWER-CALORIE SNACKS and DESSERTS

jello (1/2 c.) or low-fat pudding (1/2 c.)	70	0
Sugar-free jello, 1/2 c.	10	0
vegetable, 1	25	0
chocolate low-cal shake or hot cocoa, 8 oz.	50	0
Fudgesicle	70	0
popsicle, twin pop	70	0
frozen fruit bar	70	0
popcorn (3 c.), popped w/o fat or microwave "lite"	80	1
pretzels (38 small stick or 6 twist)	80	1
fruit, large	120	0
shredded wheat, 1/2 c.	90	0
angel food cake, sponge cake (1/12 cake)	110	0
milkshake (8 oz. fat-free milk + 1/2 c.		
unsweetened fruit)	120	0

CEREALS (1/2 CUP)

puffed wheat	35	0
corn flakes	50	0
shredded wheat, bran flakes	90	0
Grapenuts	210	0
granola	250-300	12
low-fat or nonfat	175-210	3
granola bar	235	8
low-fat	80-110	2

"ADD-ONS"

Sauces (1 Tbsp.)

Au Jus, Tabasco, hot sauce, steak sauce, picante, salsa	0	0
barbecue, catsup, mustard, teriyaki, soy, Worcestershire, sweet and sour	10-15	0
tartar	95	9
fat-free tartar	16	0

Sauces (1/4 c.)

tomato	25	0
light tomato spaghetti sauce	25-45	0-2
spaghetti (meat-free)	35-50	1
barbecue, catsup	50	1
brown gravy (mix)	30	2
brown gravy mix (nonfat)	25	0
brown gravy (homemade)	165	14
cheese	125	10
hollandaise	260	28

Dips (1/4 c.)

	Cal	Fat(g)
fat-free commercial dips	60	0
bean dip	80	4
onion dip	100	8
guacamole	115	10
cheese dip	125	10

Dressings (1 Tbsp.)

vinegar, lemon, hot sauce, picante	0	0
fat-free dressings	5-25	0
light dressings, all types	25-50	2-4
ranch, French	55	6
blue cheese, Roquefort, Italian, Russian, Caesar, oil & vinegar, etc.	70-80	8-9
light mayonnaise	50	5
mayonnaise	100	10

Condiments (1 Tbsp.)

low-calorie jelly	8-25	0
lite syrup, apple butter	30	0
sugar, honey, syrup	50	0
jelly, jam, marmalade, spreadable fruit	55	0
reduced-fat margarine	50	5
whipped butter or margarine	85	8
butter or margarine	100	10
fat-free milk	5	0
nondairy creamer, powder	30	2
nondairy creamer, liquid	20	1
half and half	20	2
fat-free, plain yogurt	6	0
sour cream	30	3
nonfat sour cream	15	0

BEVERAGES (8 OUNCES)

water, mineral water, tea, coffee, club soda, diet drinks	0	0
ginger ale	80	0
soft drinks, punch	100	0
tomato, V-8 juice	50	0
orange, grapefruit juice	100	0
grape, prune juice	200	0
fat-free milk (1/2% fat)	80	1
low-fat milk (2% fat)	120	5
whole milk (4% fat)	150	8
Carnation Instant Breakfast (with fat-free milk)	220	1
Sugar-free Carnation Instant Breakfast	160	1

Alcohol

Beer, 12 oz.		
lite	100	0
regular	150	0
wine, champagne, 4 oz.	100	0
gin, rum, vodka, 1 1/2 oz.	100	0
martini, daiquiri, 4 oz.	200	0
margarita	350-450	0
nonalcoholic beer, 12 oz.	70	0
nonalcoholic wine, 8 oz.	70	0

➢ *Fat-free does not mean calorie free!*

Quick Fat Gram Counter

Do you recognize some of your favorites? Mark the foods you eat often; then opt for lower-fat versions. You may want to highlight your best options in each grouping and keep close by for quick reference.

MEAT, FISH, POULTRY, EGGS

Beef, broiled, 3 oz. (visible fat removed)	Fat (g)	Cal.
eye of round, round steak or top round	8	180
London broil (flank steak)	8	180
porterhouse steak	8	180
Prime rib	17	250
rib eye (Delmonico) steak	10	190
T-bone steak	8	180
sirloin steak or top loin	8	180
tenderloin (filet)	8	180

Luncheon meats (1 slice)		
Louis Rich 96% fat-free Turkey Pastrami	0	25
Louis Rich Oven Roasted Turkey Breast	0	30
Oscar Mayer Turkey or Bologna	4	50
Oscar Mayer Hard Salami	3	35
Oscar Mayer 95% fat-free Smoked Cooked Ham	1	25

Seafood, 3 oz., cooked		
anchovies, canned in oil, drained, 5	2	40
Atlantic cod or Haddock	1	90
Salmon, fresh	7	150
salmon, pink, canned with bone	8	155
smoked salmon (lox)	4	100
swordfish	4	130
trout	4	125
tuna, canned in oil, drained, 1/3 c.	7	140
canned in water, drained, 1/3 c.	1	90
packaged in water, drained, 1/3 c.	1	90
shrimp, boiled, 15 medium or 12 large	1	90
breaded, fried, 11 large	10	210

Poultry, 3 oz., cooked		
chicken breast with skin, baked	8	195
no skin, baked	3	145
chicken drumstick with skin, batter fried	11	195
no skin, baked	2	75
chicken wing, no skin, baked	2	45
turkey, light meat with skin, baked	7	170
no skin, baked	3	135
turkey, dark meat with skin, baked	10	190
no skin, baked	6	160

Eggs		
1 large	5	75
Fleischmann's Egg Beaters, 1/4 c.	0	25
Healthy Choice Egg Substitute, 1/4 c.	3	60

MILK & DAIRY PRODUCTS

Milk, 1 c.	Fat (g)	Cal.
whole	8	150
2% fat	5	120
1% fat	3	100
fat-free	0	90

Cream, 1 Tbsp.		
half and half	2	20
heavy whipping cream	6	50
sour cream	3	25

Cheese		
American, cheddar or Swiss, 1 oz.	9	110
Weight Watchers American, cheddar or Swiss 2% milk pasteurized process cheese, 1 oz., 2 slices	4	100
cottage cheese, creamed, 1 c.	9	200
cottage cheese, 1% fat, 1 c.	2	160
cottage cheese, fat-free, 1 c.	0	140
cream cheese, 1 oz.	10	100
mozzarella, part fat-free, 1 oz.	5	70
Parmesan, grated, 1 Tbsp.	2	25
ricotta, 1/2 c.	16	200
ricotta, part fat-free, 1/2 c.	10	170
ricotta, low-fat 1/2 c.	6	140
ricotta, fat-free, 1/2 c.	0	80

Yogurt		
plain, 8 oz.	7	150
plain or flavored nonfat, sugar-free, 8 oz.	0	100
flavored (coffee, lemon, vanilla), 8 oz.	3	200-250
flavored, nonfat, sugar-free, 8 oz.	0	100

BREADS, GRAINS, ETC.

Breads		
bagel, 1 small	1	160
English muffin, 1	1	140
wholewheat bread, 1 slice	1	70

Cereals		
Cheerios, 1 1/4 c.	2	110
Corn Flakes, 1 c.	0	100
Raisin Bran, 3/4 c.	1	120
Shredded Wheat, 1 biscuit or 1/2 c.	0	80
oatmeal, 2/3 c. cooked	2	100
granola, 1/4 c.	5	130
Puffed Rice, 1 c.	0	50

Crackers		
Cheez-It Snack Crackers, 12	4	70
Graham crackers, 2 squares	1	60
Ritz crackers, 4	4	70
Harvest Crisps, 6	2	60
Reduced-fat Triscuits, 7	3	120

Other	Fat (g)	Cal.
pasta, 1 c. cooked	1	200
white rice, 1 c. cooked	0	225
pancakes, 4-in. plain	2	60
waffles, 7-in. plain	8	200
French toast, 1 slice	7	150
Bran muffin, large	11	350
Sara Lee Golden Corn Muffin	13	250

FRUITS & VEGETABLES

	Fat (g)	Cal.
apple, 1 medium	1	80
banana, 1 medium	1	105
fruit cocktail, canned in heavy syrup, 1/2 c.	0	90
orange, 1 medium	0	65
raisins, 1/3 c.	0	150
avocado, 1/2 medium	15	155
broccoli, 1/2 c. cooked	0	25
carrot, raw, 1 medium	0	30
corn, canned, 1/2 c.	1	65
green beans, 1/2 c. cooked	0	20
peas, 1/2 c. cooked	0	70

BEANS, NUTS & SEEDS

	Fat (g)	Cal.
kidney beans, 1/2 c. boiled	0	115
lentils, 1/2 c. boiled	0	115
cashews, dry roasted, 1/4 c.	16	200
peanuts, 1/4 c.	18	210
coconut, flaked, 1/4 c.	6	90
pistachios, dry roasted, 1/4 c.	17	195
sesame seeds, 1/4 c.	21	220
walnuts, 1/4 c.	18	190

SPREADS, OILS, DRESSINGS

	Fat (g)	Cal.
butter, 1 tsp.	4	35
whipped butter, 1 tsp.	3	30
margarine, stick & tub, 1 tsp.	4	35
diet margarine, tub, 1 tsp.	2	17
vegetable oil (corn, olive, etc.), 1 Tbsp.	14	120
vegetable oil spray, pump or aerosol	1	6
peanutbutter, 1 Tbsp.	8	95

Salad Dressings

	Fat (g)	Cal.
blue cheese or Russian, 1 Tbsp.	8	75
French, 1 Tbsp.	6	70
Italian, 1 Tbsp.	7	70
thousand island, 1 Tbsp.	6	60
light dressings, 1 Tbsp.	4-5	25-60

SOUPS

	Fat (g)	Cal.
chicken noodle, 1 c., canned	2	70
cream of mushroom, 1 c., canned	7	130
Lipton Noodle, 1 c.	2	70
Progresso Green Split Pea, 1 c.	3	150
Progresso Beef Minestrone, 1 c.	3	135
Ramen Pride Oriental Noodles & Pork Flavor, 10 oz.	8	200

SWEETS

	Fat (g)	Cal.
Cadbury's Milk Chocolate	8	150
Hershey Chocolate Kisses, 5	8	125
Milky Way Bar	11	280
Milky Way II Bar	8	190
Snicker's Bar, 2.16 oz.	14	290
Three Musketeers Bar, 2.13 oz.	9	260
angel food cake, 1/12" cake	0	125
brownie with nuts (3 x 2 x 7/8")	12	200
cheesecake, 1 large slice (5 oz.)	30	430
Hostess Ding Dong, 1	9	170
Hostess Twinkie, 1	5	160
pound cake, 1/2" slice	6	150
Almost Home Chocolate Chip Cookie	25	130
Fig Newton, 1	1	50
Gingersnaps, 4	3	120
apple pie, 1/8 pie	12	280
banana cream pie, 1/8	12	235
pumpkin pie, 1/8	13	240
chocolate pudding, 1 c.	12	385
Chocolate cake with icing	22	450
Nature Valley Granola Bar	5	120
Sara Lee Cheese Danish	8	130

FROZEN DESSERTS

Ice cream

	Fat (g)	Cal.
Breyers, 1/2 c.	8	160
Haagen Dazs, 1/2 c.	18	300
Sealtest, 1/2 c.	6	140

Other

	Fat (g)	Cal.
Fruit 'N Yogurt Bar	0	70
Fruit sorbet, 1/2 c.	0	100
Eskimo Pie, 3 oz. bar	12	180
Chocolate Pudding Pop	2	80
Ice Milk, 1/2 c.	3	120
sherbet, 1/2 c.	3	135
popsicle or fudgesicle	0	70
tofutti, 1/2 c.	12	210
fat-free frozen yogurt, 3 fl. oz.	0	80

Toppings

	Fat (g)	Cal.
chocolate syrup, 2 Tbsp.	1	90
fudge topping, 2 Tbsp.	5	125
whipped cream, 2 Tbsp.	1	16

DRY SNACK FOODS

	Fat (g)	Cal.
potato chips, 1 oz. (15 chips)	10	150
light Potato Chips, 1 oz. (15 chips)	8	150
Guiltless Gourmet Chips, 1 oz.	0	130
Orville Redenbacher's Natural Microwave Popping Corn, 4 c. popped	7	110
popcorn, air-popped, 1 c.	0	15
pretzels, 1 oz. (50)	1	111

᾽nack Attack" Tips

You're hungry. No time to compare labels! Pre-think snacks and healthy habits as listed below. The truth is, eating a healthful snack may even keep you from overeating at mealtime! Planned snacks may also increase your energy level throughout the day and keep you alert. With energy "up" and appetite "down," you can make the wisest food choices.

 Keep healthy choices on hand. Take portable snacks with you. Carry foods such as fruit, raisins, yogurt, granola bars, rice cakes and string cheese in your gym bag or briefcase. Place carrots, grapes, cherries, celery or cucumber sticks, red bell peppers, cut melon, cereal, pretzels and animal crackers in baggies.

 Choose warm beverages, sipped slowly. They fill an "empty feeling" quickly…and stay with you longer than you may think. Try flavored decaffeinated teas and coffees, warm water with lemon, soups, fat-free hot cocoa.

 Munch on "filling" foods high in water and/or fiber content; they are lowest in calories (i.e., popcorn, fruit, raw vegetables, shredded wheat, baked potato).

 Crunch and chew. Popcorn, pretzels, Cheerios, shredded wheat, Chex cereals, low-fat Cracker Jacks, low-fat granola bars, Rice Krispie bars, biscotti and rice cakes will leave you feeling satisfied.

 Make a snack attractive. Serve fruit or frozen yogurt in a pretty sherbet dish. Use a beautiful glass for your drinks.

 Eat slowly. Choose snacks that are slow to eat, and eat each piece one by one (popcorn, shredded wheat, Cheerios, Chex mix, apples, carrots, cucumber, bell pepper, etc.).

 Pause before snacking. Are you really hungry? Sometimes we eat because we're bored. Drink a tall glass of water before a snack. You'll eat less!

 Go for color. Stock your fridge with red grapes, red cherry tomatoes, red strawberries, cantaloupe, watermelon and colorful vegetables. They're filled with vitamins.

 Drink 2 quarts (64 oz.) of water a day. Add lemon or lime twists for pizzazz.

 Make healthful eating convenient and eye-appealing by planning ahead.

 Prepare snacks ahead of time as soon as you get home from shopping. Don't wait until you are hungry.

➢ *See "Snack Ideas" on p. 121 - 123.*

© 2009, *The Cooper Clinic Solution to the Diet Revolution* by Georgia G. Kostas, M.P.H., R.D., L.D., Dallas, Texas

Great Snack Ideas

FREEBIES (No Calories)

Refreshing water
    bottled or carbonated waters
    flavored, sugar-free waters
    can add sugar-free powdered flavors to water (Crystal Light
        "on the go", Lipton teas, Gatorade's Propel Fit, etc.)
Sugar-free sodas and lemonade
Crystal Light beverages and teas
Coffees, flavored, decaffeinated
Sugar-free instant teas, flavored

Teas, flavored
    herbal, decaffeinated, green tea, black tea
Sugar-free gelatin
Ocean Spray diet drinks (15 calories or less)
Fresh cranberries
Sour or dill pickles
Cucumbers, radishes, celery
Lettuce
Raw vegetables

60 CALORIES OR FEWER (No Fat)*

1 small fruit (apple, orange, etc.)	60	1/2 c. orange juice	60
1 c. cooked nonstarchy vegetables	50	1/2 c. tomato, V-8 juice	35
2 c. raw nonstarchy vegetables,		1 carrot or 1 small tomato	25
(broccoli, cauliflower, carrots)	50	1 small green salad with 1 Tbsp.	
1/2 banana (may freeze)	60	fat-free or low fat dressing	25
1/4 cantaloupe, 1/2 grapefruit	60	1 slice low-calorie bread	35
1 c. strawberries, 10 cherries, 1 c. melon	60	1 bread stick (3 1/2")	40
1/2 c. sugar-free canned or frozen fruit	50	4 pieces melba toast	40
1 small baked apple, with cinnamon	60	1 c. puffed wheat	40
1/2 c. applesauce, without sugar	50	1 rice cake or 6 mini-cakes	50
1 package low-cal dried fruit snack		1 frozed fruit juice bar	40
(apple, cinnamon, strawberry)	40	12 teddy grahams	60
1 slice, 3/4 oz., fat-free cheese	40	6 mini fat-free cookies	60
1/2 oz. (2 Tbsp.) regular cheese*	50	1 c. onion soup or egg drop soup	35
1 oz. (1 wedge) low-fat gruyere cheese*	50	1 pouch Nature Valley Fruit Crisps	50
1 oz. part-fat-free ricotta cheese*	40	Jell-O Pudding, sugar-free	50
1 oz. fat-free mozzarella (string) cheese	50	8 oz. Almond Breeze, unsweetened	60
1 mini-bar Cabot reduced-fat cheese*	50	8 oz. Progresso Light Soup	60

100 CALORIES OR FEWER (No Fat)

1 c. fat-free milk	90	1 ear corn or 1 small new potato	100
1/2 c. nonfat cottage cheese	80	1 1/2 oz. box raisins	100
(add seasonings and use as spread)		1/2 c. flavored gelatin or low-cal pudding	70
1 c. fat-free plain or unsweetened yogurt	100	1 snack-pack pudding	100
1 oz. mozzarella cheese*	75	1 small slice angel food cake (1/12 cake)	110
3 c. unbuttered popcorn or microwave light	75	1 c. homemade or canned soup	70-90
1 bread/toast or mini-bagel	75	1 packet low-cal hot cocoa mix	50-70
2 c. puffed wheat or rice	80	1 packet low-cal milkshake mix	
1 shredded wheat biscuit (or 2/3 c.)	90	(vanilla, strawberry, chocolate)	70
1 c. Cheerios	90	1 popsicle, twin pop, frozen fruit bar	70
1 c. oatsquares	90	1 Fudgsicle or fat-free frozen chocolate bar	70-100
3 graham crackers (2 in. square each)	80	1/2 c. fat-free ice milk or fruit ice	100
38 pretzel sticks (3 1/8" long)	80	1/2 c. fat-free frozen yogurt	100
1 cereal bar or low-fat granola bar (see label)*	100	1 latte' (made with 1 c. fat-free milk)	100
1 biscotti	100	1 light mocha Frappucino (Starbucks)	100
15 almonds or 4 walnut halves*	100	100-calorie snack packs (Oreos, Teddy Grahams, etc)*	100

*Snacks above are virtually fat-free; others marked * contain 2-5 grams fat on average*

© 2009, *The Cooper Clinic Solution to the Diet Revolution* by Georgia G. Kostas, M.P.H., R.D., L.D., Dallas, Texas

150 CALORIES OR LESS MINI-MEALS OR SNACKS

	Calories	Fat
grilled cheese toast made with 1 slice low-fat cheese and 1 bread slice	150	5
1/4 c. 1% cottage cheese and 1 banana	150	2
1 string cheese and 1 small apple	140	1
1 wedge Laughing Cow cheese or Cabot cheese mini-bar and 1 small pear	150	0
1/2 Tombstone Light Pizza, 8"	120	4
1/2 turkey sandwich (no mayo)	150	2
1 c. Healthy Choice Vegetable soup	120	1
1 c. 1% chocolate milk	150	1
3 Tbsp. almonds, dry roasted, unsalted	150	10
1/4 c. dry-roasted Genisoy nuts	130	4
Kashi Trail Mix Bar (w/4 g fiber)	140	5
1 c. fat-free yogurt	100	0
1 fat-free string cheese and 1 c. cereal (ie. Cheerios, Oat Squares, Shredded Wheat)	150	0
Smoothie: 1 c. fat-free milk and 1/2 frozen banana	150	0
Breakfast "grab-n-go" foods		
Instant oatmeal and grit packets, all flavors (just add hot water)	100 - 150	0 - 3
Bagel (Lender's size)	150	0

Healthy Snacks by Category

Fruit / Vegetables
Fresh fruit
Raisins
Raw vegetables

Crunchy Grains
Popcorn – microwaved (Smart Pop)
Cereals (Cheerios, Shredded Wheat, Oat Squares, etc.)
Pretzels
Soy nuts (1/4 c.)
Fat-free granola bars
Fat-free cereal bars
Fat-free Rice Krispie bars
Biscotti
Rice cakes
Graham crackers or Teddy Grahams
Fat-free or low-fat crackers (whole-wheat saltines, saltines, Harvest Crisps, Rye-Krisps, Snackwell's crackers, etc.)
Animal Crackers
Bread Sticks
Fat-free chips with salsa

Breads / Starches
Small bagels
English muffins
Bread (crunchy varieties)
Homemade bran muffins or fat-free frozen (Healthy Choice, Health Valley, Sara Lee)
Mini pizzas
Ear of corn
Small baked potato

Dairy
Fat-free milk or fat-free chocolate milk
Fat-free hot cocoa
Fat-free or low-fat yogurt
Fat-free or low-fat cheese slice on bread; or grilled cheese toast
Mozzarella cheese stick and apple
Low-fat cottage cheese with fruit
Smoothie (frozen fruit and milk)
Frozen fat-free yogurt
Chocolate fat-free pudding snacks
Latte (made with fat-free milk)

Frozen Snacks
Frozen fruit bars
Popsicles; Fudgesicles
Fat-free frozen desserts
Sorbet; fruit ice

Cookies
Vanilla wafers, ginger snaps, Fig Newtons, chocolate snaps
Fat-free cookies (Snackwell's, Health Valley)

Bakery Goods
Angel food cake
Banana bread

Mini-Meals
Sandwich (whole or half)
Soft tacos
Vegetable soup
Bean soup

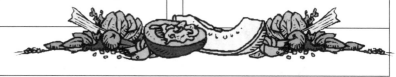

Craving The Crazy "C's"

Think about it for a second. What foods are the most tempting for you? If you're like most people, foods like cookies, chocolate…and other irresistible C's probably top your list. Put a check beside each item below that you can't pass by without at least sampling: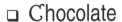

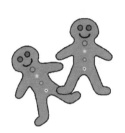

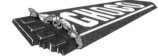

- ❑ Chocolate
- ❑ Chips
- ❑ Cookies
- ❑ Cheese
- ❑ Candy
- ❑ Crackers
- ❑ PopCorn
- ❑ Ice Cream
- ❑ Coffee drinks
- ❑ Creamy desserts

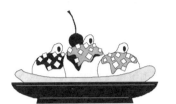

How to "Cure the Cravings"

- ❑ **Substitute other crunchy foods** such as apples, carrots, pretzels, ear of corn, dry cereals (Chex cereals, wheat or oat squares, Cheerios, etc.).

- ❑ **Enjoy lower-calorie chocolate and ice cream options.** (Single servings only!)

- ❑ **Select lower-fat cheeses,** especially presliced portions or other single servings (wedges, rounds, etc.).

- ❑ **Choose hard candy in place of chocolate candy** (Lifesavers, mints, Altoids, jelly beans). These are 3 to 10 calories each.

- ❑ **Try chocolate chews containing calcium** (20 calories each).

- ❑ **Enjoy lower-fat crackers** (Rye-Krisps, saltines, Air Crisps, Harvest Crisps).

- ❑ **Try fat-free dairy products** – hot cocoa, cold milk, smoothies, shakes, 100-calorie pudding snacks.

- ❑ **Use substitutions in your café latte** – 1/2 decaf coffee and 1/2 steamed fat-free milk.

- ❑ **Buy unbuttered or "light" popcorn** such as Orville Redenbacher's Smart Pop. Yes!

- ❑ **Wait 10 minutes**: An impulse may pass.

Cheese, Please

Cheese

Of course, you can eat cheese! It is a nutritious food, containing calcium, vitamin A, protein, many B vitamins and other key nutrients. However, to keep fat in check, check out cheeses by label, and limit the amount you eat. Keep in mind the following suggestions:

√ Choose **fat-free, low-fat, light, medium-fat** (reduced-fat or 2% milk) or **cholesterol-free** cheeses. Choose cheese with no more than 4-7 grams of fat per ounce.

√ Limit **high-fat** cheeses to smaller portions (1/2 - 3/4 oz.), or eat them only occasionally. Popular high-fat cheeses contain 1 tablespoon of butterfat (10 g fat) per 1 ounce cheese, which is typically equal to one slice.

√ Eight slices of traditional cheese contain 8 tablespoons of butterfat...equal to one stick of butter!

√ Soy cheese provides a way to consume more soy and less fat!

TIPS

√ Grate cheese to use less (1 oz. = 3 Tbsp.)

√ Choose sharp cheese to use less (feta, blue cheese, gorgonzola, asiago, jalapeno, etc.)

Fat-Free Cheeses (no fat)

Contain a trace amount of fat & 30-50 cal. per oz.

Alpine Lace Free 'n Lean cheeses - slices, cream cheese, cheese spreads
*Borden fat-free cheese and singles
Borden fat-free cottage cheese
Frigo fat-free ricotta cheese
Guiltless Gourmet Nacho Cheese Spread
Healthy Choice cheeses
*Kraft Free Singles—American, Cheddar
Kraft Healthy Favorites
Lifetime fat-free cheeses
Philly-free cream cheese
President's Fat Free Crumbled Feta
Smart Balance Cheddar
*Smart Beat fat-free slices

* individually wrapped

Low-Fat Cheeses (25% fat)

Contain 1-3 gm fat and 40-70 cal. per oz. or per slice

Borden Lifeline slices *(1 slice = = .66 oz. = 35 calories)*
Boursin Light
*Cabot 50% Reduced fat Cheddar mini-bar *(.75 oz. portion)*
Cabot 75% Reduced fat Cheddar
Cottage cheese *(1-2% fat)*
Galaxy Veggie Slices - Swiss, American, Mozzarella, Provolone
Health Valley string cheese
Hoop or Pot cheese
Kraft Light 'N Lively slices *(1 slice = .75 oz. = 35 calories)*
*Kraft Light Singles and 2% singles
*Laughing Cow (fat-free milk) - Gruyere cheese wedges or mini-bonbel rounds *(.75 oz. portions)*
Lifetime low-fat cheeses with sterols
Lite Jarlsberg, reduced fat, sliced
Philadelphia Light Cream Cheese
Ricotta, part fat-free
Sargento Moo Town Snackers Light String Farmers Cheese
Sargento Preferred Light Mozzarella
Smart Beat American Sandwich Slices
Soyakaas (soy) Cheddar, Mozzarella, Monterray Jack
Tofu (from soybeans, cholesterol-free)
Weight Watchers American or Mozzarella slices
   (1 slice = 1 ounce = 50 calories)
Veggie or soy cheese slices

Reduced-Fat Cheeses (50% fat)

Contain 4-7 g fat and 70-90 cal. per oz.

Alpine Lace Reduced fat Swiss, Cheddar,
    Provolone, Monti-Jack Lo
Alpine Lace Muenster (low sodium)
Alouette Light Spreadable
Bonbel
Borden Light American
Brie (low-fat milk)
Cabot 50% Reduced fat Cheddar, Jalapeno,
    Pepper Jack or Cheddar/DHA Omega 3
Camembert (Domestic)
Chavrie Goat's Milk Cheese
Edam
Feta
Fondue cheese
Formagg
Kings Choice Light Havarti
Kraft Cracker Barrel Light

*Kraft 2% Milk Sharp Cheddar, Colby,
    Monterey Jack, Mozzarella, Swiss
Land-O-Lakes Light Swiss
Lucerne 2% Sharp Cheddar
Mozzarella
Neufchatel (to replace cream cheese)
New Holland Lower-Fat Havarti
Parmesan
Pizza cheese (Mozzarella)
Polly-O Twists (Mozzarella & Colby)
Port du Salut (low-fat)
Rondele - Lite Soft Spreadable Cheese
Sargento Light Cheddar, Swiss, Mozzarella
String Cheese (Mozzarella)
Velveeta Light Singles, Kraft *(1 slice = .75 oz. = 35 cal.)*
Velveeta 2% Milk Cheese
Weight Watchers Cheddar

* individually wrapped

High-Fat Cheese (90% fat)

Contain 8-10 g fat per 1 oz. (100-110 cal. per oz.)

American (including slices)
Bleu cheese
Boursin
Brick
Brie
Cheddar - natural or processed
Colby
Co-Jack
Cracker Barrel (Kraft) - all types
Cream cheese
Fontina

Gjetost
Golden Image (Kraft)
Gouda
Gruyere
Havarti
Jarlsberg
Limburger
Longhorn
Manchego
Monterey Jack
Muenster

Parmesan
Port
Port du Salut
Provolone
Queso blanco white cheese
Romano
Roquefort
Scandic (mini-cholesterol)
Stilton
Swiss

Note:

1. *Sodium content of cheeses:*
   1 oz. processed cheese = 400 mg sodium
   1 oz. natural cheese = 200 mg sodium
   1 oz. natural Swiss, gruyere, ricotta = 100 mg sodium
   Special "low-sodium" cheeses are now available: cheddar, colby, gouda, jack, Swiss, cottage, etc.
2. *1 oz. low-fat cheese = 1 oz. "lean meat" based on protein, calories and fat.*
3. *1 oz. low-fat cheese = 3/4 oz. high-fat cheese, based on calories and fat.*

Chocolate & Ice Cream

Richer **Chocolate** Choices	Cal.	Fat (g)
chocolate chips, 1 oz.	150	8
chocolate kisses, 6 pieces	150	10
chocolate fudge, 1 oz.	150	10
brownie, 1 small	150	6
cream-filled chocolate cookies, 2	150	6
chocolate pudding, 1/2 c.	150	6
chocolate icing, 2 Tbsp.	170	7
Milky Way Lite, 1.6 oz.	170	5
chocolate cookies, 2	180	7
chocolate milk, 1 c.	230	10
M & M's, plain, 1.7 oz. package	240	10
chocolate cupcake with icing	280	10
chocolate bar, 2 oz.	300	15
chocolate cake with icing, 1 slice	425	21

Richer **Frozen Dessert** Choices	Cal.	Fat (g)
sugar-free choc-coated ice cream bar	150	11
ice cream sandwich	170	8
chocolate-coated ice cream bar	175	10
sugar-free ice cream sandwich	180	6
soft-serve ice cream, 1/2 c.	180	6
Tofutti, 1/2 c.	220	1-12
Dove choc ice cream bar, 3 fl. oz.	270	17
very rich specialty ice cream, 1/2 c.	300	8
chocolate ice cream, 1/2 c.	165-300	10-20
fudge brownie sundae, 10 oz.	1150	57

TRY Tasty Lighter **Chocolate** < 120 cal < 5 g fat		
Chocolate Andes Crème de Menthe thins, 1	25	1
Tootsie roll, 2 1/2" x 3/8"	30	1
After 8 Mint	30	1
Viactive Chocolate Calcium Chews, 2	40	0
Snackwell's Devil's Food cake cookie	50	0
Snackwell's Cookie Cake, Choc Mint	50	0
Hershey's miniatures or nuggets, 1	50	3
Hershey's Bites, Almond Joy, 4	50	3
Low-calorie hot cocoa, 1 c.	50	0
Tootsie Pop, 1	60	1
Junior Mints, 6 or York Bites, 6	60	1
Chocolate Teddy Graham crackers, 12	60	2
Chocolate fat-free sugar free snack pack pudding (Jell-O, Hunt's, Hershey's), 1/2 c.	60	1
Quaker Chocolate Crunch Rice Cakes, 1	60	1
Pepperidge Farm Bordeaux cookies, 2	70	4
Hershey's Sweet Escape, 1 snack bar	80	3
Swoops (Reese's, Almond Joy, York), 3	90	5
Chocolate "snap" cookies, 4	100	3
Kudos M & M Bar, 1 bar	100	3
Hershey's Tastetations, 15	100	2
Hershey's 100 cal Snacsters	100	4
Weight Watchers brownie	100	3
Hostess 100 cal Choc Cupcake, 3 pack	100	3
Oreo Thin Crisps, 100 cal pack	100	2
Reduced Fat Oreos, 2	100	3
Fudge topping or chocolate syrup, 1 Tbsp.	60	2
Smucker's Light Fudge Topping, 1 Tbsp.	35	0
Cool-whip Chocolate, 2 Tbsp.	25	1

TRY Tasty Lighter **Frozen Dessert** < 120 cal < 3 g fat		
popsicle, sugar-free (2-bar)	15-35	0
juice bars (read labels)	50-100	0
Creamsicle, sugar-free	25	1
Cascacian Farms Frozen Fruit Jce bar	40	0
Fudgsicle, no sugar added	40	1
Weight Watchers Chocolate Mousse bar	60	1
Blue Bunny Health Smart Bar	60	0
popsicle, 2-bar	70	0
Fudgsicle	70	1
Dole or Dreyer's fruit bar, no sugar added	70-80	0
Weight Watchers choc fat-free dessert, 1/2 c.	80	0
Healthy Choice Fudge Bar	80	1
Jell-O chocolate pudding pop, 1	80	2
Blue Bell chocolate fat-free fudge bar	80	0
Blue Bell chocolate fat-free frozen dessert, 1/2 c.	80	0
Skinny Cow's Low Fat Dipper bar	80	3
Breyers Double Churned 98% fate free, 1/2 c.	90	1
Weight Watchers Chocolate Treat Bar	90	0
Eskimo Pie Pudding bar	90	2
Haagen-Daas Raspberry & Vanilla bar	90	0
"Skinny Cow" fat-free fudge bar	90	0
fat-free frozen yogurt, 1/2 c.	100	0
fruit ice, fruit sorbet, or Blue Bell Sherbet, 1/2 c.	100	0
ice milk, 1/2 c.	100	3
diet ice cream, 1/2 c.	100	0
Haagen Daas Frozen Yogurt bar	100	1
Klondike Slim a Bear Ice Cream Sandwich	100	1
Starbuck's Frappuccino bar, 2.5 oz.	120	2
Healthy Choice Tin Roof Sundae	120	2
Hole Fruta! Pure Fruit Sherbet, 1/2 c.	130	1
"Skinny Cow" low-fat ice cream sandwich	130	2

Lower-Calorie Foods by Brand Name

Grocery Shopping? This list of healthful food options will save you a lot of time and calories!

LUNCHEON MEAT (1 oz.)	Cal.	Fat (g)
Boar's Head		
Turkey, ham, beef	30	0
Corned beef/brisket	40	2
Louis Rich		
Chicken or turkey breast (smoked		
or oven-roasted, 96%-98% fat-free)	30	<1
Turkey ham, pastrami or turkey bacon	60	2
Hormel Light 'n Lean		
Lemon-peppered smoked breast of turkey	30	1
Ham, cooked or smoked	25	1
Rotisserie-smoked chicken	10	1
Turkey pastrami, 8 rounds	40	2
Healthy Choice		
Turkey breast, ham	30	1
Chicken breast, 6 slices	50	0
Frank, 97% fat-free	50	1
Extra lean low-fat ground beef, 3 oz.	90	2
Plantation		
Turkey breast, smoked or oven-cooked	30	0
Turkey pastrami	40	2
Hillshire Farm Deli Select		
Smoked chicken & roasted ham	30	0
Smoked ham, 97% fat-free	30	1
Food Club		
Corned beef, smoked beef	40	2
Ham, turkey, chicken	45	2
Carl Buddig, 4 extra-thin slices		
Pastrami	40	2
Smoked beef	45	2
Smoked chicken, smoked turkey	50	4
Oscar Mayer (97% Fat-free)		
Chicken	25	<1
Smoked cooked ham, 1 slice	25	1
Corned beef, smoked beef, turkey bologna	30	1
Bacon, 2 slices	60	5
Sara Lee Light		
Chicken, turkey, beef, pork, ham	30-35	0-1
Ham, 3 varieties	40-45	0-2
Corned beef/brisket	35-40	2
Beef pastrami	50	3

MEATLESS OPTIONS		
Green Giant Harvest Burgers, 1	140	4
Morning Star Farms		
Meatless Chicken Patties, 4	170	10
Better 'n Burgers, 1	70	0
Breakfast Links, 2	60	3
Breakfast Strips, 2	60	5
Light Life		
Smart Deli Roast Turkey	80	0
Smart Dogs	45	0

TUNA AND FISH	Cal.	Fat (g)
Bumble Bee tuna (pack), 7 oz.	180	3
Chicken of the Sea tuna		
Chunk Light in Spring Water, 6 1/2 oz.	185	3
Star Kist tuna		
Solid white in spring water, 6 1/8 oz.	175	2
Healthy Choice Breaded Fish Filet, 1	180	4
Mrs. Paul's Healthy Treasures Fish Filet, 1	170	3
Gorton's Grilled Filets, 1	130	6
Lobster Delight, 1/2 package	60	0

EGG SUBSTITUTES		
Egg Beaters (1/4 c. = 1 egg)	25	0
Second Nature Eggs (1/4 c. = 1 egg)	35	0
Papetti Foods All Whites (3 Tbsp.)	25	0

CHEESE		
Alpine Lace Reduced fat		
Swiss or Cheddar (1 oz. = 1 1/3 slices)	70	5
Borden		
Fat-Free American, Swiss (1 oz.)	40	0
Liteline Slices (1 slice = 3/4 oz. = 35 cal.) -		
Swiss, sharp cheddar, Colby, American	50	2
American-Sodium Lite (1 slice = 3/4 oz. = 35 cal.)	50	2
Cabot		
75% Reduced fat Cheddar, 1 oz.	60	3
50% Reduced fat Cheddar, Jalapeno, Pep Jack, 1 oz.	70	5
50% Reduced fat cheese, mini bars, 3/4 oz.	50	3
Kraft		
Fat-free cream cheese (1 oz. = 2 Tbsp.)	25	0
Light cream cheese (1 oz. = 2 Tbsp.)	60	5
Light Neuchaftel (1 oz.)	70	6
Light mozzarella, shredded or block (1 oz.=1/4 c.)	80	4
2% milk cheeses:		
Swiss, American, sharp cheddar	70	4
(1 slice = 3/4 oz. = 50 cal, 5 g fat)		
Parmesan (1 oz. = 3 Tbsp.)	80	5
Velveeta Light (1 oz.)	70	4
Kraft Free (1 oz.)	45	0
Laughing Cow (Reduced Calorie)		
Mini-Bonbel Rounds, 3/4 oz.	50	3
Gruyere Cheese Wedges, 3/4 oz. wedge	50	3
Healthy Choice, 1 oz.		
Fat-free cream cheese, 2 Tbsp.	25	0
American Slices, 1 slice	25	0
Shredded nonfat cheddar, 1/4 c.	45	0
Nonfat mozzarella string cheese, 1 oz.	45	0
Frigo Fat-free ricotta, 1/2 c.	40	0
Food Club Mozzarella, part fat-free, 1 oz.	80	5
Precious		
Ricotta, low-fat, 1/2 c.	140	6
Ricotta, fat-free, 1/2 c.	80	0

COTTAGE CHEESE (1/2 Cup)	Cal.	Fat (g)
Borden Nonfat	70	0
Weight Watchers (1% fat)	80	1
Breakstone, fat free	80	0
Sc.hepps (1% fat)	80	1

BREAD (1 Slice)

	Cal.	Fat (g)
Very thin sliced bread (reduced-calorie or "light"):		
Pepperidge Farm, Orowheat, Lightstyle, Earth Grains, Less (white or wholewheat), **Country Hearth** diet sliced, **Mrs. Baird's, Nature's Own** 100% wholewheat	40-50	0
Stella D'Oro Zwieback toast, 3 sticks	60	0
Kangaroo Pita Salad Pocket	80	1
Thomas' English Muffin, Lt Multi-Grain	100	1

BAGELS

	Cal.	Fat (g)
Small, 2 oz.	160	1
Large, 3-5.5 oz. (deli-style)	250-400	2

PIZZA

	Cal.	Fat (g)
Tombstone Light		
Supreme, 8-in. (1/2 pizza)	250	9
Vegetable, 12 in. (1/2 pizza)	220	6
Healthy Choice Supreme French Bread Pizza	340	6

MARGARINE (1 Tablespoon)

	Cal.	Fat (g)
"Liquid oil" listed as first ingredient:		
Benecol or **Promise Activ** spread	70	8
Benecol Light or **Promise Activ Light**	50	5
Shedd's Spread	90	10
I Can't Believe It's Not Butter	90	10
Fleischmann's Light	40	4.5
Fleischmann's Premium Blend	70	8
Brummel & Brown yogurt/margarine spread	50	4
Smart Balance Omega-3 Plus spread	60	7
Smart Squeeze Non-fat margarine	5	0

BUTTER SUBSTITUTES

	Cal.	Fat (g)
Butter Buds, Molly McButter sprinkles	12	0
I Can't Believe It's Not Butter pump spray	0	0

COOKING OILS (1 Tablespoon)

	Cal.	Fat (g)
Olive, corn, sunflower, safflower, canola, enova	120	14

COOKING SPRAY OILS (per spray)

	Cal.	Fat (g)
Pam, Baker Joy, Weight Watchers, Mazola, etc.	2	0

SOUR CREAM (2 Tablespoons)

	Cal.	Fat (g)
Land O' Lakes fat-free sour cream	30	0
Daisy Light low-fat sour cream	60	5

MAYONNAISE (1 Tablespoon)	Cal.	Fat (g)
Weight Watchers		
Light mayonnaise	25	2
Fat-free mayonnaise	12	0
Kraft		
Miracle Whip Light	35	3
Miracle Whip Free	15	0
Light Mayonnaise	50	5
"Free" Mayonnaise	10	0

SALAD DRESSINGS (1 Tablespoon)

	Cal.	Fat (g)
Annie's Fat-free Italian Garlic/Honey	8	0
Brianna's Fat-free Lemon Tarragon	17	0
Kraft Fat-free		
Caesar or Italian	15	0
Bleu Cheese, French or Thousand Island	20	0
Catalina, Ranch or Honey Dijon	25	0
Good Seasons (No oil)		
Zesty Herb or Honey Mustard	6-10	0
Creamy Italian, fat-free	8	0
Girard's Fat-free Raspberry or Caesar	25	0
Hidden Valley Fat Free		
Bleu Cheese or Italian Parmesan	10	0
Caesar, French or Honey Dijon	25	0
Light Ranch	40	3
Ken's Steakhouse Lite dressings		
Sweet Vidalia Onion, Blue Cheese,. fat-free Italian, Vinaigrettes	15-35	0-2
Marie's Fat-free Italian Vinaigrette or Zesty Ranch	15	0
Newman's Own Lite Balsamic, Sesame Ginger, or Raspberry Walnut Vinaigrette	25-35	2
Seven Seas		
Italian, fat-free	4	0
Italian	30	3
Creamy Italian, 1/3 less fat	45	4
Lite Ranch	50	5
Spectrum		
Sweet Onion/Garlic, fat-free	8	0
Fat-free Creamy Garlic	10	0
Weight Watchers		
Caesar, fat-free	10	0
Creamy Cucumber, fat-free	18	0
Creamy Italian, fat-free	30	0
Ranch, French, or Honey Dijon	40	0
Creamy Italian, fat-free	12	0
Wish Bone		
Bleu Cheese or Red Wine Vinaigrette, fat-free	15	0
Just 2 Good low-fat Ranch or French	20	1
Thousand Island, fat-free	20	0

SALAD SPRAYS (10 sprays)

	Cal.	Fat (g)
Wishbone, Ken's Light, etc.	10	1

BEVERAGES	Cal.	Fat (g)
Herb Teas; all teas, 8 oz.	0	0
Sugar-Free Soft Drinks, 12 oz.	0	0
Lipton Tea		
all flavors, sugar-free, instant, 8 oz.	2	0
Crystal Light all flavors, 8 oz.	4	0
Country Time Lemonade, unsweetened, 8 oz.	4	0
Kool-Aid (all flavors with Nutrasweet), 8 oz.	4	0
Lite-Line (all flavors with Nutrasweet), 8 oz.	6	0
Tang, sugar-free, 8 oz.	7	0
Tropicana Light n Healthy Orange Juice, 8 oz.	50	0
Ocean Spray		
Cranapple Juice, low-calorie, 6 oz.	30	0
Light grape juice & other varieties, 8 oz.	40	0
Minute Maid Light Lemonade, 8 oz.	15	0
Gatorade G2, 20 oz.	70	0
Propel Fitness Waters; all flavors, 8 oz.	10	0

HOT COCOA OR SHAKES

	Cal.	Fat (g)
Carnation Diet Hot Cocoa, 1 packet	50	0
Swiss Miss Lite, 1 packet	50	0
fat free with marshmallows	40	0
Nestle, 1 packet	70	0
no sugar added, reduced calorie w/calcium	50	0
fat-free with marshmallows	40	0

CHIPS, POPCORN, SNACKS

	Cal.	Fat (g)
100 cal chip pks-**Sunchips, Pringles, Cheetos,** etc.	100	0
Burnes & Ricker Bagel Crisps (1 oz. = 5 crisps)		
Regular	130	4
Fat-free	100	0
Guiltless Gourmet		
Baked tortilla chips (1 oz. = 20 chips)	110	1
Black bean or pinto bean dips (1 oz.)	25	0
Fat-free queso (1 oz.)	25	0
Frito Lay		
Baked Tostitos Tortilla Chips (1 oz. = 13 chips)	110	1
Baked Potato Chips (1 oz. = 15 chips)	120	2
Baked Cheetos Mini-Bites (.75 oz. = 24 pieces)	100	3
Health Valley Fat-Free Puffs		
Cheese or Caramel Corn Puffs (1 oz. = 50 puffs)	100	0
Louise's Fat-Free Potato Chips, no salt		
(1 oz. = 30 chips)	110	0
Pringles, Light fat-free (1 oz. = 15 chips)	70	0
Hain's Mini rice cakes (6 flavors), 6-8 cakes	60	0
Quaker Quakes Mini rice cakes (4 flavors) 6-8 cakes	60	0
Rold Gold Pretzels (1 oz. = 10 pretzels)	110	0
Healthy Pop Jolly Time, 5 c.	100	0
Orville Redenbacher Smart Pop, 2 c.	70	1
Weight Watchers microwave popcorn, 1 oz.	90	1
Vic's Corn Popper, low-fat		
White Cheddar (1 oz. = 2 1/2 c.)	110	3
Caramel (1 oz. = 1 c.)	110	0

CEREAL & GRANOLA BARS (1)	Cal.	Fat (g)
Carnation Breakfast Bar	150	6
Fiber One Bar	150	5
Health Valley Fat-Free Granola Bar	140	0
Healthy Choice Fat-Free Granola Bar	100	0
Kashi TLC Bars (avg values)	150	5
Kellogg's Low-Fat Crunchy Granola Bar	80	1
Rice Krispie Treat	90	2
Smart Start Healthy Heart bar	150	3
Nature Valley Granola Bar		
Chewy low-fat bar	110	2
Wholegrain low-fat fruit bar	80	1
Quaker Chewy Granola Bars, avg. values	100	2
Simple Harvest Wholegrain bar	140	3
South Beach Cereal Bar	120	0

DIPS (2 Tablespoons)

	Cal.	Fat (g)
Land O' Lakes Fat-free dips		
Ranch, French Onion, Salsa	30	0
Kraft		
Green onion, Avocado, French onion, Ranch	60	4
Hummous, all brands	60	2
Wegmans Tzatziki	30	3

SOUPS

	Cal.	Fat (g)
Amy's Organic Soups (10.5 oz. can)		
Chunky Tomato Bisque	240	7
Butternut Squash	200	5
Campbell's (10 1/2 oz. can)		
Won Ton	100	3
Beef Mushroom, Chicken Gumbo, Chicken with Stars, Chicken with Rice, Old Fashion Vegetable, Vegetarian Vegetable	150	5
Clam Chowder (Manhattan Style), Chicken Vegetable, Chicken Noodle, Cream of Potato, French Onion, Vegetable Beef	175	6
Alphabet Vegetable, Clam Chowder	200	8
Gold Label Select (carton)		
Italian Tomato	180	1
Golden Butternut Squash	180	3
Lipton Cup-A-Soup (1 packet)		
Chicken Noodle	50	1
Lipton Cup-A-Soup Lite (1 packet), all flavors	45	1
Progresso Soups (18.5 oz. can)		
Home Style Vegetable & Rice	60	0
Italian Style Vegetable	60	0
Savory Vegetable Barley	60	0
Southwestern Style Vegetable	60	0
Healthy Choice Soups, 15 oz.		
Chunky Beef Vegetable	220	2
Chunky Chicken Noodle/Veg.	320	8
Chili with Beans/Ground Turkey	400	10
Spicy Chili with Beans/Ground Turkey	440	10

Health Valley Soups/Beans	Cal.	Fat (g)
5-Bean Soup, 15 oz.	200	0
3-Bean Chili, 10 oz.	180	0
Organic Black Beans/Tofu Wieners, 15 oz.	320	6
Organic Lentils/Tofu Wieners, 15 oz.	340	6
Western Black Beans/Veg., 15 oz.	210	2
Hearty Lentils/Veg., 15 oz.	240	2

FRUIT

Food Club "Light," 1/2 c.		
Fruit Cocktail, Cling Peaches and Peaches	50	0
Pear Halves or Pineapple	60	0
Libby's "Light," 1/2 c.		
Fruit Cocktail, Peaches and Pear Halves	50	0
Featherweight, 1/2 c.		
Apricots (water packed); mandarin oranges	35	0
Grapefruit segments	40	0
Applesauce, peaches, fruit cocktail, fruits for salads (all water packed)	50	0
Sliced Pineapple	70	0
Weight Watchers Dried Fruit Snack, 1 packet		
Dried apples, dried peaches, dried pineapple and dried strawberries	25-50	0
Mott's or **Lucky Leaf**, 1/2 c.		
Applesauce, sugar-free	50	0
Nature Valley Fruit Crisps, 1 pouch	50	0

SWEETS, EXTRAS

SUGAR-FREE JELLY (1 Teaspoon)
Knott's Light Fruit Spread	8	0
Smucker's Low Sugar	25	0
Polaner's Sugar-free Spread	10	0

SYRUP (1 Tablespoon)
Aunt Jemima Light or **Butterworth's** Light	30	0
Maple Groves Sugar-free syrup	10	0

PANCAKE MIX
Aunt Jemima Light Buttermilk, 2	130	2
Hungry Jack Extra Light, 2	120	2

WAFFLES
Kellogg's Special K, 1	80	0
Kashi Go Lean, 1	80	1

NON-DAIRY CREAM TOPPINGS (1 Tablespoon)
Dream Whip	8	0
Cool Whip, La Creme	16	1
Fat-Free Cool Whip, regular or chocolate	6	0

FROZEN DESSERTS (see p. 126)
Weight Watchers		
Ice Milk, all flavors (4 oz., 1/2 c.)	120	4

	Cal.	Fat (g)
Ice Cream Treats, all flavors, 1 bar	100	7
Fat-Free Frozen Dessert Bars, 1 bar	30-90	0
Ice Cream Sandwich, 1 bar	130	8
Hot Fudge Sundae, 1	160	4
Blue Bell		
Diet ice cream, all	100	0
Fat-free frozen yogurt, 1/2 c.	120	4
Fat-free fudge bar, 1	80	0
Cream pops, 1	60	1
Mini light sandwich, 1	80	2
Frozen bars		
All Flavors, 1 bar	70	0
Sugar-free, 1 bar	15-35	0
Dreyer's		
Frozen yogurt, 1/2 c.	110	4
Fat-free dessert, 1/2 c.	100	0
Dannon Frozen yogurt	110	0
Dole		
Fruit and Juice Bars, 1	70	0
Fruit and Yogurt Bars, 1	60	0
Sorbet, 1/2 c.	70	0
Welch's Fruit Juice Bar	25	0
Creamsicle, sugar-free bar, 1	25	1
Fudgesicle bar, 1	70	1
Sugar-free bar, 1	35	0
Jell-O Pudding Pops, 1 bar	80	2
Borden		
Eskimo Bar, sugar-free, 1 bar	150	11
Eskimo Bar, nonfat, 1 bar	130	7
All Natural Ice Milk (4 oz., 1/2 c.)	100	2
Orange sherbet, 1/2 c.	100	1
Klondike Light		
Ice Cream Sandwich (Slim a Bear)	100	1
Chocolate Bar	110	6
Haagen-Daas		
Frozen Yogurt Bar	100	1
Healthy Choice, 1/2 c.		
Frozen Desserts, all flavors	130-140	2
Ultra Slim-Fast		
Frozen Dessert, 1/2 c.	100	0
Fudge Bar, 1 bar	70	10
Breyer's		
Slow Churn, 1/2 c., all flavors	100	4
Blue Bunny, 1/2 c.		
Frozen yogurt, low-fat	115	3
Skinny Cow		
Low-fat Dipper Bar	80	3
Fat-free Fudge Bar	90	0
Ice Cream Sandwich	130	2
TCBY Yogurt, 1/2 c.		
Sugar-free, nonfat	72	0
Nonfat	100	0
Regular	120	1

CAKES/PIES/PASTRIES	Cal.	Fat (g)
Hostess, 100 cal packs (3 cupcakes)		
Chocolate, Carrot or Golden Cupcakes	100	3
Pepperidge Farm Desserts Light		
Apple 'N Spice Bake, 1 slice	170	2
Fudge Brown, fat-free	120	0
Sara Lee Free & Light, 1 slice		
Apple Danish	130	0
Pound Cake	70	0
Apple Crisp	150	2
Apple Pie	190	4
Pillsbury Lovin' Lites		
Fudge Brownie Mix (1/24)	100	2
Blueberry Muffin Mix (1/12)	100	1
Weight Watchers		
Strawberry Cheesecake, 4 oz.	180	4
Apple Pie, 3.5 oz.	165	4
Brownie, 1	100	3

GELATINS, PUDDINGS	Cal.	Fat (g)
Jell-O with Nutrasweet, all flavors, 1/2 c.	8	0
Hunt's, Hershey's, Jell-O fat-free puddings, all flavors, 1/2 c.	60-100	0

COOKIES	Cal.	Fat (g)
Entenmann's		
Fat-free cookies, 1	80	0
Health Valley		
Fat-Free Apricot Cookies, 3	75	0
Nabisco		
Devil's Food Cakes, 1	70	1
Fig Newtons, 2	120	2
Nilla Wafers, 7	120	4
Reduced fat Oreos, 3	140	4
100-calorie Snack Packs (**Oreo, Chips Ahoy, Teddy Grahams, Ritz bits, Wheat Thins**, etc.)	**100**	**3-6**
SnackWell's		
Cookie Cakes, Chocolate Mint or Black Forest, 1	50	1
Mini Chocolate Chip Cookies, 6	60	1
Oatmeal Raisin or Chocolate Sandwich Cookies, 1	60	1
Devil's Food or Double Fudge, 1	50	0
Cinnamon Grahams, 9	50	0

	Cal.	Fat (g)
Sunshine		
Animal Crackers, 13	120	3
Teddy Grahams, 1/2 oz.	60	2

CRACKERS	Cal.	Fat (g)
Blue Diamond Nut Thins, 16	65	1 Kashi
TLC Bars (avg values)	150	5
Devonshire Melba Rounds, 5	50	0
Hain Ryecrackers, 6	60	1
Health Valley		
Rice Bran crackers, 3	50	2
Whole-Wheat Crackers, 1 oz.	80	1
Nabisco		
Fat-free saltines, 5	50	0
Saltines, regular or wholewheat, 5	60	2
Triscuits, regular, unsalted or low-fat, 3	60	2
Old London Onion Rounds, 5	50	0
Pepperidge Farm tiny goldfish, 22	60	2
Sunshine Oyster & Soup Crackers, 16	60	1
Snackwell's		
Cheese Crackers, 18	60	1
Wheat Crackers, 5	50	0
Ralston-Purina Rykrisps, 2	40	0
Wasa Crispbreads, all types, 1	45	0
100-cal packs (**Goldfish, Ritz, Wheat Thins**, etc.)	100	5

YOGURT	Cal.	Fat (g)
Blue Bunny Lite 85, 6 oz.	80	0
Yoplait		
Light, fat-free, sugar-free, 6 oz.	95	0
Lucerne, fat-free, 8 oz.	120	0
Dannon		
Premium low-fat, plain, 6 oz.	110	3
Lite & Fit w/ non-fat, 6 oz.	100	0
Lite & Fit Smoothie, 7 oz.	80	0
Fage, non-fat, plain, 8 oz.	100	0

NOTE:

1. Check "Gourmet Foods", "Diet Foods", "Organic" and "Health Foods" sections at your grocery store, along with regular food sections, for special low-calorie, low-fat, low-sugar, low-sodium products.
2. Check for your local brand names. Take a grocery store tour with a dietitian in your city.
3. New specialty foods arrive every week. Keep checking labels & finding new products.
4. Check www.calorieking.com for more foods.

Grocery Shopping Tips

The key to eating balanced meals and snacks at home is to stock up with low-calorie, nutritious foods that you really enjoy. Shopping doesn't have to be overwhelming! Take note of my following grocery shopping tips—and remember to resist those temptations in the store so you won't be tempted again at home.

1. **Make a shopping list** from your eating plan and stick to it. Avoid buying unnecessary and high-calorie foods. Do not try to shop from memory on the spur of the moment.

2. **Shop after a meal when you are not hungry** or at a time of the day when you are least susceptible to food cues. Hunger pangs often lead to overbuying and high-calorie foods.

3. **Shop once a week on a regular schedule.** The less time spent in a grocery store, the better. Plus, you'll save money.

4. **Avoid tempting shopping aisles.**

5. **Shop at "inviting" stores** with beautiful, fresh produce. This makes the right food irresistible!

6. **Buy low-calorie snacks.** Avoid high-fat, sugary foods.

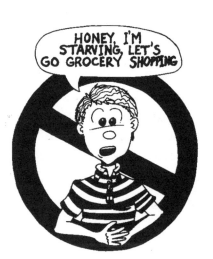

7. **If you are tempted by a high-calorie "junk food," stop and think.** Select a lower-calorie substitute. If you must have the "junk food," buy a very small quantity.

8. **Put grocery bags in your trunk** to avoid snacking on the way home.

9. When home, **put foods away immediately—out of sight!**

READ FOOD LABELS

1. Look for **SUGAR** as: sugar, corn syrup, maple syrup, molasses, honey, dextrin, sorghum, brown sugar, sorbitol, mannitol, sucrose, fructose, lactose, dextrose, galactose, glucose, maltose, mannose

2. Look for **SALT** as: salt (sodium chloride), MSG (monosodium glutamate), sodium bicarbonate (baking soda), brine, sodium propionate, sodium alginate, sodium hydroxide, sodium sulfite, sodium saccharin, etc.

3. Look for **FATS** as: butter, oil, shortening, lard, hydrogenated fats, beef fat, cream, bacon, mayonnaise, dressing

    Choose unsaturated oils (olive, canola, safflower, corn, sunflower, soybean). Avoid coconut and palm oils, saturated fats and partially hydrogenated fats and oils added to many commercial products.

Step 5
Get Moving!

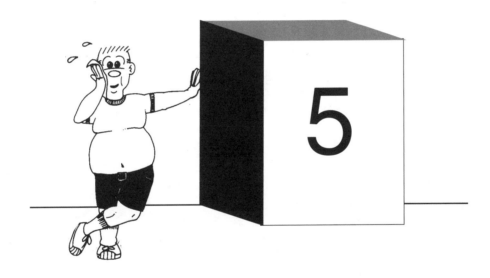

Step 5

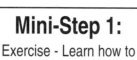

Mini-Step 1:
Exercise - Learn how to begin and fit it in.

Mini-Step 2:
Create your
"Balanced Fitness Plan."

Rather take a "magic pill" than exercise? Start moving, and once you do, you'll realize how *good* walking or another favorite activity makes you feel! It lifts your spirit, gives you a sense of accomplishment and aids tremendously in weight loss.

Perhaps you've been inactive for a long time or need to move your exercise program up a notch. This step is for you! We'll explore new research that shows the power of exercise in promoting health and preventing disease, and we'll look at other significant benefits an active lifestyle offers.

I often hear people say they don't have time to fit in fitness. If you're struggling in this area, try some of my "Fitting in Fitness" tips (p. 141-142), as well as some of my solutions to "roadblocks to fitness" on p. 152-153.

Are you ready for some action? Proceed to the specific exercise programs outlined on p. 145, and notice how your body begins to become conditioned as you gradually increase the intensity of your workout. I encourage you to incorporate the strengthening and stretching exercises (see p. 147-149) to keep your muscles fit. Do you want to get the most from your workout? I'll show you how on p. 140.

ACTION STEPS

① Determine your roadblocks to fitness, and find solutions that will keep you on your feet—and off the couch!

② Establish your own motivation techniques and ways to maintain an active lifestyle.

③ Design your own seven-day exercise plan (p. 144).

④ Balance your program with aerobic activity, strength training and stretching. Try all of these types of exercise and see how different each makes you feel.

© 2009, *The Cooper Clinic Solution to the Diet Revolution* by Georgia G. Kostas, M.P.H., R.D., L.D., Dallas, Texas

Why Exercise?

"I can now mow my lawn without stopping to rest every 15 minutes!"

"Exercise is a time-giver, not a time-taker. It's an energy-giver, not an energy-drainer."

"Becoming more active changed my fat distribution. I lost inches in my waist and hips!"

"Exercise is my play-time daily."

"Exercise is the best stress-buster I've found!"

"It's the only way I can re-energize my body, refresh my spirit, renew my mind and refocus all at one time."

"I put in time but get more back because I don't tire as early at night. It's the best time and energy investment I know."

U. S. Surgeon General's Reports to the American people:

"Accumulate 30-60 minutes of moderate activity most days of the week."

© 2009, *The Cooper Clinic Solution to the Diet Revolution* by Georgia G. Kostas, M.P.H., R.D., L.D., Dallas, Texas

Benefits of Exercise

Study after study has shown that exercise is a vital part of successful weight-loss—and a healthy lifestyle. If you want to experience a better quality of life, **GET MOVING NOW!** The benefits are numerous, ranging from physiological to psychological:

BENEFITS

1 **Weight Control:**
- burns calories and fat
- speeds metabolism
- decreases appetite — naturally
- promotes fat-burning
- builds muscle, which increases metabolism
- reduces stress and boredom, which can lead to excessive eating
- motivates better eating
- changes your appetite, so you desire more light, low-fat foods

2 **Physiological (Cardiovascular):**
- improves cardiovascular health and circulation
- increases HDL-cholesterol blood levels
- decreases cholesterol, triglycerides and blood pressure
- improves muscle tone, agility and strength
- increases stamina and endurance
- increases resistance to stress and illness
- builds stronger bones to prevent osteoporosis

3 **Psychological:**
- builds self-confidence and a positive attitude
- reduces emotional stress and depression
- increases alertness
- enables a sense of well-being and enjoyment of life
- helps you feel and look your best

4 **Social:**
- opens up a new world of friends
- creates a new recreational interest

EXERCISE IS NOT A CHOICE - IT'S A MUST!

© 2009, *The Cooper Clinic Solution to the Diet Revolution* by Georgia G. Kostas, M.P.H., R.D., L.D., Dallas, Texas

Mix It Up

What types of exercise should you do for maximum results? It depends on what you hope to accomplish.

 Aerobic Exercise *Provides cardiovascular endurance and fat-burning benefits.*

> *Examples:*
> - **Vigorous activities:** race-walking, biking, jogging, swimming, aerobic dance, dancing, spin classes, jumping rope, stair climbing machine, vigorous tennis, martial arts, etc.
> - **Moderate activities:** brisk walking, yardwork, vacuuming/mopping, car-washing, basketball shooting, etc.
> - **Lifestyle (light) activities:** walking, shopping, sight-seeing, golf, laundry, light gardening, frisbee throwing, playing with children or pets.

The results from any aerobic activity depend on your intensity. If lighter, go longer. The lighter the intensity, the longer you need to exercise to match the caloric expenditure of a shorter, more vigorous activity. Spend 30 minutes (vigorous) to 45 minutes (moderate/light) per workout. A 30-minute moderate activity can be split into three 10-minute segments.

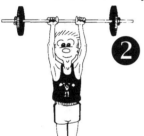

Strength Training *Provides muscle tone and endurance, muscular strength, bone density and a faster metabolism (from muscle).*

> *Examples:* Calisthenics, resistance exercises (push-ups, abdominal crunches, free weights, weight machines, etc.).

 Flexibility/Stretching *Provides muscle agility, protection from injury, relaxation.*

Before and after exercise, and after the warm-up, always stretch your muscles slowly.

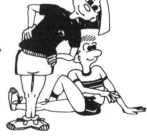

 Remember, it all begins with that first step!

For the best results with fitness, weight loss and weight maintenance, combine aerobic and strengthening and stretching exercises. Consider hiring a fitness specialist to design the best customized program for you.

AEROBIC FITNESS GOALS FOR WEIGHT LOSS

F **F**requency: 4-5 times per week

I **I**ntensity: moderate to vigorous

T **T**ime: 30-45 minutes per workout

For best weight-loss results, burn 200-300 (average 250) calories per day.
(See *Calorie Expenditure Tables*, p. 154-155.)

LANDMARK STUDIES AT THE COOPER INSTITUTE HAVE SHOWN:

1 **Small steps, big results**. Even the smallest improvement in cardiovascular fitness is worthwhile, significantly reducing your risk of heart disease, hypertension, stroke and cancer. You don't have to run a marathon to be healthy! Brisk walking 30 minutes a day, five days a week will improve fitness and reduce by 55% your risk of a heart attack, stroke, cancer or diabetes.

2 **Pace yourself**. Walk fast or slow…15 miles a week…and you'll reap the same heart-healthy benefits, a better HDL cholesterol and an 18% reduced risk of coronary heart disease.

3 **Pick up your pace.** A 12-minute mile burns 53% more calories than a 20-minute mile and promotes greater overall fitness and aerobic conditioning.

4 **Split it up.** Whether you exercise for 30 minutes straight or split it up into three 10-minute segments, you still benefit your health, burn calories and can lose weight.

5 **Be proactive.** You can cut your death risk in half if you move from being "sedentary" or "low-fit" to "moderately fit." Good health does not require "super-fitness"!

6 **10,000 steps a day.** Sedentary people take an average of 5,000-6,000 steps daily. Studies have shown that 10,000 steps a day at a moderate (brisk) pace, as measured by a pedometer or step-counter,* will meet the Surgeon General's recommendation for physical activity needed daily for health benefits. A brisk-30 minute walk (2 miles) gives you 5,000 steps!

I recommend AcuSplit's step-counter. Call (800) 444-5764, ext. 3161 or (800) 538-9750 to order.

EACH STEP COUNTS!

10,000 steps a day: for heart, overall health and improved or "basic" fitness

15,000 steps a day: for weight loss, heart health and "moderate" fitness

20,000 steps a day: for maximum fat-burning and a "high" level of fitness

---

 Note: Always check with your physician before beginning an exercise program, especially if an injury or health condition exists.

Recent Research: "A step in time saves lives and weight"

1. **Walking is the key to maintaining weight loss for five years or longer**. Forty-nine out of every 50 people in the National Weight Control Registry database of thousands who lost at least 30 pounds walk daily.

2. **Women who walk briskly for at least three hours a week reduce their risk of heart disease by up to 40%**. These brisk walks have the same effect as 15 to 20 minutes of more vigorous daily exercise. Even previously sedentary women who start walking experience substantial reductions in heart attack and diabetes risk (The Nurses' Health Study of Harvard University).

3. **Older people who give up a sedentary lifestyle and start taking hour-long walks three times a week have better memory and judgment ability** (University of Chicago).

4. **A 12-year study of 60- to 80-year olds demonstrates that daily, moderate-intensity, two-mile walks reduced one's death rate by half** (University of Virginia).

5. **Three 10-minute walks can increase fitness and decrease body fat just as well as one 30-minute walk** (research in Great Britain).

It's Never Too Late

"I guess I just forgot to get old," says Fan Benno-Caris, 90. At 70, Fan started a speed-walking class. Within 3 years, she won bronze and silver medals in the National Senior Olympics, and five gold medals in the Texas State Senior Games! Since then, she has competed internationally, breaking 5 World Records and 7 US National Records for 5K and 10K race walks, winning 5 gold medals and 3 silvers in World Champion competitions, 5 gold medals and 4 silvers in National events, and 12 gold medals in Texas competitions. At age 85, Fan was asked to join the US Women 70-74 year old team, helping them win "the gold" at the World Championship event! When Fan set the World Record for the difficult 3K Indoor Walking competition in 2004, she even broke her own best time. Fan carried the Olympic Torch in 2002; in 2005, she was named Ms. Texas Senior America. Her life is full of achievement...and continual goals!

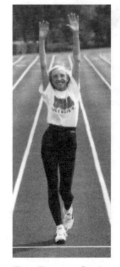

Fan Benno-Caris
90-years-young!

An author and motivational speaker, Fan "walks the talk," preaching about the benefits of an active lifestyle, goals and "winning." Fan's life is full of vigor, fun and laughter; she is passionate about many things...a champion of life itself!

"I tell people that the secret to life is to never stop moving," she says. "Unfortunately, most people, as they get older, give themselves permission to stop moving. But movement is essential. It puts oxygen in your body and gives you energy."

Author's Note: Four weeks after being Fan's walking buddy, we sped up our pace from 15 minutes a mile to 13 minutes a mile. As she approached her 12-minute mile, I couldn't keep up and was forced to drop out...and Fan was twice my age! It's never too late to get fit!

Exercise Heart Rate: Hit Your Target!

How much aerobic exercise do you need to get cardiovascular, health and fitness benefits? This is a commonly asked question—and it depends on your goals.

You exercise more comfortably, safely and efficiently when you exercise at the appropriate intensity, called your **target heart rate (THR).** At least 20 minutes will build aerobic conditioning; 30 to 45 minutes will promote weight loss. How do you know what intensity is best for you? The Cooper Clinic recommends exercise at a THR of 55%-85% of your maximum heart rate (MHR), as listed below. Are you exercising at this level?

Two methods tell you if you are getting the most from your workout:

1 **Simplest way:** If you are "exerting" but not "overdoing," and can carry on a conversation while exercising, most likely you are exercising right on "target"! Use the modified Borg Scale below to rate your level of intensity. Strive to exercise at perceived levels 2-5.

Borg Rating of Perceived Exertion (RPE) Scale (Modified)

This scale rates the level of exertion you are experiencing from 0 (rest) to 10 (extreme effort):

10	Very, Very Hard
8	Very Hard
6	Hard
5	Somewhat Harder
4	Somewhat Hard
3	Moderate
2	Light
1	Very Light
0	No Exertion

5 Somewhat Harder
4 Somewhat Hard   = Target Intensity
3 Moderate   (55 - 85% MHR)
2 Light

Copyright 1992, Gunnar Borg. Reprinted with permission. Adapted from *Medicine and Science in Sports and Exercise,* 1982, Vol. 14, No. 5, pg. 377-381.

2 **Technical way:** Measure your heart rate by checking your pulse or by using a heart monitor as shown below.

Age	Recommended Target Heart Rate (THR)*		Maximum Heart Rate (MHR) (unsafe)
	Beats Per 10 Seconds	Beats Per Minute	
20	18-28	110-168	200
30	17-27	102-162	190
40	17-26	102-156	180
50	16-24	96-144	170
60	15-23	90-138	160
70	14-21	84-126	150

*Recommended THR is 55%-85% of MHR.

For maximum benefit, exercise at your target heart rate!

How To Take Your Pulse

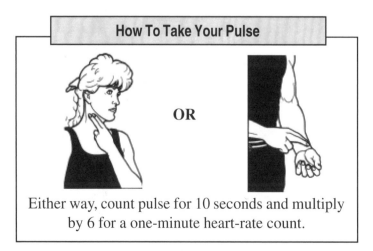

OR

Either way, count pulse for 10 seconds and multiply by 6 for a one-minute heart-rate count.

Fitting in Fitness

Even before you know where or how to begin an exercise program, the most important thing is simply to **MOVE DAILY**! Step up to the challenge. Identify what you can do from the list that follows:

STEP 1: **Ease into exercise.** Find ways to add more lifestyle activity to your daily routine. Which will you try? ☑

- ☐ Sit instead of lying down, as you read, watch TV, open mail, etc.
- ☐ Stand instead of sitting when talking on the phone.
- ☐ Walk instead of driving. You can make many of your local errands fun on foot or bike!
- ☐ Take stairs instead of elevators.
- ☐ Pick up your walking pace.
- ☐ Stoop, bend, reach, stretch—use your muscles. ("Use it or lose it.")
- ☐ Park your car as far as possible from your destination.
- ☐ Choose the farthest phone, bathroom or path between two points.
- ☐ "Walk and talk." Visit with a friend or family member on foot.
- ☐ Make an after-dinner walk part of your lifestyle.
- ☐ Clean your closet, vacuum or mop; do yard work or home repairs; wash your car; sweep.
- ☐ Use coffee or lunch breaks at work to climb staircases or walk long hallways.
- ☐ Stretch at your desk. Do arm, neck and shoulder rotations.
- ☐ Make your own list of ways to move more daily.

STEP 2: **Establish a regular exercise program.** Which can you do? ☑

- ☐ Set up a personal daily routine of walking, biking, swimming, jogging, etc., at a set time.
- ☐ Join a dancing class, spin class, walking club or team sport. Groups are motivational.
- ☐ Find an exercise partner. Meet at a designated time daily.
- ☐ Involve yourself in active hobbies—gardening, carpentry, dancing, etc.
- ☐ Try your hand at a new recreational sport—tennis, volleyball, badminton, ping-pong, bowling, racquetball, golf, etc. Take lessons!
- ☐ Meet with a personal trainer or certified fitness specialist to create a game plan that fits your needs.
- ☐ Become a mall-walker. Leave your charge card at home!
- ☐ Set goals and rewards for yourself. Write them down and keep a daily progress record.

1. Make **SMART** goals:

   Specific   **M**easurable   **A**chievable   **R**ewarding   **T**imely

   Example: Walk 2 miles in 36 minutes at 7 a.m., Monday, Wednesday, Friday and Saturday in my neighborhood, listening to my favorite music and news station.

2. Write down **realistic** short- and long-term goals (weekly, monthly, quarterly, yearly). *Examples: (a) Be consistent with my aerobic activity 4 times a week and strength-train 3 times a week for the next 6 weeks. (b) Participate in 2 benefit walks/races in my community this year. (c) Plan an active vacation (hiking, biking, etc.). (d) Gain 5 pounds of muscle in one year to restore what I've lost.*

STEP 3: **Find ways to "work in" your workout.**

☐ Choose convenient activities you enjoy.

☐ Exercise while doing something routine. For example: (1) Walk on your treadmill as you watch the daily news; (2) Listen to TV or tapes as you walk or bike (book tapes are great!); (3) Read as you stationary bike; (4) Pair up with a friend to "walk and talk"; (5) Have meetings "on foot."

☐ Go slow at first and avoid strain. Increase your goals weekly.

☐ Develop your plan of action. (See p. 143-144.)

☐ Strive for sustained exercise of at least 20 minutes at the right intensity to reap the fullest cardiovascular benefits and 30-45 minutes to burn body fat stores for the most consistency.

☐ Set aside a regular time daily for exercise, and keep with it! Aim for morning!

☐ Set a goal to burn 200-250+ calories a day (see p. 154-155).

☐ Keep a daily activity log (see sample, p. 40) and monitor your progress.

☐ Involve friends and family.

☐ Focus on benefits you feel.

☐ Step over stumbling blocks. Although vacations and work schedules can change your routine, try your hardest to include a daily activity so you won't step out of your routine. Have a backup plan to include a different type of activity on these days.

☐ Reset your time priorities. You must forego one activity daily to make room for physical activity.

☐ Make time for physical activity as a stress-reducer. (Kids call it "recess" or "play.")

STEP 4: **Balance your program for best results.** (See p. 143.) What's your next move?

☐ aerobic activity
    ☐ more time   ☐ more intensity
    ☐ more distance   ☐ more variety

☐ warming up/cooling down, five minutes before and after exercise (see p. 147.)

☐ strength training, 2-3 times a week, 20-30 minutes each time (see p. 148-149.)

☐ stretching, 2-3 times a week, 5-10 minutes each time (see p. 147.)

☐ hiring a qualified trainer

WARNING

**NOT BEING ACTIVE
IS LIKE
SMOKING A PACK
OF CIGARETTES
A DAY**

Guidelines for a Balanced Fitness Plan

A balanced fitness plan includes several components: **aerobic activity, strength training, flexibility** and a **warm-up/cool-down before and after exercise.** Each of these activities benefits the body differently. Together, they maximize fat-burning, overall fitness and health. I recommend combining:

1. **AEROBIC ACTIVITY**
   - 4-5 times per week for weight loss
   - 30-45 minutes is optimal per session
   - Borg Exertion level 2-5 (see p. 140); heart rate at 55%-85% MHR

   Beginners:
   - Start slowly: 3 times per week, 20-30 minutes per session.
   - As your fitness level improves, add more days per week and increase your minutes per session. Go further, longer, faster and/or more frequently to keep improving fitness.

2. **STRENGTH TRAINING**
   - 3 times per week, 20-40 minutes each time.
     Beginners: Start at 2 times per week.
   - Do weight machines or free weights at a gym with guidance from a personal trainer.
   - Strength-train at your home with guidance from a personal trainer.
   - Start with light weights or a low setting on weight machines. Do a set of 10-12 repetitions. Repeat.
   - See diagrams on p. 148-149 on how to build muscular strength and endurance.

3. **FLEXIBILITY**
   - Stretch before and after you exercise, each time you exercise, and after the warm-up and cool down.
   - Stretch 3-5 minutes and only after the muscle is warmed up to prevent injury.
   - See diagrams on p. 147, or attend a stretch class.

4. **WARM-UP/COOL-DOWN**
   - Warm-up (pre-exercise): Walk, cycle or walk in place slowly 3-5 minutes to warm up. This prevents injury, increases endurance and helps you ease into exercise comfortably. Lightly stretch. Hold for 10 seconds. (See diagram on p. 147.)
   - Cool-down (post-exercise): Slow down your intensity level for 3-5 minutes after completing your desired aerobic activity. Stretch and hold for 20-30 seconds (see diagram on p. 147). This slows your heart rate gradually (safely) and relaxes your muscles. You'll feel rejuvenated!

> **The following page shows you how to design your own favorite fitness plan based on these guidelines.**

Program By: Colette Cole, MS, Personal Trainer & Fitness Coordinator, Cooper Fitness Center, Dallas, TX
Consultations available; call 972-233-1782, ext. 4400.

Designing Your Balanced Fitness Plan

Aerobic Activity, Strength Training, Stretching and Warm-up/Cool-down

Here is a sample balanced exercise "game plan." Use it as your guide.

GENERAL EXERCISE PLAN

Day 1	Day 2	Day 3	Day 4	Day 5	Day 6	Day 7
Aerobic Activity* *Borg: 4-5* *30 minutes* Strength Train Stretch	Aerobic Activity *Borg: 3-4* *>30 minutes*	Aerobic Activity *Borg: 4-5* *30 minutes* Strength Train Stretch	RELAX	Aerobic Activity *Borg: 4-5* *30 minutes* Strength train Stretch	Lifestyle Activity+ *Borg: 2-3* *>45 minutes*	RELAX

Borg 4-5 = very brisk pace; Borg 3-4 = brisk pace; Borg 2-3 = fairly brisk pace

***Aerobic Activity** ("heart-healthy" exercise):* walking/jogging, biking (indoor/outdoor), swimming, aerobic classes (dance, step, spinning, etc.), vigorous tennis, stair climbing, aerobic machines (treadmill, rowing, stair climbing machine, etc.) *Also, see Dr. Cooper's Aerobic Exercise Plans, p. 145.*	**+Lifestyle Activity** (less structured exercise): long walks, bike rides, hiking, dancing, shopping, yard work, lawn mowing, cleaning car, gardening, raking leaves, vacuuming/sweeping/mopping, active hobbies, etc. *These activities should be continuous and done at a brisk pace.*

EXAMPLE

Day 1	Day 2	Day 3	Day 4	Day 5	Day 6	Day 7
Warm-up Bike *Borg: 4-5* *30 minutes* Cool-down Strength Train Stretch	Warm-up/ Walk *Borg: 3-4* *45-60 minutes* Cool-down	Warm-up/Step Aerobic Class/Video *Borg: 4-5* *30+ minutes* Cool-down Strength Train Stretch	RELAX	Warm-up Swim *Borg: 4-5* *30 minutes* Cool-down Strength Train Stretch	Lifestyle Activity: Yardwork or walk in park *Borg: 2-3* *60 minutes*	RELAX

Fill in each day with your exercise plan. Make sure you have a balanced program for the week.

☑ MY EXERCISE PLAN

Day 1	Day 2	Day 3	Day 4	Day 5	Day 6	Day 7

Moving From Sedentary to Fit

Dr. Cooper's Progressive Aerobic Exercise Plans

To build aerobic fitness, progress gradually with these plans.

WALKING PROGRAM

WEEK	DIST. (miles)	FREQ. (times/wk.)	TIME (min.)
1	2	3x	36
2	2	3x	34
3	2	4x	32
4	2	4x	30
5	2.5	4x	39
6	2.5	5x	38
7	2.5	5x	37
8	3	5x	46
9	3	5x	45
10	3	5x	44
11			
12			

JOGGING PROGRAM

WEEK	ACTIVITY (type)	DIST. (miles)	FREQ. (times/wk.)	TIME (min.)
1	Walk	2	3x	34
2	Walk	2.5	3x	42
3	Walk	3	3x	50
4	Walk/Jog	2	4x	25
5	Walk/Jog	2	4x	24
6	Jog	2	4x	22
7	Jog	2.5	4x	20
8	Jog	2.5	4x	26
9	Jog	2.5	4x	25
10	Jog	3	4x	31
11	Jog	3	4x	29
12	Jog	3	4x	27

Legend

- ☐ progressive fitness
- ▨ moderate fitness (for overall health)
- ▨ optimal fat-burning (for maximum weight loss)

FREQ = Frequency

DIST = Distance

SWIMMING PROGRAM

WEEK	DIST. (yards)	FREQ. (times/wk.)	TIME (min.)
1	300	4x	12
2	300	4x	10
3	400	4x	13
4	400	4x	12
5	500	4x	14
6	500	4x	13
7	600	4x	16
8	700	4x	19
9	800	4x	22
10	900	4x	22
11			
12			
13			
14			

STATIONARY CYCLING PROGRAM

LOAD	SPEED (mph/rpm)	FREQ. (times/wk.)	(min.)
1.5	15/55	5x	6
1.5	15/55	5x	8
1.5	15/55	5x	10
2.0	15/55	5x	12
2.0	15/55	5x	14
2.0	15/55	5x	16
2.0	15/55	5x	18
2.0	15/55	5x	20
2.5	17.5/65	5x	18
2.5	17.5/65	5x	20
2.5	20/75	5x	20
2.5	20/75	5x	22.5
2.5	20/75	5x	25
3.0	25/75	5x	30

Dr. Cooper says "moderate fitness" is:

Walking 2 miles in -

- less than 30 minutes, 3 times a week

- 30 - 40 minutes, 5 - 6 times a week

Calories Per Session

- 200 - 300 initially
- 400 - 600 as you become more fit

➢ For more of Dr. Cooper's recommended exercise plans, see his books. The above are from *The Aerobics Program for Total Well-being*, 1983.

➢ Precede any workout with a 5 minute warm-up; follow with a 5 minute cool-down.

- **Benefits**—Improved fitness level; increased cardiovascular endurance; stronger muscles and bone; more energy; more fat-burning; increased fitness level; a faster metabolism at 6-12 weeks; body composition improvements; and visible improvements in your pace, strength, endurance, inches lost.

- **Add Intensity to Add Results**—The higher the intensity of your exercise session, the more calories you'll burn.

    As your cardiovascular fitness improves, you will see a gradual decrease in your exercising heart rate and perceived exertion. It's time to step up the intensity of your aerobic activity to raise your heart rate to its target zone. For example, walk on a treadmill and increase your speed (mph) or incline (% grade) to increase the intensity. If walking outdoors, take a path with small hills when possible. "Pushing" yourself a little promotes fitness and takes you to the next level of overall fitness. Also, alternating fast/slow paces over a 30- to 45-minute brisk walk speeds fitness gains.

- **Fat Loss**—You'll lose ½ pound of fat each week when you burn approximately 1,500 calories a week (200-300 calories daily) from becoming active 3-4 hours a week.

Pick Up Your Pace to Burn 33-50% More Calories!

- Go from 3.5 mph to 4.5 mph and burn 33% more calories.
- Go from 3.5 mph to 5.0 mph and burn 50% more calories.
- Researchers have discovered that walkers can burn just as many calories as runners doing the same speed when they go above 4.5 mph.

You Don't Feel Like Exercising Today?

Tell yourself:

"Exercise is the best part of my day."

"Every little bit helps."

"Something is better than nothing."

"I'll feel great when it is over."

Stretching Exercises for Total Body Flexibility

1) Upper Torso/Arms

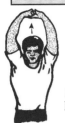

Interlock fingers above head. Push palms upward and stretch until reaching point of tightness and hold.

2) Chest/Shoulders/Arms

Grasp hands behind back. Slowly lift arms to comfortable tightness and hold.

Always check with your physician before starting any exercise program. Stop if muscle or joint pain occurs while doing any exercise. Consult your physician before continuing this exercise.

3) Upper Back/Shoulders/Arms

Grasp elbow with opposite hand, gently pulling elbow in toward head and hold. Repeat with opposite arm.

4) Upper Torso/Shoulders/Arms

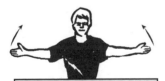

Bring arms up and out from sides. Gently pull arms back until you feel tightness in the chest, shoulder and arm muscles.

The following exercises will indeed help improve your flexibility. They emphasize safety and should be done before and after vigorous activity, and always after a warm-up and cool-down.

GUIDELINES
- Stretch slowly to a point of tension, not pain.
- Do not bounce.
- Do not stretch a muscle if there has been a recent sprain/strain, bone injury or sharp joint pain or back injury. (See your physician for appropriate treatment and exercises.)
- Before aerobic or strength training exercise: Hold 10 seconds.
- After aerobic exercise: Hold 20-30 seconds.
- Do one set of each exercise.

5) Upper Leg

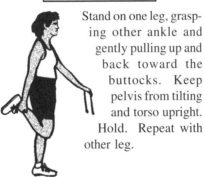

Stand on one leg, grasping other ankle and gently pulling up and back toward the buttocks. Keep pelvis from tilting and torso upright. Hold. Repeat with other leg.

6) Upper and Lower Leg

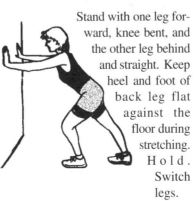

Stand with one leg forward, knee bent, and the other leg behind and straight. Keep heel and foot of back leg flat against the floor during stretching. Hold. Switch legs.

7) Lower Torso/Hips/Buttocks/Upper Leg

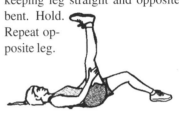

Sit with one leg straight in front, crossing other leg over. Place hand on the hip and gently pull inward until point of tightness. Hold. Repeat with other leg.

8) Buttocks/Upper and Lower Leg

Lie on back. Grasp thigh behind the knee, and gently pull towards chest, keeping leg straight and opposite leg bent. Hold. Repeat opposite leg.

9) Lower Back/Upper and Lower Leg/Buttocks

Sit on floor with one leg bent, knee to the chest, the other leg straight. Lean forward reaching out toward the toes. Hold. Repeat with the opposite leg.

10) Lower Back/Buttocks/Upper Leg

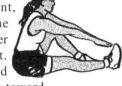

Lie on back. Grasp below and behind knees and pull thighs in toward the chest. Keep back flat. Hold.

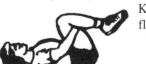

Source: Colette Cole, MS, Cooper Fitness Center, Dallas, Texas
Illustrations: Jay Colt Weesner, The Cooper Institute, Dallas, Texas

© 2009, *The Cooper Clinic Solution to the Diet Revolution* by Georgia G. Kostas, M.P.H., R.D., L.D., Dallas, Texas

Strengthening Exercises for Strong Muscles & Bones

1a) Wall Push-Up (for Beginners)

Place your hands wider than shoulder-width apart, even to shoulder height, and your feet away from the wall. By bending your elbows, lean your body toward the wall to a 90° angle at the elbow joint. Push back up to straighten your arms. Keep your back straight and your abdominals tight.

GUIDELINES

- Perform each exercise slowly.
- Begin with a weight you can lift; 10-12 repetitions with proper form.
- Rest 45-60 seconds between sets.
- Exhale while you lift; inhale when bringing weight down.
- Proper form is more important than increasing weight with improper form.
- *Beginners:* Start with one set each. As the exercise becomes easier, increase the number of sets to 2, then 3.

4) Bent-Over Row (Back)

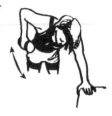

Support your body weight with one hand on a table, chair or stable object at approximately hip height. Holding the weight, pull your arm back, keeping your elbow close to your body and the palm of your hand facing inward. Pinch your shoulder blades together, keep your back straight and your abdominals tight. Bring your arm back down toward the floor, keeping a pinch in your shoulder blades. Switch arms.

1b) Push-Up (Intermediate)

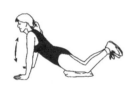

Same as above; but keep your knees on the floor. Use a pillow under your knees.

2) Flat Bench Fly (Chest)

Lie on a flat bench or surface holding weights above your chest. Slightly bend your elbows to a 90° angle and lower arms toward the floor until your elbows are even with your shoulders. Reverse the movement until the weights are above your chest.

5) Arm Extension (Triceps)

Support one hand and one knee on a flat surface. Lift and hold your elbow by your side and even with your shoulder height. Start with your hand directly below your elbow and extend your arm back, straightening your elbow. Keep your back straight and your abdominals tight. Switch arms.

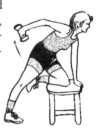

1c) Push-Up (Advanced)

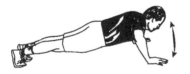

Place your hands wider than shoulder-width. Keep your back and knees straight with your feet together. Start with your elbows straight (not locked), and lower your body until there is a 90° angle in your elbow. Keep your abdominals tight, and move up and down slowly.

3) Lateral Raise (Shoulders)

Stand with your chest out and your knees slightly bent. Hold the weights by your side with your elbows slightly bent and raise them to shoulder level only. Slowly lower them until the weights are back at your side.

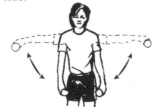

6) Arm Flexion (Biceps)

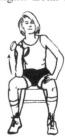

Sit on the edge of a chair with your back straight. Lean forward with your legs slightly spread. Place your elbow on your thigh holding the weight. Slowly lower and straighten your elbow with your palm facing away from your thigh. Bring the weight back toward your chest. Switch arms.

Always check with your physician before starting any exercise program.

STOP

Stop if muscle or joint pain occurs while doing any exercise. Consult your physician before continuing this exercise.

Source: Colette Cole, MS, Cooper Fitness Center, Dallas, Texas
Illustrations: Jay Colt Weesner, The Cooper Institute, Dallas, Texas

7) Squats (Legs)

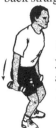

Stand with your feet hip-width apart, keeping your weight on the heels. Keep your back straight, abdominals tight and knees slightly bent. Lower your torso by bending your knees forward (not to extend past the edge of your toes) and your hips back as if sitting in a chair. Don't go lower than the diagram shows. Hold dumbbells to advance the exercise.

8) Step-Ups (Legs)

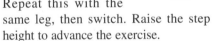

Stand with your back straight, chest out and abdominals tight. Face a step 6 to 15 inches tall. (The height of the step depends on your fitness level and height.) Place one foot on the center of the step so your knee is directly over your ankle. Lift the opposite leg and place it on the step, then return it to the floor. Repeat this with the same leg, then switch. Raise the step height to advance the exercise.

9) Heel Raises (Calf)

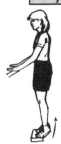

Stand on the edge of a step or stable object on the floor. Raise your heels up, then lower, stopping even with the step. Stand on one foot to advance the exercise.

10) Crunches (Abdominals)

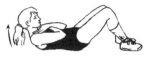

Lie on your back. Bend both legs 70-90° so the soles of your shoes are flat on the floor, and place your hands crossed over your chest. Keeping your neck aligned with torso, slowly lift your upper body until low back is flat on floor, and slowly relax. Repeat.

11) Back Extension (Low Back)

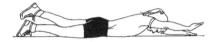

Lie face-down on the floor, with legs straight and both arms straight above your head, palms facing down. Slowly lift your right arm and left leg off the floor as comfortably as you can. Keep your knees and elbows as straight as possible. Repeat. Switch to left arm and right leg. (Keep your hips, trunk and forehead flat on the floor throughout exercise.

Just a Note:

Home Options:
There are many choices in home exercise equipment that are inexpensive and yet very effective. Some examples are Swiss balls, medicine balls, balance boards, power balls, dyna-discs and exercise tubing. The balls, boards and discs aid the development of core strength, joint stability, mobility, motor skills, and improved balance and posture. Be sure to seek the guidance of a personal trainer educated in postural alignment and body mechanics before using this equipment.

Don't wait to weight train! See for yourself . . . Lifting weight lifts your spirits!

Exercise to Prevent Osteoporosis

Osteoporosis (bone loss) has become a major health concern in America due to an increasing number of bone injury cases each year. It is estimated that osteoporosis affects two in five women and one in five men. Bone fractures caused from osteoporosis occur in half of all women and one-third of all men. And the consequences can be devastating. Studies show that people who fracture a hip have a 50% chance of not being able to walk without help, 25% chance of needing long-term care and a 10%-20% chance of dying in the first six months after injury. For more details on osteoporosis and what you can do to prevent it, read the following responses to commonly asked questions.

Q: What is osteoporosis?

A: Osteoporosis is the abnormal thinning of bones. Thinner, weaker bones break more easily. Although this disease process occurs more in women, an increasing number of men are developing this disease as we live longer. The following lifestyle factors decrease the chances of bone loss and are totally within our control: physical activity, ample calcium intake (see p. 217-218), limited caffeine and alcohol, not smoking and avoidance of certain medications. Risk factors beyond our control include: a small body build, being underweight, gender (female), fair skin, excess exercise, surgical or early menopause or amenorrhea, and a family history of osteoporosis.

Q: What can I do to help prevent the deterioration of bone tissue?

A: Most importantly, change the lifestyle risk factors you *can* control—and the sooner, the better. Women reach peak bone mass density at about age 30-35 and gradually begin to lose bone at about age 35. The more bone you start with, the less chance of a future bone injury or osteoporosis. Start early. Start young. This is critical!

Q: How much bone loss can one expect each year after age 35?

A: Approximately 1% bone loss per year for women. That's why from ages 35-65, a woman may lose 30% of her backbone and/or femur and, therefore, becomes vulnerable for falls and breaks.

Q: Why is physical activity so important in the prevention and treatment of osteoporosis?

A: Exercise increases bone density. The more the mechanical load or weight placed on the bone, the more bone density is increased.

Q: What specific activities should I do?

A: Weight-bearing activities are the key. These are upright exercises that involve gravity, movement and muscle-pull on the bone, such as walking, aerobic dance, jogging, stepping and strength training. Swimming and biking are not preferred activities because they do not put weight-bearing or "load" on the muscles and bones. Physical activity also improves muscle strength and balance, which are important factors in preventing falls. To increase bone mass, your exercise program should be specific for the desired area you wish to improve. For example, strength training on your arms only will have no effect on your trunk or legs; and vice-versa. A good strength-training program should include all major muscle groups (for balance). Consult a personal trainer who is educated on specific exercise prescriptions for the prevention of and treatment of osteoporosis. The strengthening exercises on p. 148-149 provide a beginning program for stronger bones and muscles. A trainer will help you progress further, faster.

For more information, read: Strong Women, Strong Bones by Miriam Nelson, M.D., G.P. Putnam's Sons, 2000; and Women's Health & Fitness Guide by Michele Kettles, MD, Colette Cole and Brenda Wright, Human Kinetics, 2006.

On a personal note, I can tell you that the author improved her own bone density dramatically in one year by following Colette Cole's strength-building protocol and adding more calcium!

Stay Motivated to Move!

A routine is one of the best ways to stay motivated to exercise daily. Make these incentives a part of your routine.

- **Keep it simple.** Simply move! Find ways to move daily.

- **Keep it fun.** Think of moving as your time out, thinking time, recess.

- **Think small.** Every little step helps! Don't set the bar too high.

- **Make time.** Set work limits. Get out and walk!

- **Make every activity count.** Move briskly. Go faster or further to challenge yourself. Put extra effort into cleaning your floors, windows, laundry, etc. Read your mail while on a stationary cycle. Do abdominal crunches during TV commercials. Stretch while on the phone, or do step-ups for strong calves. Hand-deliver items at work.

- **Have a change of pace...vary the intensity of your workouts.** One day push yourself a little harder (pick up your pace), and the next day keep a brisk but comfortable pace. Changing the intensity gets you fitter, faster and improves your endurance.

- **Enjoy a change of space.** A change of scenery is inspiring. Enjoy a walking trail, bike path, park, scenic area, beautiful neighborhood, lake, school track, gym, spin class, water aerobics class, etc.

- **Keep it interesting.** Cross-train. Vary your activities. It's more fun, and you'll work different muscle groups.

- **Add pep to your step…**with daily walking anywhere, whether in the grocery store, to and from your car, etc.

- **Strength-train.** You'll feel toned and possess a new sense of inner and outer strength.

- **Step up!** Take the stairs everywhere! You burn 1 calorie per 5 steps. Fifteen steps make a staircase: That's 3 calories per staircase! Take stairs up and down four round-trips a day, and you'll lose 2.5 pounds a year.

  - **Be comfortable.** Wear good walking shoes and loose clothing suitable for brisk walking or the activity you've chosen.

    - **It's never too late.** At any age, fitness and strength are attainable. Many people are fitter at ages 50-70 than 20-40.

      - **Fit activity into your life.** Do it with a friend for accountability. Join a club for social support.

        - **Anticipate interruptions.** Vacations, weekends, business travel, visitors, holidays, sick days, extra hectic days. Don't let a few days "off track" turn into weeks. Try your back-up plan and get back on track ASAP. Don't get caught in the trap of negative self-talk ("I'm bad. I didn't exercise.") Just thinking about exercise is a step in the right direction.

- **Be creative and flexible.** Opportunities to move are everywhere!

- **Be sociable.** Join a friend or groups in classes/ on teams for fun activities. You'll be energized by social companionship.

- **Think "benefits."** Reflect on the rewards from being active.

- **Home exercise.** Buy a workout video—or, if you know you'll not use it for a catch-all— spring for a treadmill.

How to Overcome Barriers to Exercise

Let's be honest: We've all had those moments when exercise was one of the least important (or most undesirable) items on our "to do" list. Exercise is a choice and a "must," and nobody can *make* you do it but yourself! The next time you confront one of the following obstacles, fight back with the solutions provided below. Identify which works best for you.

BARRIER	SOLUTIONS
Not enough time (too busy)	• Reset priorities. • Have a set time daily to exercise. • Exercise before work or a lunch break. • Walk dog twice a day (whether you have one or not!). • Increase activity in daily lifestyle: mow, rake, garden, mop, clean home, etc. • Start your day with exercise for consistency. • Split it up into two 15-minute brisk walks a day. • Schedule "walk and talk" visits/meetings with others.
Family responsibilities	• Share duties; get family involved with exercise. • Walk, bike, play tennis and volleyball together.
Inconvenient or inaccessible gym/facilities	• Get home equipment; go to the mall, local recreation centers, school track, neighborhood, YMCA, pools, classes, trails, parks, stairwells, long corridors, parking lots, etc.
Too tired	• Exercise earlier in the day—it will likely give you needed "pep."
Too out of shape	• Go slow. Take one day/step at a time.
Don't like to sweat	• Set up fan on bike/treadmill; swim; mall-walk; enjoy water-aerobics. • Split it up (three 10-minute walks).
Not enough energy	• It gives you energy and time back. See yourself as a recreational athlete.
Lack of interest	• Try a new activity; exercise while reading, watching TV, visiting with friend(s), walking a dog. • Make it fun—consider it "play time" (like kids!). • Get the right shoes and comfortable clothes to walk.
Home distractions	• Change into workout clothes before you leave work. Be "ready to go" for exercise en route (park, gym, school/track, mall), or exercise as soon as you arrive home or before going in! • Keep shoes/clothes in car for use anytime.

BARRIER	SOLUTIONS
Excessive expectations	• Get real. Be reasonable and realistic with your goals and program. • Don't let a slip-up in your routine make you give up. Just move (and lose!).
Weather (cold, hot, rain)	• Gyms, malls and indoor classes/equipment override the weather! • At home: try exercise videotapes, stairs, etc.
Bored	• Vary your program: walk, bike, kick-box, etc. • Listen/watch your favorite programs (radio, TV, video) while exercising. • Join recreational classes and teams. Ideas: dancing, bowling, softball teams, Spin classes, tennis lessons, water aerobics, volleyball groups, etc. • Create recreational physical activities such as gardening, horseback riding, dancing, volksmarching groups, hiking or biking groups; weekend charitable walks and races.
Travel a lot	• Use hotel/airport long corridors and stairwells and exercise facilities; walk malls; sight-see on foot; use hotel pool. • Have a personal trainer show you exercises for easy packing: exercise bands, ankle weights, aqua weights.
Not prepared	• Keep gym bag/shoes in car trunk at all times. • Sleep in workout clothes. The next morning, hop out of bed, into your shoes and out the door! (OK, brush your teeth first!) • Be prepared daily to exercise!

WHY EXERCISE?

According to a 1997 Discovery Health Media poll
(www.discoveryhealth.com), people exercise for the
following reasons:

22% to feel good physically

16% aerobic/cardio fitness

11% to control/lose weight

7 % to stay healthy

6 % to build strength/stamina

5 % to look good

*"Do what you can, with what
you have, with where you are."*

--Theodore Roosevelt

EXERCISE CALORIES

To calculate the exercise calories you expend per hour, find your "exercise" in the left column and your "weight" in the right column. In the place where they intersect is the figure indicating the **calories burned per hour**. For example, if you aerobic dance for 1 hour and weigh 125 pounds, you will expend 285 calories.

Activity	Weight (in pounds)				
	110	125	150	175	200
Aerobic dancing	250	285	340	395	450
Archery	225	255	305	360	410
Baseball	225	255	305	360	410
Basketball	415	470	565	660	750
Bowling	180	205	245	285	325
Calisthenics (vigorous)	225	255	305	360	410
Cross country skiing					
-moderately hilly	595	675	810	945	1080
-indoor machine (11 mph)	330	375	450	525	600
Cycling					
-outdoor (5.5 mph)	195	220	260	305	350
-outdoor (9.4 mph)	300	340	410	475	545
-outdoor racing (19 mph)	505	575	690	805	920
-Schwinn Aerodyne	510	580	695	810	925
-stationary (mod tension)	330	375	450	525	600
Golf					
-w/ Cart (90-120 minutes)	145	165	200	230	265
-no Cart (90-120 minutes)	185	210	255	295	340
Handball/Squash	635	725	870	1015	1155
Hiking – 4 mph, 20 lb. pack	355	405	490	570	650
Horseback Riding	225	255	305	360	410
Ice Skating	275	300	350	390	425
Nordic Ski Machine					
Heavy (18 mph)	1100	1250	1500	1750	2000
Medium (11 mph)	330	375	450	525	600
Light (6 mph)	225	255	305	360	410
Racquetball	550	625	750	875	1000
Roller Skating/Blading	275	300	350	390	425
Rope Skipping (100 skips/min)	560	640	765	895	1020
Rowing (sculling or machine)	620	705	845	990	1130

 © 2009, *The Cooper Clinic Solution to the Diet Revolution* by Georgia G. Kostas, M.P.H., R.D., L.D., Dallas, Texas

Activity	Weight (in pounds)				
	110	**125**	**150**	**175**	**200**
Running (Jogging)					
5:30 min/mile (11 mph)	870	985	1185	1380	1575
6:00 min/mile (10 mph)	755	860	1030	1200	1375
7:00 min/mile (8.5 mph)	685	780	935	1090	1245
7:30 min/mile (8 mph)	655	745	890	1040	1190
8:00 min/mile (7.5 mph)	625	710	850	990	1135
8:30 min/mile (7 mph)	603	685	825	960	1100
9:00 min/mile (6.5 mph)	580	660	790	920	1050
10:00 min/mile (6 mph)	535	605	730	850	970
11:00 min/mile (5.5 mph)	470	530	640	745	850
11:30 min/mile (5.25 mph)	405	460	550	645	735
12:00 min/mile (5 mph)	375	425	510	600	680
Scuba Diving	355	405	490	570	650
Snow Skiing – Downhill	300	340	410	480	545
Softball	225	255	305	360	410
Stair Climbing (moderate)	515	600	750	850	960
Stairmaster (machine)	595	675	810	945	1080
Step Aerobics - 120 steps/min	550	625	750	875	1000
Swimming - 45 min/mile	385	435	525	610	700
- 60 min/mile	300	335	405	475	540
Table Tennis (moderate)	200	225	270	315	360
Tennis - Doubles	225	255	305	360	410
- Singles	325	370	445	520	600
Treadmill - 12 min/mile	375	425	510	600	680
- 13.5 min/mile	330	375	450	525	600
Volleyball - Competitive	435	495	595	700	800
- Recreational	165	185	225	260	300
Walking/Race Walking					
12:00 min/mile (5 mph)	435	495	595	700	800
Walk/Jog Combination					
13:30 min/mile (4.5 mph)	330	375	450	525	600
Walking					
15:00 min/mile (4 mph)	300	345	415	480	550
17:00 min/mile (3.5 mph)	250	285	345	400	450
20:00 min/mile (3 mph)	225	255	310	360	410
30:00 min/mile (2 mph)	145	165	200	230	265
Weight Training/Lifting (Light)	270	310	370	430	500

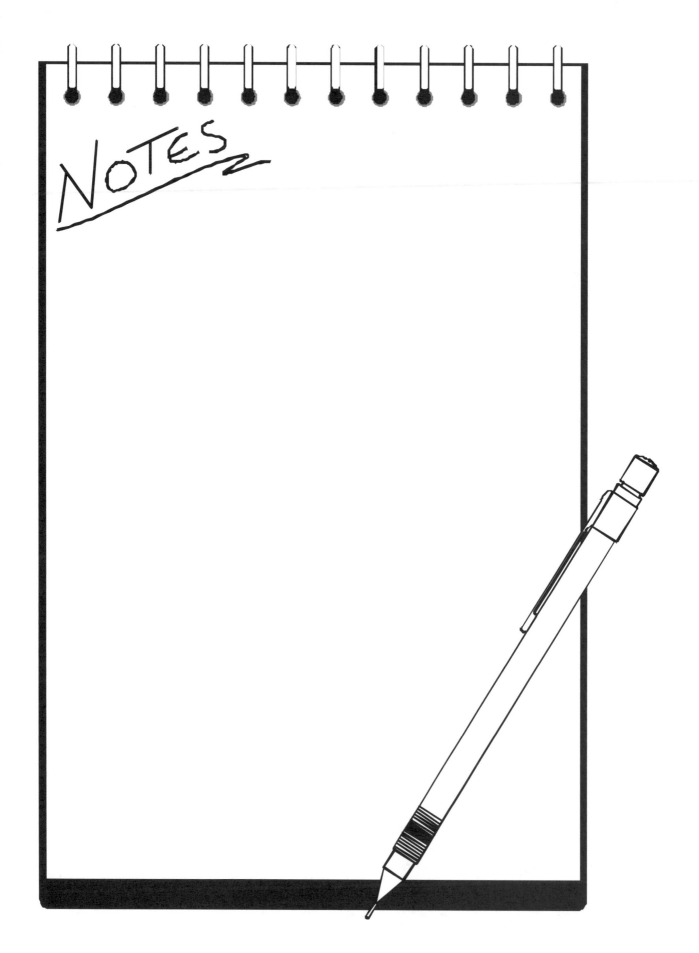

NOTES

Step 6
Flee from Fat

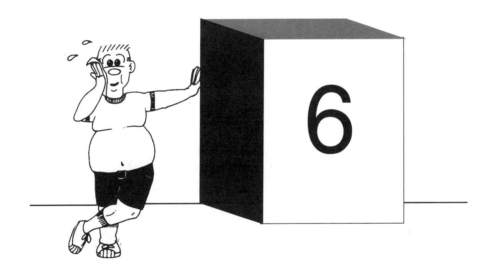

Step 6

Mini-Step 1:
Learn what type and how much fat you eat.

Mini-Step 2:
Discover 3-4 new ways to eat less fat.

This section gives you the low-down on fat. Take note: If you eat the right amount and type of fat each day, not only will you lose weight more quickly and keep it off, but you will lower your blood cholesterol and triglyceride levels and reduce your risk of heart disease and cancer. In this section, I'll help you discover:

- the different types of fats you eat
- fats in your blood
- 15 ways to eat less fat
- …and just about everything else you should know about fat!

Yes, I know, "remove" and "reduce" sound daunting—but if you can *replace* unhealthy habits with healthy ones, you'll soon realize that you aren't giving up a thing. In fact, you'll be gaining a better quality of life.

ACTION STEPS

① Eat 10 fish, poultry and vegetarian meals this week.

② Try something new this week—more oatmeal, beans, salmon, soy. You choose. Make it a habit.

Fats, Cholesterol & Heart Disease

How can you protect your heart? Eat the right type and amount of fat! This reduces artery inflammation and lessens the development of atherosclerosis, or "hardening of the arteries," the disease process that underlies most heart attacks. Elevated blood fats deposit on artery walls, become oxidized and harden as plaque, narrowing the vessel opening and restricting blood flow. If a piece of plaque breaks off, a blood clot forms and may "plug" a blood vessel, acutely impairing blood flow. This leads to heart attacks and strokes. Reduce your risk! Here's how:

Lifestyle Factors That Reduce Heart Disease:

- A healthy weight
- Aerobic exercise, 30+ minutes, 3-5 times weekly
- Healthy, balanced, low-fat eating, rich in plant foods; seafood 2 times a week
- Less abdominal fat (women's waist < 35 inches, men's < 40 inches)

- Healthy blood pressure (<120/80)
- Normal cholesterol, triglyceride and blood sugar levels; large LDL particle size
- High HDL cholesterol
- Normal c-reactive protein level (measures inflammation)
- Normal homocysteine level

- Not smoking
- Treating depression
- More vitamin D
- Less salt
- Less alcohol
- 1/2 - 1 aspirin daily
- Stress management; ample sleep

♥ Small Habits, Big Results ♥

Do this:	To lower your heart attack risk by:
☐ Eat seafood twice a week	40%
☐ Consume 5 fruits/vegetables daily	30%
☐ Eat 3 wholegrain foods daily	20-25%
☐ Consume 20 grams of fiber daily	28%
☐ Eat beans (dried) 4x a week	19%
☐ Eat 1.5 cups cooked oatmeal daily	12%
☐ Have no more than 1-2 alcoholic drinks daily	9%
☐ Exercise regularly (30 min, 5 days/wk)	14%
☐ Walk briskly 3-5 hours weekly	35%

Lose 10 lbs. and Cholesterol drops 25 points!

How Much Can Your Diet Lower LDL Cholesterol?

Recommendations of National Cholesterol Education Program		Lowers LDL by
Saturated fat	< 7% of calories (=20-30 g/day)	8-10%
Dietary cholesterol	< 200 mg/day	3-5%
Weight reduction	Lose 10 pounds	5-8%
Soluble fiber	5-10 g/day	3-5%
Plant sterols and stanols	2 g/day	6-15%
Dietary Cumulative Estimated Total:		**20-30% ♥**

Matches impact of medications!

♥ Means 50% less risk of heart attack!

With diet, exercise and weight loss, you may lower LDL by 50%!

 Try as many recommendations above as possible . . . the collective benefits add up!

What Types of Fats Are In Our Foods?

Too much unhealthy saturated or trans fat can lead to heart disease. How much and what *types* of fats are healthy?

Read below. Our **blood fat goals** are **high HDL**, and **low LDL, total cholesterol and triglycerides**. (See p.161)

Eat More

Monounsaturated Fats

mainly come from plants. They uniquely help *lower LDL and total blood cholesterol, while keeping HDL high.* Sources:
- olive oil, peanut oil, canola oil
- peanuts, almonds, pecans
- avocado, olives

Polyunsaturated Fats

usually come from plants and seafood. They *lower blood cholesterol and LDL, but may lower our HDL.* Sources:
- safflower, corn, sunflower, soy, flax, cottonseed oils
- soft tub margarines made from these oils with "liquid oil" listed as first ingredient and **no trans fats**
- non-hydrogenated ("natural") peanutbutter, where oil separates out
- seafood, especially salmon (Omega 3's)
- flaxseeds, walnuts, most nuts

Omega 3's

are polyunsaturated fats and seafood (EPA, DHA*), marine plants (DHA), plant oils, flax, soy and walnuts (ALA*), fish oil supplements and new foods with DHA or ALA added. *They promote heart health in various ways*.* Eat:
- two 6-oz servings of oily fish weekly - i.e. salmon, mackerel, sardines, or
- 4 servings of less oily fish weekly - i.e. white tuna (fresh or canned), rainbow trout, cod, bass, flounder, cod, halibut, haddock, shrimp, and
- flax seeds, canola oil, soy, walnuts or DHA & ALA-enriched foods daily. (See pg. 164.)

* **EPA** (eicosapentaenoic acid) & **DHA** (docosahexaenoic acid) *reduce heart disease, arrythmias, blood clotting, arterial wall inflammation and plaque build-up.* **DHA** *also promotes eye and brain health.* **ALA** (alpha-linolenic acid) *fights inflammation and perhaps cancer and heart disease.*

Eat Less

Saturated Fats

are found in meat and dairy, commercial pastries and snack foods. *They raise blood cholesterol and triglycerides.* Sources:
- meat fat in beef, lamb, pork, sausage, bacon, hot dogs.
- dairy fat in butter, whole milk, cheese, cream, sour cream, ice cream
- coconut and palm (kernel) oils; chocolate
- "hydrogenated" or "hardened" vegetable oils (in peanutbutter, stick margarine, crackers, commercial bakery products, etc.); also called **trans fats**

Dietary Cholesterol

is a fat-type substance in dairy, meat and desserts that can *raise blood cholesterol.* Sources:
- butter, cream, cheese, ice cream, sour cream, whole milk
- sausage, cold cuts, beef, ham, pork, lamb, bacon, hot dogs, burgers, fatty meats
- bakery products made with these foods
- egg yolks, liver and organ meats

Omit

Trans Fats

are the most harmful. *They raise LDL and total cholesterol, and lower good HDL!* These fats form from high heat or food processing when liquid oils turn to solids from "hydrogenation" (added hydrogen). They are found in:
- hard margarines, crackers, cookies, chips, purchased snack foods and desserts
- fast foods, fried foods, microwave popcorn
- foods with "hydrogenated" fats

Many restaurants now ban trans fats!

Fats in Blood

If you've been eating *too much* fat or the *wrong type* of fat—and it's easy to do if you don't read your food labels or eat out often—you now know 1) fats add calories and 2) fats affect your body chemistry, particularly your blood levels of two main circulating fats: total cholesterol (and its component HDL & LDL cholesterols) and triglycerides.

Definitions

LDL: is "low-density lipoprotein" or "bad" cholesterol that deposits in arteries. Saturated fats raise LDL levels. **We want LDL to be low**. Each 1 point decrease in LDL decreases heart disease risk by 1-2%!

HDL: stands for "high-density lipoprotein" and refers to the "healthy" cholesterol. HDL removes fat deposits in arterial walls through reverse cholesterol transport, whereby HDL transports LDL out of the arteries! **We want HDL to be high**.

Triglycerides: are fats that deposit in arteries and increase heart disease risk. Anytime we overeat fat, sugar, alcohol or calories, the surplus calories convert to triglycerides. **When we lower triglyceride levels, good HDL goes up!**

Desired Blood Levels*

* Cooper Clinic recommendations

Total Cholesterol	<	200
HDL Cholesterol	>	45+ men, 55+ women
LDL Cholesterol	<	130 (100 is ideal)
Cholesterol-to-HDL Ratio	<	4.0 (men)
	<	3.0 (women)
Triglycerides	<	150 (120 is ideal)

(< = less than) (> = more than)

How To Change Blood Levels:

To Raise HDL

- ♥ Exercise aerobically - 3 to 5 days a week, 30 to 45 minutes each time (approx 15 miles walked/jogged weekly)
- ♥ Do not smoke
- ♥ Lose weight, if needed
- ♥ Eat monounsaturated fats
- ♥ Lower triglycerides
- ♥ Eat fish (Omega 3's)

To Lower LDL & Total Cholesterol

- ♥ Lose weight, if needed
- ♥ Exercise aerobically - 3 to 5 days a week, 30 to 45 minutes per time
- ♥ Eat monounsaturated fats
- ♥ Limit foods rich in saturated fat and cholesterol
- ♥ Eat more fresh produce, oats, wholegrains, beans, nuts, seafood
- ♥ Eat plant foods with anti-oxidants to prevent cholesterol oxidation, and with flavonoids to thin blood (see p. 164)
- ♥ Eat foods with stanols/sterols

To Lower Triglycerides

- ♥ Exercise aerobically - 3 to 5 days a week, 30 to 45 minutes per time
- ♥ Lose weight, if needed
- ♥ Reduce saturated fats
- ♥ Eat more seafood (Omega 3's)
- ♥ Limit alcohol (≤2 drinks/day)
- ♥ Limit sugar and sweets

Cholesterol & Saturated Fat in Foods

How can you eat less total fat, saturated fat and cholesterol? Choose wisely!

Daily Limits:	
Cholesterol:	100-300 mg
Saturated fat:	10-20 grams, or advised by physician or registered dietitian
Total fat for weight loss:	30-40 grams fat (women) or 50-60 grams fat (men)
Total fat to maintain weight:	50 grams fat (women) or 70 grams fat (men)

FOOD *	Serving Size	Cholesterol (mg)	Saturated Fat (g)	Total Fat (g)
Egg**	1	213	1.5	6
Liver, beef**	3 oz.	370	3.5	9
Beef, pork, lamb (lean cuts) *see www.beef.org*	3 oz.	75	3.5	8
Veal (lean)	3 oz.	90	2.5	5
Chicken, Turkey (light meat without skin)	3 oz.	60	1.3	3
Fish	3 oz.	45	.1	2.5
Oysters, clams, crab**	3 oz.	120	.1	2.1
Shrimp (15 medium), lobster**	3 oz.	95	.2	1.0
Frankfurter, all beef	1	32	6.5	17
Cold cuts	3 oz.	75	6.5	21
Cheese, American or cheddar	1 oz.	25	6.0	9
Cheese, Light (2% fat)	1 oz.	20	2-4	4-6
Cheese, mozzarella (part fat-free)	1 oz.	15	3.0	5
Cheese, cottage (1% fat)	1 c.	5	1.5	2
Cheese, ricotta (part fat-free)	1 c.	40	6.0	10
Cream cheese (2 Tbsp.)	1 oz.	30	5.0	10
Milk, whole	1 c.	35	5.0	8
Milk, fat-free	1 c.	5	0	0
Yogurt, low-fat	8 oz.	15	2.5	6
Yogurt, nonfat	8 oz.	5	0.0	0
Ice cream	1 c.	55	8.0	18
Ice milk	1 c.	15	3.0	6
Butter	1 Tbsp.	35	7.0	10
Margarine, tub	1 Tbsp.	0	1-2	10
Promise Activ Spread (with sterols)	1 Tbsp.	25	1.5	8
Promise Light Activ Spread (with sterols)	1 Tbsp.	<5	1.0	5
Smart Balance Fat-free Squeeze Margarine	1 Tbsp.	6	0	0
I Can't Believe It's Not Butter spray	1 spray	0	0	0
Vegetable Oil	1 Tbsp.	0	0-2	14
Nuts	1 Tbsp.	0	0-2	5

** Not all foods are high in both cholesterol and saturated fat. Cut down on foods containing large amounts of **either**.*
** It is OK to eat shellfish (they contain no saturated fat), and 3-4 eggs weekly, and organ meats once weekly.

How To Meet Daily Limits:			
	Fat (g)	Sat fat (g)	Chol (mg)
6 oz. lean meat/fish/poultry	6-18	7	150
1 oz. low-fat cheese	4-6	2-4	25
6 tsp. unsaturated oils/fats (ie. oil, margarine, dressings)	30	0	0
fruit, vegetables, grains, beans	0	0	0
fat-free dairy products	0	0	0
Totals:	40-54	9-11	175
Goals are met	**≤60**	**10-20**	**≤300**

15 Ways to Eat Less Fat

☑ **Choose Lean Protein**:
- ☐ 4 to 6 oz. *daily total* of lean meat, poultry, seafood, low-fat cheeses.
- ☐ Vary protein sources weekly: 3-4 chicken, 3-4 fish, 3-4 lean meat, 3-4 bean or all-vegetable meals/week.
- ☐ Choose from 29 lean beef cuts such as filet, tenderloin, flank, top round, top sirloin (see www.beef.org); choose extra lean ground beef with 15% fat. For lean beef recipe ideas see *The Healthy Beef Cookbook*, by R. Chamberlain & B. Hornick.

☑ **Reduce Fat**:
- ☐ Add less fat to foods: 3 to 6 tsp. (= 1-2 Tbsp.) daily of soft tub margarine, oils, mayonnaise, dressings, etc.
- ☐ Eat fewer high-fat foods: snacks, fatty meat, hot dogs, sausage, ice cream, whole milk, fried foods, greasy foods, donuts, sweet rolls, candy bars, desserts, crackers, fast food, mayonnaise, salad dressings, creamy or cheese toppings.
- ☐ Choose specialty, low-fat products such as light margarines; low-fat and fat-free salad dressings and mayonnaise; nonfat yogurt; fat-free milk; nonfat and low-fat cheeses; tuna in water; "lite" frozen dinners; "butter" pump sprays, and spray salad dressings.
- ☐ Cook with less fat: broil, bake, grill, steam, boil, stir-fry. Use vegetable sprays and butter substitutes (i.e., Olive Oil Pam, Canola Oil Pam, I Can't Believe It's Not Butter spray, etc.)
- ☐ Read food labels. Select foods with 0-3 grams fat per 100 calories. Look for the American Heart Association's heart check mark logo on some foods (see www.heartcheckmark.org).

☑ **Eat More Plant Foods:**
- ☐ Choose at least 10 complex carbohydrate foods each day (fruit, vegetables, bread, cereal, wholegrains, starches, beans). These foods are fat-free, high in fiber and very "filling"—ideal for weight.
- ☐ Let 3/4 of your plate contain plant foods (vegetables, starches, fruit, beans) and 1/4 of your plate contain protein (entree).
- ☐ Eat more all-vegetable meals (salads, soups, baked potatoes, pasta, vegetables, beans).

☑ **Be Fat Savvy Eating Meals In or Out:**
At Restaurants:
- ☐ Split entrees. Get dressings and sauces on the side and add conservatively. Order grilled, baked, broiled, boiled, steamed foods.

At Home :
- ☐ Collect 8-10 great low-fat recipes you enjoy. Buy a low-fat cookbook that lists the nutrient analysis per recipe. Keep recipes simple, with 5-6 ingredients at most. Choose easy, convenient, quick recipes. (see Appendix B for cookbook ideas and recipes online.)
- ☐ Eat spicy foods—you won't miss fattening sauces. Add salsa, cilantro, ginger, Italian spice blends, etc.
- ☐ Choose low-fat treats and toppings:
  - ☐ top baked potatoes with yogurt, cottage cheese, salsa, marinara, butter sprinkles or sprays
  - ☐ top salads with spray dressings, yogurt, cottage cheese, salsa, balsamic vinegar, lemon
  - ☐ for snacks, try wholewheat bagels, fruit, "lite" popcorn, pretzels, popsicles, frozen nonfat yogurt, ice milk, Cheerios, homemade Chex cereal mix, wholegrained crackers or toast.

> See Step 4 for more on "Fats" and
> Step 10 for "Cooking Tips"

Heart Healthy Foods & Ingredients that Reduce Cholesterol Levels

☑ **Which will you try?**

Soluble Fiber Foods

(10-15 g/day) *Choose 1 daily:*
- ☐ 1/2 c. oat bran, cooked
- ☐ 1 1/2 c. oatmeal, cooked
- ☐ 2 pkts. Quaker Take Heart or Weight Control Instant Oatmeal
- ☐ 3 c. Cheerios
- ☐ 1/2 c. beans, peas, lentils
- ☐ 1 Tbsp. sugar-free Metamucil (psyllium)
- ☐ 2 tsp. Konsyl powder (psyllium)
- ☐ Others: broccoli, cauliflower, eggplant, Brussel sprouts, apples, oranges

Wholegrains

(3 servings daily)
- ☐ 1 c. oat cereal
- ☐ 100% wholewheat bread or cereal
- ☐ 1 c. Kashi cereals
- ☐ 1/2 c. brown rice
- ☐ 5 Reduced-fat Triscuit crackers
- ☐ 100% wholewheat or corn tortilla
- ☐ 3 cups popcorn
- ☐ 1 c. cooked Barilla Plus pasta

Fiber-rich Foods

(25-30 g daily)

Here's how:
- ☐   2 large fruit (6-8 g)
-   + 2 c. vegetables, cooked (8 g)
-   + 3 wholegrain bread slices (6 g)
-   + 1/2 c. beans or high-fiber cereal (6-8 g)
-   = **TOTAL: 20-30 g**, or
- ☐ 1/2 c. Gen. Mills Fiber One cereal (14 g)
- ☐ Quaker Instant Wt Control oatmeal pkt (6 g)
- ☐ La Tortilla Factory WW low carb tortilla, large (14 g) or small (8 g)
- ☐ Kashi Go Lean bar (6 g)

Monounsaturated Fats

(1 Tbsp. daily)
- ☐ olive oil, canola oil, peanut oil
- ☐ almonds, peanuts, pistachios
- ☐ olives, avocado
- ☐ most nuts, 2 Tbsp. per day

All foods in this column lower LDL & total cholesterol.

Omega-3 Fatty Acids

(7 g weekly)

Seafood - eat 2 times weekly, especially salmon, tuna, swordfish, haddock, sardines
- ☐ 6 oz. Salmon or Mackerel (3.7 g)
- ☐ 6 oz. Tuna steak or Striped Bass (1.6 g)
- ☐ 3 oz. Tuna, white, canned (0.3 g)
- ☐ 6 oz. Snapper, Flounder, Cod, Sole, Halibut, most white fish (1 g)
- ☐ or daily fish oil supplement (i.e., Cooper Complete Advanced Omega-3)
- ☐ or 1 tsp. cod liver oil daily

Plant sources (with ALA Omega-3) -
- ☐ 1 Tbsp. flax oil (7 g)
- ☐ 1 Tbsp. ground flaxseed (1.6 g)
- ☐ 1 Tbsp. canola oil (1.6 g)
- ☐ 1 Tbsp. soybean oil (1g)
- ☐ 2 Tbsp. walnuts (1 g)

DHA Omega-3 fortified Foods:

(we need .16 g DHA daily)
- ☐ 8 oz. Tropicana Healthy Heart Orange Juice (.05 g)
- ☐ 1 c. Silk Plus Omega-3 soy milk (.03 g)
- ☐ 1 c. Horizon Organic Milk Plus DHA (.03 g)
- ☐ 1 oz. Cabot Low-fat Cheddar cheese w/ Omega-3 (.03 g)
- ☐ two 4-oz. cartons Yoplait Kids yogurt (.03 g)
- ☐ 1 Horizon Omega-3 egg (.2 g)

ALA Omega-3 fortified Foods:
- ☐ 1 Tbsp. Promise Activ or Activ Light spreads (.55 g)
- ☐ 1 Tbsp. Smart Balance Omega Plus or I Can't Believe It's Not Butter Mediterranean spreads (.4 g)
- ☐ 3/4 c. Health Valley Organic Golden Flax cereal (1 g)
- ☐ 3/4 c. Nature's Path Flax Plus Raisin Bran (.6 g)
- ☐ 1 c. Kashi Go Lean Crunch Honey Almond flax cereal (.5 g)
- ☐ 1 c. cooked Hodgson Mill Organic Wholewheat Pasta w/Flax (.6 g)
- ☐ 1 c. cooked Barilla Plus Pasta (.2 g)
- ☐ 1 Tbsp. Smart Balance Omega-3 Peanutbutter (.5 g)
- ☐ 1 Tbsp. Spectrum Organic Omega-3 Soy Mayonnaise (2 g)
- ☐ 1 Tbsp. Hellman's Canola Mayonnaise (1 g)

Omega-3's improve heart, eye and brain health, and reduce triglycerides, blood pressure and inflammation.

Stanols/Sterols

(2 g daily total)

Eat 2 servings at meals daily to lower cholesterol 20 points in 6 wks! 1 serving =
- ☐ 1/2 bottle Promise Activ SuperShot
- ☐ 1 Tbsp. Promise Activ spread or Promise Active Light
- ☐ 2 Tbsp. Benecol or Benecol Light spread
- ☐ 2 Tbsp. Smart Balance Omega Plus Spread
- ☐ 8 oz. Minute Maid Heart Wise OJ
- ☐ 1 Coco Via (chocolate) bar
- ☐ Nature Valley Healthy Heart granola bar
- ☐ Bayer Aspirin Plus, 1 caplet (.4 g)
- ☐ Choles-Off or Red Yeast Rice tablets
- ☐ Benecol Smart Chews (order online)
- ☐ 8 oz. Kroger Active Lifestyle Milk
- ☐ 3 slices Orowheat Wholegrain & Oat Bread
- ☐ 1 oz. Lifetime Low-fat Cheese

Fruit & Vegetables

(5+ daily)

Choose from each grouping daily:
- ☐ 5+ colorful fruit and vegetables
- ☐ greens
- ☐ "red" foods (grapes, berries, tea)
- ☐ onions, leeks, garlic, shallots
- ☐ citrus, apples, bananas, cherries
- ☐ cruciferous vegetables, eggplant, carrots

Antioxidants & phytochemicals in these foods prevent plaque in arteries; flavonoids in "red" foods & onion family are natural blood thinners & clot-busters.

Foods with Folic Acid

(400-800 mcg daily)

These lower homocysteine:
- ☐ greens, beans, orange juice, asparagus, broccoli
- ☐ fortified cereals, bread, rice
- ☐ supplement (with vitamins B6 & B12)

Nonfat or Low-fat Dairy

(2-3 daily)

Choose foods with Vitamin D.
- ☐ 1 oz. milk, yogurt
- ☐ 1 c. Kroger Active Lifestyle Milk
- ☐ 1 oz. low-fat (1-2% fat) cheeses
- ☐ 1 oz. Cabot 50% less & 75% less fat cheeses (Cheddar, Pepper Jack, Jalapeno)

© 2009, *The Cooper Clinic Solution to the Diet Revolution* by Georgia G. Kostas, M.P.H., R.D., L.D., Dallas, Texas

Step 7
Master Eating Out
and Special Occasions

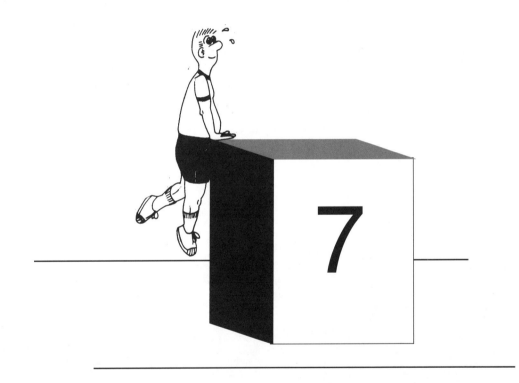

Step 7

Mini-Step 1:

Eating out does not mean over-eating! Try these behavorial strategies.

Mini-Step 2:

Learn how to order 500-700 calorie meals out at salad bars, fast food places, etc.— your key to "eating out" success.

Gathering with friends and family for a special celebration is part of our lifestyle—and eating goes along with it. With this step you'll learn how to develop strategies for special situations such as parties, entertaining, weekends, travel, holidays, vacations, and most importantly, dining at restaurants. The good news: You can become an expert at cutting down on calories at any social function!

If you're like most Americans, eating out is a way of life. What are your wisest selections of . . . entrees? ethnic foods? fast foods? salad bar items? desserts?

The "Meals Out" comparison chart may benefit you more than any single chart in this book! Check it out. I provide examples of typical meals that pack in roughly 2,000 calories/100 fat grams. Then I list variations that can dramatically reduce the calorie count to 500-700 and fat grams to 25 or fewer. Talk about worthwhile! With this knowledge, you'll feel empowered to lose weight, even when dining out.

ACTION STEPS

① Plan a new strategy for handling food at a special occasion, vacation, weekend, holiday. Repeat what works.

② Practice ordering a 500-700 calorie meal out. Also, try splitting an entree with one person and sharing a dessert with several others.

③ Become more savvy at salad bars. Skip prepared salads with mayonnaise such as potato or tuna salad. Instead, load up on fresh fruits and veggies and use dressings sparingly.

④ Replace alcohol with a low-calorie beverage such as a club soda mixed with juice.

Managing Special Occasions

Special situations easily trigger eating and may disrupt your good eating goals. How do you handle eating in restaurants, entertaining friends or relatives, parties, traveling, vacations, holidays, weekends, binges, snacks, celebrations? The key, I'm convinced, is to develop strategies. How?

1. **Anticipate** an eating situation and how you will take control of it. Rehearse an imagined scene. Be optimistic and picture yourself successfully eating in a planned manner and enjoying it. Re-enact your "preview." Enjoy your success.

2. **Plan alternative activities**. What can you do in various eating situations to avoid overeating? Think of several ideas in advance, then practice them. For example, drink more water before eating; take a before-dinner walk; plan a dinner conversation.

3. **Learn to relax**. Practice relaxation techniques such as imagery, exercise before eating, or enjoy other activities that calm you and help you control your eating urges. What relaxes you? A shower? Classical music? What about a manicure? Be creative.

4. **Pre-plan meals and snacks**...and follow your decision.

5. **Rethink social events** as a time for people—not just food and drink.

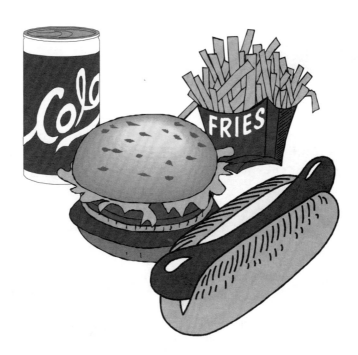

Entertaining & Parties

FOR THE HOST

If you are hosting, here are some ways to make the event a success for everyone:

1. **Present food creatively.** A festive table means more than calories.

2. **Offer low-calorie options,** such as raw vegetables and fresh fruits, a cottage cheese or yogurt dip, salads, baked or broiled meats, sauces on the side. Guests can decide for themselves whether they want the "extras." You don't have to serve only "diet foods." Serve smaller portions of your favorite rich foods and larger portions of lighter foods.

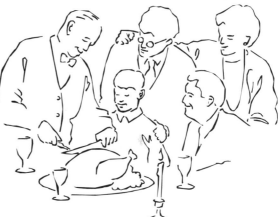

3. **Cut desserts** into different size portions. Let your guests choose their portions.

4. **Prepare the least tempting foods first** and the most tempting last. You will have less time to snack on your favorite things.

5. **Have everything ready early** so you can relax and get ready at a leisurely pace.

6. **Give away leftovers** (without being pushy).

7. **If you receive food gifts**, wrap them up and freeze them to serve to future guests.

FOR THE GUEST

Perhaps you've been invited to a party. Since you aren't in the driver's seat, what can you do to stay on the health bandwagon?

1. **Never arrive hungry.** Curb your appetite with a small, healthy snack (such as an apple) before going to a party. Don't use the excuse, "I've starved all day!" Your body doesn't see it that way.

2. **Focus on the people—not the foods.** Talk more and eat less. Make it a point to carry on a conversation with at least 10 people individually.

3. **Take something "light,"** such as a raw vegetable plate, fruit plate, popcorn, low-fat cheese, crackers, pretzels, etc. Your host will appreciate your gesture, and you will be sure to have something nutritious to eat.

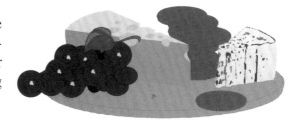

4. **Set ground rules before you go out.** Decide to eat one mini-serving of everything, or skip certain foods such as chips, butter, "loaded" potatoes, olives, nuts, etc.

5. **Drink water, club soda, low-calorie beverages.** Having something in your hand at a party such as a drink may help you feel more comfortable. In addition, it keeps a hand too occupied to reach for more food! Avoid high-calorie drinks such as alcohol, Frappuccino, eggnog or punch.

6. **Minimize food contact.** Never stand near a food table to talk.

7. **Scan a buffet table and decide what you want.** Then fill a plate just *once*. No seconds except vegetables! Sit away from the food table.

8. **Serve yourself.** Do not accept food from others.

9. **Eat slowly.** The quicker you finish, the more your host may tempt you with seconds. In 20 minutes, second helpings seem less appealing.

10. **Plan responses to insistent hosts.** For example: "No, thank you...everything was delicious, but I can't eat another bite." Or, "No, thank you. But I would enjoy a glass of water."

11. **Remind yourself** that refusing food does not mean rejection and, conversely, that eating and overeating does not mean "I like you."

12. **Don't tell anyone you are "dieting."** You might be encouraged to "forget the diet—it's a special occasion!" Besides, most people don't notice if you skip rich dishes.

13. **Request a small serving or half of a serving.** When you verbalize your commitment, you will not back down!

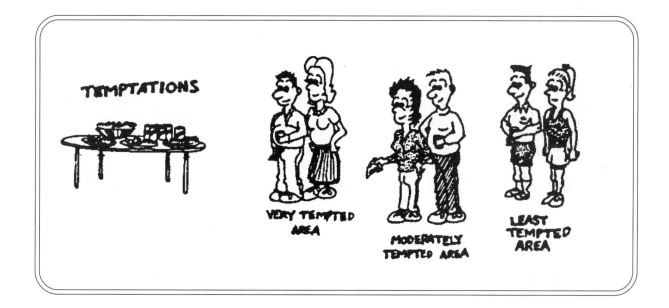

ating Out Skills

If you have gone to all-you-can-eat buffets all of your life, you will need to make some changes in order to maintain a healthy weight. Likewise, if you have become used to rich, cream-based foods, you will need to select alternative entrees. Below are 19 tips to help you master the art of dining out the healthful way.

1. **Choose restaurants** that have the type of foods you want.

2. **Learn to enjoy the company** more than the food.

3. **Decide ahead of time** what you will order. (Pick up a menu beforehand if you can!) Write down your selection. This prevents temptation.

4. **Share entrees** to save 250-750 calories (and several dollars!). Or take the other half of your order home for tomorrow.

5. **Ask for "double vegetables"** and **"half the entree."**

6. **Order salad dressings on the side.** Use 1-2 Tbsp.

7. **Ask how foods are prepared.** Request substitutes (i.e., margarine instead of butter, baked fish or chicken instead of breaded and fried, baked potato instead of fried, clear soup instead of a creamy one, onion soup without the bread and cheese topping, steamed vegetables without sauces, etc.).

8. **Start meals with volume:** water, diet drinks, salads, raw vegetables, clear soup, hot tea. (Or start with a snack like this at home.)

9. **Avoid fried or creamed foods, thick gravies, cheese sauces or sugar glazes.** If you have no choice, remove the crust, or push the sauce aside and eat the food underneath.

10. **Order meat and fish broiled or baked, poultry without skin, veal, lean cuts of beef** (such as a filet, top sirloin, flank, London broil, shishkabob). Assume butter, and ask for entrees without butter or sauces. You could also ask for them on the side and use sparingly.

11. **Omit fat-filled foods such as chips or fries.** If the restaurant will substitute, request fruit, soup, tomato slices, etc.

12. **Ask to remove bread and butter, chips, crackers, etc., from the table.** Or, move food to the far end of the table, away from you to avoid a hand's reach.

13. **Drink water, tea, diet drink, club soda or coffee** as a beverage. Sip slowly throughout the meal.

14. **Choose hot tea or decaffeinated coffee as an appetizer.** Hot liquids empty from the stomach slowly, and you'll feel less hungry.

15. **If you're ordering a hamburger,** get a 1/4-pound size with *double* tomato, double lettuce, pickles, onion, mustard. Skip mayonnaise, cheese, bacon, sauces.

16. **At salad bars, try these suggestions:**

- Choose lettuce greens, cucumbers, radishes, carrots, green pepper, onions, beets, mushrooms, bean sprouts, cauliflower, tomatoes, beans, peas, broccoli. These are low-calorie ingredients. (Try juice from a three-bean salad as dressing.)

- Avoid thick, creamy salad dressings, croutons, cheese toppings, seeds, nuts, olives, avocado, bacon bits, creamed items. They are high in calories and in fat.

- Limit prepared salads—pasta, potato, coleslaw, chicken or tuna salad, marinated vegetables, etc. Most of these also are high in fat.

17. **Decide ahead of time to pass up dessert,** despite what others do. Instead, sip on water, coffee or tea. If the others are willing and you *really* want to try a dessert, see if they will split it four ways. (Only eat your fair share!)

18. **Take home leftovers of large portions.** Add an extra vegetable "to go," and you'll be set for a complete meal tomorrow.

19. **If you overeat,** have your own compensating strategy for the next day: an "all vegetable" day, soup day, exercise day, mini-meal day or two-meal day. Don't make this a regular practice.

Menu Words to Know

Choose	Avoid
Broiled, grilled	Fried, buttered
Poached, steamed	Gravies, sauces
Stir-fried	Au gratin
Marinara sauce	Cheese or cream sauces
Piccata (lemon-wine sauce)	Casseroles, pot pies
Tomato sauce	Pesto sauce
Red or white clam sauce	Parmigiana
Wine sauce	Marinated

A Word About Alcohol

Many people enjoy having a glass of wine with a meal—and in moderation, this may be fine. But keep in mind that alcohol is full of calories, virtually devoid of nutrients, may slow down fat-burning and typically weakens one's eating willpower. For these reasons, many often find it best to avoid alcohol altogether when managing their weight.

Recent studies have shown that a *moderate* intake of alcohol may have a positive effect on heart health, but consuming more than this has a negative impact, increasing one's risk of high blood pressure, elevated triglycerides, and certain types of cancer (breast and colon). What is "moderation"? One serving a day for women and two servings a day for men. The box below defines a "serving size", which is approximately 100 calories.

1 serving =	5 oz. wine
	1.5 oz. liquor
	12 oz. beer or light beer

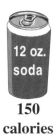

150 calories

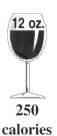

250 calories

See how quickly alcohol calories add up!

Beverage	Serving Size	Calories
Light beer	12 oz. can	100
Beer	12 oz. can	150
Dry wine (red or white)	6 oz. glass	125
Sweet wine	6 oz. glass	270
Champagne	6 oz. flute	160
Bloody Mary	10 oz. glass	125
Rum and Diet Coke	6 oz. glass	100
Gin and Tonic	6 oz. glass	180
Martini	4 oz. glass	250
Cosmopolitan	4 oz. glass	215
Mojito	8 oz. glass	350
Daquiri	8 oz. glass	450-850
Margarita	12 oz. glass	550-650

How can you enjoy a drink without gaining weight? Drink occasionally. Invest in smaller serving glasses. Limit yourself to one drink (women) or two (men). Plan ahead by including the beverage in your day's total calories. Pay close attention to **serving sizes** - just as food portion sizes have increased in recent years, so have alcohol serving sizes. Your best bet is to choose beer, wine, or liquor mixed with a no or low calorie mixer such as diet soda or tomato juice. Sweet and sour mixes, juices or sweet liqueurs add a lot of calories.

Alternatives: I recommend ordering bottled water, diet soft drinks, club soda with a twist of lime, tomato or V-8 or cranberry juice, iced tea, flavored water, sugar-free fruit flavored seltzer, other low-calorie drinks or club soda mixed with juice. These alternatives may spare you from a "spare tire"!

Eating Out Menu Tips

To make it easier for you to select from a menu, become very familiar with this list—or take it along with you the next time you dine out! Treat it like a dear friend!

FOOD	CHOOSE	LIMIT
APPETIZERS	Broth, bouillon, consommé, gazpacho, tomato juice, V-8 juice, fruit, fruit cup, fruit juice, raw vegetables, shrimp or crab cocktail, oysters on the half shell	Cream soups, chowders, fried foods, nachos, potato skins
SALADS	Fresh fruit, vegetable with salad dressing on the side, raw vegetables, chef's salad with turkey or chicken (omit cold cuts)	Potato salad, macaroni salad, Jell-O salad, coleslaw, taco salad with guacamole
MEATS	Baked, roasted or broiled: fish, poultry (chicken, turkey, Cornish hen); lean cuts of beef, veal, lamb, pork, tenderloin steaks (filet, T-bone, top sirloin). Poached or boiled eggs; cottage cheese	Fried, breaded, with gravy or sauce or combinations (stew, casseroles, hash, etc.). Fried or scrambled eggs; eggs benedict
SANDWICHES	Chicken, turkey, tuna or lean roast beef on wholewheat bread with lettuce and tomato, without mayonnaise	Luncheon meats (cold cuts), sausage, hot dogs, hamburgers, fried meat
POTATOES, STARCHES	Baked, boiled, mashed potatoes (with condiments on side); corn, rice, pasta with marinara or tomato sauce	Fried, au gratin, scalloped, hash-browned, with meat or cream cheese sauces
VEGETABLES	Raw, boiled, steamed, baked; or vegetable plate as a meal	Fried, creamed, au gratin, with sauces or gravies
BREADS	All plain breads and rolls, English muffins, breadsticks, crackers, graham crackers (preferably whole grains)	Sweet rolls and muffins, coffee cake, Danish pastry, doughnuts, garlic bread
FATS	Margarine, salad dressing, mayonnaise (limited amounts)	Butter, cream, sour cream, gravy, sauces, olives, nuts, avocados, fried foods, bacon
DESSERTS	Fresh fruit, sherbet, angel food cake, nonfat frozen yogurt, sorbet, ice milk, fruit ice, popsicles	Pies, cakes, custards, puddings, cookies, sweetened fruits, ice cream
BEVERAGES	Coffee, tea, skim milk, buttermilk, diet drinks, water	Chocolate milk, regular soft drinks, milk shakes, lemonade, alcohol
MISCELLANEOUS	Chicken fajitas, soft chicken tacos, cheese pizza, bean soups	Sausage pizza, greasy or fried dishes

Note: Order all foods without butter or margarine, mayonnaise, gravy, sauces, salad dressing, etc. Add your own "on the side" topping to control portions.

© 2009, *The Cooper Clinic Solution to the Diet Revolution* by Georgia G. Kostas, M.P.H., R.D., L.D., Dallas, Texas

Meal Comparisons

How quickly those calories add up when we eat out! It's easy to consume more calories in one meal than we typically need in a day. My top 5 recommendations: (1) *Avoid appetizers completely*, unless you select fruit, vegetables, tomato soup, sliced tomatoes, a salad, shrimp cocktail, or hot tea; (2) *Split an entree* or *take 1/2 home*; (3) Ask for "*double vegetables*"; (4) Always *order dressings and sauces "on the side"*; (5) *Select seafood and poultry* dishes primarily. Most appetizers are loaded with fat and calories, as you'll see below.

Take a look at the meal comparisons I've provided. Most meals out contain 2,000 calories and 100 grams of fat! See how you can transform a 2,000-calorie meal into one with 500 to 700 calories (and no more than 25 fat grams)—and still get a delicious array of food!

STEAK HOUSE

Instead of:

	Cal	Fat (g)
16-oz. rib-eye (cooks to 12 oz.)	1050	75
1 baked potato,	300	0
"loaded" w/ 1 Tbsp. butter,	100	5
1 Tbsp. sour cream,	30	3
1 Tbsp. cheese	35	3
1 dinner roll	80	1
w/ 1 tsp. margarine	35	4
tossed salad	25	0
w/ 4 Tbsp. dressing	320	32
4 oz. wine	100	0
Total:	**2075**	**123**

Try This:

	Cal	Fat (g)
6-oz. filet steak (tenderloin)	360	18
1 small baked potato or 1/2		
large potato, w/	150	0
1 tsp. margarine*, chives	35	4
1 Tbsp. sour cream	30	3
tossed salad	25	0
w/ 1 Tbsp. light dressing**	50	5
Water	0	0
Total:	**650**	**30**

* add salsa or soy sauce = 0 cal, 0 g fat, or
   add 1 Tbsp. cheese = 35 cal, 3 g fat
**1 Tbsp. regular dressing adds 80 cal, 8 g fat

MEXICAN RESTAURANT

Instead of:

	Cal	Fat (g)
30 large chips	750	45
with salsa	0	0
2 large beef enchiladas	1000	70
1 serving Spanish rice	300	12
1 serving refried beans	350	18
1 Margarita	450	0
Total:	**2850**	**145**

Note:
A basket of chips = 1200-1500 calories, 75-90 g fat!

Try This:

	Cal	Fat (g)
3 soft corn tortillas; salsa	200	0
Fajitas (1/2 order):		
2 flour tortillas	200	5
4 oz. chicken (no oil)	200	6
pico de gallo, lettuce,	0	0
tomato, onion		
1/2 c. borracho beans (1/2 order)	120	1
Water or tea	0	0
Total:	**720**	**12**

Note:
1. Skip guacamole and sour cream. Ask for "no oil" with chicken.
2. Taco salads with picante sauce = 670 cal, 40 g fat.

TEXAS-STYLE

Instead of:	Cal	Fat (g)		Try This:	Cal	Fat (g)
6 oz. barbecue beef brisket	600	42		4 oz. barbecue chicken breast (remove skin)	210	5
1/2 c. fried okra	200	12		1 med. corn on the cob	100	2
1 fried pie	300	15		w/ 1 tsp. margarine	35	4
3/4 c. potato salad	430	38		1/2 c. coleslaw	180	7
12 oz. soft drink or beer	150	0		1 large dinner roll	160	2
				water	0	0
Total:	**1680**	**107**		**Total:**	**685**	**20**

ITALIAN RESTAURANT

Instead of:	Cal	Fat (g)		Try This:	Cal	Fat (g)
typical serving lasagna	1200	50		2 cups spaghetti (no oil)*	400	0
1 slice buttered garlic bread	200	12		w/ meat-free tomato sauce	150	10
tossed salad	25	0		2 slices Italian bread (no butter)	160	2
w/ 2 Tbsp. Italian dressing	160	16		tossed salad	25	0
1 piece cheesecake	350	23		w/ 1 Tbsp. Italian dressing	80	8
6 oz. red wine	150	0		1 serving berries or fruit	60	0
				water	0	0
Total:	**2085**	**102**		**Total:**	**875**	**20**

Note: 4 cups pasta often served; ask for "no oil"

FRENCH RESTAURANT

Instead of:	Cal	Fat (g)		Try This:	Cal	Fat (g)
6 oz. Chicken Kiev	500	33		6 oz. Chicken in Rosé Sauce	350	16
1 c. cream of celery soup	150	10		1/2 c. sautéed fresh vegetables	65	4
1/2 c. wild rice	150	5		watercress & romaine salad	15	0
1/2 c. sautéed mushrooms	45	4		w/ 1 Tbsp. French or Ranch dressing	55	6
1 dinner roll	80	1		1 slice French bread (3")	70	1
w/ 1 tsp. margarine/butter	35	4		fresh seasonal fruit plate	100	0
Caesar salad (w/ croutons, cheese) and	200	13				
4 Tbsp. dressing	320	32				
Chocolate soufflé	320	22				
Total:	**1800**	**124**		**Total:**	**655**	**27**

SEAFOOD RESTAURANT

Instead of:	Cal	Fat (g)
6 oz. fried fish w/ batter (3 pieces)	400	23
3 hush puppies	150	7
1/2 c. coleslaw	180	10
1 large order French fries	475	25
12 oz. soft drink	150	0
Total:	**1355**	**65**

Try This:	Cal	Fat (g)
8 oz. baked or broiled fish w/ lemon, no butter*	240	3
1/2 c. broccoli w/ margarine	60	4
1/2 c. rice w/ margarine	150	4
1 wholewheat roll	80	1
water	0	0
Total:	**530**	**12**

*add 100 cal, 10 g fat if 1 1/2 Tbsp. lemon-butter used

CHINESE RESTAURANT

Instead of:	Cal	Fat (g)
1 eggroll	200	12
3 c. sweet & sour pork w/ vegetables	1450	80
1 c. fried rice	370	12
1 fortune cookie	30	2
6 oz. sake (rice wine)	240	0
Total:	**2290**	**106**

Try This:	Cal	Fat (g)
2 c. chicken chow-mein (lunch portion or 1/2 dinner)*	500	16
3/4 c. steamed rice (1/2 portion)	160	0
1 fortune cookie	30	2
Jasmine Tea	0	0
Total:	**690**	**18**

*Any stir-fried dish w/vegetables & chicken, shrimp or beef will be approx. 500-600 cal, 10-20 g fat. Evening portions will be larger (4 cups). Eat half, and take the rest home.

FAST-FOOD RESTAURANT

Instead of:	Cal	Fat (g)
1 quarter-pound cheese-burger	525	30
1 small order French fries	220	12
regular chocolate shake	350	8
Total:	**1095**	**50**

Try This:	Cal	Fat (g)
1 roast beef sandwich (medium, i.e., Arby's)	350	15
1/2 small order French fries	110	6
tossed salad with	25	0
1 Tbsp. light dressing**	20	2
water	0	0
Total:	**505**	**23**

** 1 Tbsp. regular dressing = avg. 80 cal, 8 g fat

PIZZA

Instead of:

	Cal	Fat (g)
4 pcs. 12" pepperoni pizza	940	40
2 beers (24 oz.)	300	0
Total:	**1240**	**40**

Try This:

	Cal	Fat (g)
2 pcs.12" cheese pizza w/ mushrooms, green pepper, onion	400	14
tossed salad	25	0
w/ 1 Tbsp. French dressing	55	6
water or iced tea	0	0
Total:	**480**	**20**

OTHER WAYS TO MAKE A RESTAURANT MEAL LESS THAN 500 CALORIES:

1

Steak Dinner	Cal	Fat (g)
6-oz. filet steak	360	18
1 small baked potato or 1/2 large	150	0
w/ 2 pats margarine & chives	70	8
tossed salad	25	0
w/ 1 Tbsp. French or ranch dressing	55	6
water	0	0
Total:	**660**	**32**

Steak Dinner Revised	Cal	Fat (g)
3-oz. filet steak*	180	9
1 small baked potato or 1/2 large	150	0
w/ 1 pat margarine & chives	35	4
tossed salad	25	0
w/ 1 Tbsp. French or Ranch dressing	55	6
water	0	0
*split with a friend or take 1/2 home		
Total:	**445**	**19**

2

Dinner of Appetizers	Cal	Fat(g)
5 jumbo boiled shrimp w/ 2 Tbsp. cocktail sauce	100	0
salad w/ 1 Tbsp. dressing	100	8
soup (1 c. vegetable)	100	5
large bread or roll without butter	100	1
Total:	**400**	**14**

See p. 180 for websites of restaurants that list nutrient analysis of their foods.

ADDITIONAL TIPS

If you do eat more calories and fat at a restaurant, eat lightly at the next meal. Let your week balance the fat. If you eat out frequently, ask for an all-vegetable meal 3-4 times a week. Ask to split an entree. Note that entrees contain the most calories and fat. Think of eating out as mealtime, not "splurge" time.

Eating Out : Are You Calorie Savvy?

Recent surveys show that we are eating out more and more. Most Americans consume five or more meals out a week that averages an extra 250 calories a day. That could put on 25 pounds a year! Gaining a sense of "higher-calorie" and "lower-calorie" options enables us to blend food selections so that our overall calorie intake is reasonable . . . just "go heavy on the light foods, and light on the heavy foods." Learn when to share portions (entrees, desserts, appetizers, rich foods) and when to "double up" (on veggies).

EXTRAS: APPETIZERS, DESSERTS, SNACKS

√ Best choices

Be selective with "extras" (appetizers, desserts, snacks). Any alone can equal the calories of an entire meal. Keep these "sides" at 100 - 200 calories. Sharing is the easiest way to cut calories!

Appetizers

	Amount	Cal	Fat (g)		Amount	Cal	Fat (g)
fried onion	1 large	1700	81	buffalo wings	12	700	50
Mexican chips	1 basket	1250	73	chicken wings	2	150	8
cheese fries	2 cups	1200	85	chicken fingers, fried	2	100	7
potato skins, loaded	8 pieces	1260	95	cream soup	1 cup	250	15
	2 pieces	315	24	√ vegetable soup	1 cup	100	5
chili con queso dip	1/2 cup	250	20	√ gazpacho	1 cup	50	0
and chips	12 chips	300	18	√ French onion soup	1 cup	150	9
fried zucchini	1/2 cup	200	12	√ fruit cup	1 cup	100	0
fried cheese	1 stick	200	20	√ shrimp w/ cocktail	5 large	50	0
cheese nachos	1 order	810	48	sauce			
	3 nachos	200	12	*√ try to keep between 100 - 200 cal.*			

Desserts / Pastries

	Amount	Cal	Fat (g)		Amount	Cal	Fat (g)
fudge brownie sundae		1130	57	√ nonfat frozen yogurt	1 cup	200	0
cheesecake	1 thick slice	630	47	√ poached pear	1	170	0
rich vanilla ice cream	1 cup	540	35	√ fresh fruit	1 cup	50-100	0
apple pie	8 oz. slice	540	28	√ biscotti	1	100	2
Starbucks cinnamon				√ Altoid mint	1	3	0
scone	1	530	26				
Cinnabon cinnamon							
roll	1	670	34				

Snacks

	Amount	Cal	Fat (g)		Amount	Cal	Fat (g)
Movie theater popcorn				Big Gulp giant cola	44 oz.	510	0
buttered, large	22 1/2 c.	1575	112	Pizza	1 lg. slice	500	20
small	7 cups	490	35	Deli bagel	1 large	300	0
without butter	7 cups	400	27	➤ *See p. 120-123 for more ideas.*			

  © 2009, *The Cooper Clinic Solution to the Diet Revolution* by Georgia G. Kostas, M.P.H., R.D., L.D., Dallas, Texas

TYPICAL ENTREE CHOICES

Try to keep your entire meal at 500 - 700 calories, 25 or less grams of fat. Note that by sharing entrees or taking half home, many more food options fit in!

Mexican

	Cal	Fat (g)		Cal	Fat (g)
√ Tacos, chicken (2)	420	30	Tostada	650	37
√ Beef fajitas	615	24	Cheese enchiladas (2)	830	60
Chile con Carne	375	17	Taco salad in taco shell	1065	70
√ Tamale	415	25	√ without shell, guaca-	518	32
Quesadilla	475	33	mole, sour cream		
Tacos, beef (2)	500	35	Arroz con pollo	1200	74
Mexican chips (25)	625	36			

Italian

	Cal	Fat (g)		Cal	Fat (g)
√ Veal Picatta	300	21	Pasta Primavera	550	32
√ Chicken Parmigiana	400	25	Manicotti with meat	560	32
√ Veal Parmigiana	500	30	Chicken Cacciatore	600	42
√ Pasta e Fagioli	600	22	Ravioli with meat	750	37
√ Spaghetti w/ tomato sauce	850	17	Calzone	850	38
(3 1/2 c.)			Cannelloni, beef	890	50
Tomato/Mozzarella Salad	275	23	Spaghetti w/meatballs (3 1/2 c.)	1155	39
Garlic bread (1/4 loaf)	515	25	Fettucini Alfredo	1200	78
Caesar salad	520	45	Lasagna	1200	50

Chinese

	Cal	Fat (g)		Cal	Fat (g)
√ + Szechwan shrimp (4 c.)	927	20	√ + Kung Pao chicken (5 c.)	1620	75
√ + Chicken chow mein (5 c.)	1000	30	Fried rice (2 c.)	740	24
√ + Beef and broccoli (4 c.)	1175	45	BBQ spare ribs, pork	1225	78
√ + General Tso's chicken (5 c.)	1600	60			

+ *ask for 1/2 order to consume 500-800 calories*

Greek

	Cal	Fat (g)		Cal	Fat (g)
√ Spinach pie with feta	450	23	Humus, 1/2 c.	325	18
√ Gyro	520	17	Moussaka	630	48
Greek salad with feta	250	22			

TIP

Choose "healthy," "lite" and similar menu items.

American

	Cal	Fat (g)		Cal	Fat (g)
√ Broiled chicken (no skin, 6 oz.)	240	7	Loaded baked potato	620	30
√ Broiled fish filet (with butter)	250	7	Chicken fingers (5)	620	34
√ Grilled chicken sandwich (no mayo)	300	8	Prime rib (cooked, 6 oz.)	650	55
			Chicken pot pie	680	37
√ Turkey sandwich, deli, no mayo	320	6	Hamburger	500-700	30-50
√ Roast beef (cooked, 6 oz.)	320	14	Blackened redfish (w/ 3 Tbsp. butter)	700	45
√ BBQ chicken (1/4 of chicken, with skin*)	350	20	Patty melt	770	50
			Tuna salad sandwich (11 oz.)	835	56
Fried chicken* (1 chicken breast)	325	18	Ham & cheese croissant	850	40
T-bone, porterhouse, sirloin (cooked, 6 oz.)	380	18	√ Pancakes (4) with 1/4 c. syrup and 2 Tbsp. margarine	940	29
Fried fish filet*	400	16	Fried seafood platter	970	50
√ Ham & cheese deli sandwich	600	23	Prime rib (precooked, 16 oz.)	1280	94

√ *Best choices fall between 500 and 700 calories and include the total meal.*
* *Trim skin/crust to trim off 100 calories and 10 g fat*

The following restaurant's websites list the nutrient content of their menus:

Applebees	www.applebees.com
Bob Evans	www.bobevans.com
Chili's	www.chilis.com
Olive Garden	www.olivegarden.com
Outback Steakhouse	www.outback.com
Perkins	www.perkinsrestaurant.com
P. F. Changs	www.pfchangs.com
Red Lobster	www.redlobster.cbord.com
Sbarro's	www.sbarro.com

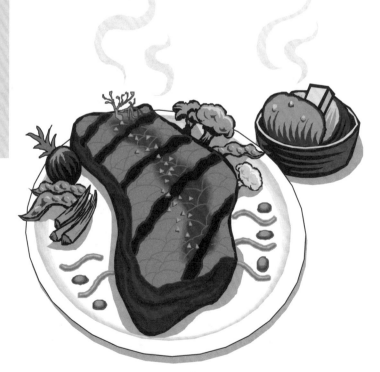

Salad Bars

Select salads sensibly! My top picks are fresh fruits and veggies. You can load up on these without adding many calories. Plus, they are packed with nutrients. Go easy on selections with mayonnaise.

0 - 10 Calories

	Amount	Cal	Fat (g)
Artichoke hearts	2	10	0
Bean sprouts	3 Tbsp.	7	0
Beets	2 slices	8	0
Broccoli	1/4 c.	6	0
Celery (3-inch stick)	2	4	0
Cucumber	4 slices	2	0
Carrots	1/4 c.	6	0
Cauliflower	1/4 c.	6	0
Green or red pepper	3 slices	6	0
Mushrooms	2 Tbsp.	3	0
Lettuce, all types	1 c.	8	0
Olives	2 large	10	2
Onion	1 slice	2	0
Radishes	2 whole	5	0
Tomato	2 slices	5	0

5 - 25 Calories

	Amount	Cal	Fat (g)
Chick-peas	2 Tbsp.	35	0
Garbanzo beans	2 Tbsp.	35	0
Kidney beans	2 Tbsp.	35	0
Raisins	1 Tbsp.	25	0

30 - 50 Calories

	Amount	Cal	Fat (g)
Bacon bits (real or imitation)	1 Tbsp.	35	2
Cheese (all types grated)	1 Tbsp.	35	3
Coleslaw	1/4 c.	50	5
Fresh fruit	1/2 c.	50	0

60 - 80 Calories

	Amount	Cal	Fat (g)
Cottage cheese	1/4 c.	55	3
Egg	1	80	5
Sunflower seeds	1 Tbsp.	50	5
Three-bean salad	1/4 c.	50	3

100 Calories

	Amount	Cal	Fat (g)
Avocado	1/4	90	9
Canned fruit	1/2 c.	100	0
Chicken, crab and tuna salad	1/4 c.	100	5
Croutons	1/4 c.	100	6
Macaroni and potato salad	1/4 c.	100	5

Salad Dressing

	Amount	Cal	Fat (g)
Lemon juice, vinegar	1 Tbsp.	0	0
Picante sauce (salsa)	1 Tbsp.	0	0
French, ranch	1 Tbsp.	55	6
Bleu cheese, Italian, Thousand Island, Russian, Caesar	1 Tbsp.	80	8
Reduced-calorie and fat-free dressings	1 Tbsp.	6-30	0-4
Cottage Cheese (as dressing)	1/4 c.	55	3

Miscellaneous

	Amount	Cal	Fat (g)
√ Breadsticks	2	45	5
√ Crackers	4	60	2
Cornbread	1 piece	180	6
√ Soup - broth or tomato-based	1 c.	100-200	5-10
Soup - creamy or cheese-based	1 c.	200-350	7-20

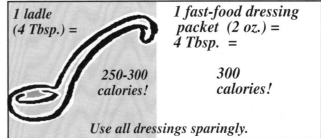

1 ladle (4 Tbsp.) = **250-300 calories!**

1 fast-food dressing packet (2 oz.) = 4 Tbsp. = **300 calories!**

Use all dressings sparingly.

TIP

- If you are sulfite-sensitive, ask your waiter about the salads before ordering.
- Even the smallest Caesar salad contains 500 cal. Ask for dressing on the side.

Fast Foods

People often assume that fast-food restaurants are "forbidden"—but it just isn't so. Fast food is part of the American lifestyle. We used to say "as American as apple pie." Today we hear "as American as a Big Mac and Coke!"

I do want to encourage you to make wise selections at fast-food restaurants. Begin by asking for the nutritional content of their foods. (You can also find this information in this book's Appendix C or on the Internet for each fast-food chain.) Studies show that the average fast-food meal costs you 1,200 calories! It usually is high in fat, cholesterol and sodium (salt). You can change this. Here's how:

10 BEST CHOICES (all made without mayonnaise)

	CAL	FAT (g)
1. Grilled chicken sandwiches	300	8
2. Small burgers	300	10
3. Small cheeseburgers	350	15
4. New Subway 6-inch lighter sandwiches/no cheese	300	5
5. Small roast beef sandwiches	350	15
6. Chicken or veggie pitas (order without dressing)	300-500	10-20
7. Small soft tacos, any type	175	10
8. Bean burritos	400	12
9. 2 slices of cheese or veggie pizza	500	20
with a big salad and 1 Tbsp. dressing	600	30
10. Salad with 1 Tbsp. dressing on the side	100	10
and topped with grilled chicken	250	15

10 FAST-FOOD ORDERING TIPS

1. "Know before you go." Select a meal with 15-25 g fat, 500-700 calories. (See Appendix C for fast-food nutrition values, and mark your best options.)

2. Skip mayonnaise, sauces, bacon; ask for double tomatoes, double lettuce, onion, pickle, mustard.

3. Ask for light dressings on salads or request regular dressing "on the side." Use sparingly. A typical 2-oz. packet of dressing contains 4 Tbsp. and 350 calories. Use half of this amount.

4. Drink water, 1% milk, juice, tea and sugar-free soft drinks. Skip soft drinks (150-250 calories) and shakes (300-400 calories), or split a shake.

5. Omit fried foods.

6. Order a small nonfat frozen yogurt. Skip the ice cream, pies, sweets, desserts.

7. Remove the skin or crust from rotisserie and fried chicken, and you'll remove 150-200 cal and 5-10 g fat.

8. At salad bars, eat lots of lettuce, greens, tomatoes, carrots, green peppers, celery, cucumbers, mushrooms. Limit dressings, ham, croutons, pasta or potato or rice salads, cheese, nuts, seeds, marinated vegetables.

9. Carry fresh fruit with you from home to have as dessert.

10. Select a baked potato. Top with cottage cheese, picante sauce, 2 Tbsp. grated cheese and/or sour cream or chili.

500-Calorie Fast-Food Meals

Here are a few new ideas that keep fast-food options high and calories low.

FAST-FOOD MEALS

Burger	Cal	Fat (g)
McDonald's cheeseburger	310	12
2% milk	120	5
Fresh fruit (from home)	60	0
Total:	**490**	**17**

Sandwich	Cal	Fat (g)
Arby's Roast Beef (regular)	320	13
Garden Side Salad	35	0
2 Tbsp. Light Buttermilk Ranch Dressing	50	0
Total:	**405**	**13**

Pizza	Cal	Fat (g)
2 slices Pizza Hut's Thin n' Crispy ham, (medium)	360	12
Salad	25	0
2 Tbsp. ranch dressing	110	12
Total:	**495**	**24**

Chili	Cal	Fat (g)
Wendy's chili (small)	220	6
6 crackers	70	2
2% milk	120	5
Side Salad	25	0
1 Tbsp. French or ranch dressing (or 1 pkt. Fat-free Ranch = 80 cal, no fat)	55	6
Total:	**470**	**19**

Wrap	Cal	Fat (g)
Chick Fil-A's Chargrilled Chicken Cool Wrap, no dressing	390	7
Fresh fruit cup (medium)	60	0
Total:	**450**	**7**

Chicken Sandwich	Cal	Fat (g)
Burger King's Grilled Chicken Whopper, no mayo	410	7
1/2 small order French fries	120	6
Total:	**530**	**13**

See web addresses for fast-food restaurants on p. 283.

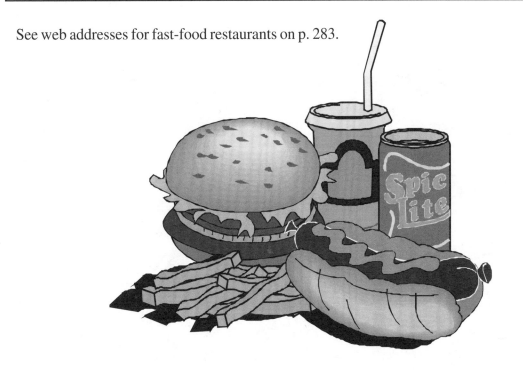

© 2009, *The Cooper Clinic Solution to the Diet Revolution* by Georgia G. Kostas, M.P.H., R.D., L.D., Dallas, Texas

Healthy Travel and Vacations

When you travel, do you quit your healthy eating and exercise programs? Let me encourage you to make both part of your new lifestyle, whether you're at home or on the road. Here are my recommendations for keeping on track.

TIPS

1. Choose a restaurant that allows more food choices than a fast-food chain serving only fried foods, hot dogs and shakes.

2. Take an ice chest in your car filled with water, diet drinks, fruit, cut-up veggies, or even a picnic lunch. Avoid high-calorie foods like potato chips, nuts, cookies and candy.

3. When traveling in the car, stop for lunch at a restaurant or picnic area. Don't eat in the car. You won't enjoy it as much, and you may eat more.

4. When you stop for a meal, take a walk or stretch. Get 10 minutes of exercise if you can.

5. Decide in advance to skip the peanuts on a plane. Drink a lot of water (8 to 10 cups) so you won't get dehydrated and fatigued. Take a snack with you (raisins, bagel, pretzels, fruit).

6. Order a "vegetarian," "low-calorie" or "seafood" meal 24 hours before your flight.

7. Balance one rich meal with one all-vegetable meal daily such as a vegetable plate, soup and salad; or a baked potato and salad.

8. Don't center all your activities around eating as the main pleasure of the trip.

9. Take your exercise clothes and use them! You can jump rope in your hotel room, take brisk walks, "stair-walk" in stairwells, and stay at hotels with exercise facilities or club affiliations.

10. Avoid vending machine snacks. Carry a healthy alternative snack, and keep it handy for a quick "pick-me-up."

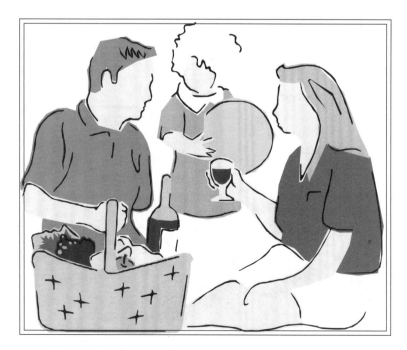

Weekends

Many clients tell me that weekends are challenging for them. They do so well during a structured workweek, but when Saturday hits, they lose control! If you are one of these people, consider the following:

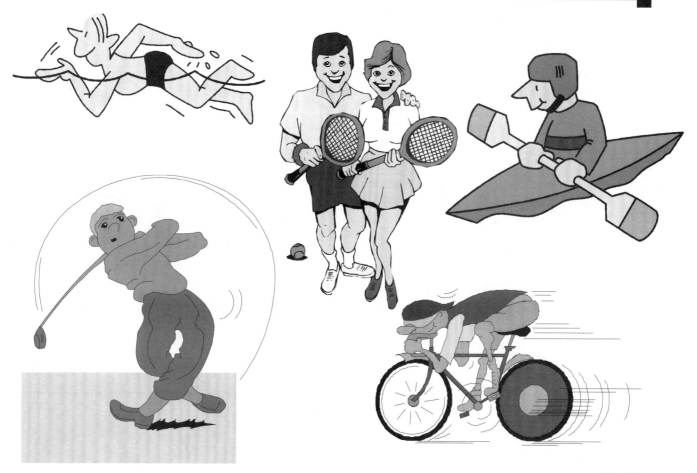

STRATEGIES

1. **Before the weekend arrives, plan fun activities** that do not involve eating.

2. **Break the habit of gaining 5 pounds over the weekend** and having to lose that "extra" weight before Friday. Adjust your eating and exercise on weekends to fit your schedule. Keep healthy foods on hand to help you eat well and not gain weight.

3. **Do not use food as your form of relaxation or recreation.** Plan special recreational activities, social time, hobby time and "downtime" to relax.

4. **Determine not to "let go" of your eating program.** Practice your strategies!

5. **Eat more fruit and vegetables at home** to balance out richer meals.

6. **Exercise recreationally.** In other words, dance, play golf or tennis, swim, take long walks and bike rides, etc. Join a weekend exercise group as a fun way to meet people and keep up with your program!

Holidays

Do you gain 5-10 lbs over the holidays? Eating traditions, limited time, heightened emotions, and more tempting food exposure easily lead to extra pounds over the holidays—particularly from Thanksgiving through Christmas. What a tough way to begin the new year! If you have battled the bulge in holidays past, challenge yourself this year to focus on your new lifestyle and to implement the following strategies:

1. Plan ahead.

- Choose foods that, for you and your family, are an essential part of a particular holiday. You don't have to completely give up something that has been a tradition for generations! Cut back on other foods. Eat larger portions of lighter foods; smaller portions of heavier foods.
- Plan food preparation, the holiday meal itself and use of leftovers. Make the most tempting foods last to spare yourself!
- Holiday time is often an emotional time. Plan activities to avoid emotion-related eating (as from loneliness, loss, happiness, etc.). Decorate for the holidays. Attend special holiday events, musicals, etc. Avoid eating alone if possible. (If you know of someone else who may be eating alone, have him or her over for your own celebration!)
- Keep food stored out of sight.
- Get involved in fun activities/hobbies that are not centered solely around food (i.e., picture albums, slides, card games, ping-pong, volleyball, basketball, walks, bike rides, window-shopping, talking).
- Don't wait to eat healthful until after the holidays. Enjoy a few "extras" and be sensible.
- Plan relaxing times for yourself. Enjoy the time away from your regular routine to read, work on hobbies, enjoy music, call a friend, etc.
- Remember, giving your time and attention to someone says "I love you" much more effectively than giving or eating food.
- If you get fatigued, nap instead of snack. Also, use exercise to boost your energy.

2. Stay active.

- Continue exercising throughout the holidays…it is a great stress-reducer. If you don't have time for even 30 minutes, try to work in at least 15. Remember that you can get the same health benefits by breaking a 30-minute session into two 15-minute bouts.

3. Be in control at parties.

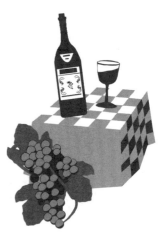

- Never arrive hungry. A small snack beforehand can save you hundreds of calories later. Exercising beforehand cuts your appetite, too.
- Focus on the people, not on the food. Plan to speak to each guest if possible.
- Position yourself far away from the food.
- Survey the food before that first bite. Choose two or three items you like most. Eat these and just sample small portions of other foods.
- Skip the appetizers and alcoholic drinks—they are loaded with calories! Save your calories for the main meal.
- Drink five glasses of water per party.
- Eat slowly—you'll eat less. Sip slowly on beverages.
- Set a time to stop eating.
- Wait 20 minutes after eating before considering "seconds." Chances are, you will not want more food.

4. Take control at home.

- Be generous—give away food gifts! Don't stockpile candy and other "goodies."
- Avoid making excessive quantities of food. Freeze leftovers immediately or give them away.
- Keep low-calorie favorites on hand within easy reach.
- Serve special low-cal beverages and foods to you and your guests (spiced tea, fruit, popcorn, Chex mix, etc.).
- Give away fruit baskets and breads.
- Do not make high-calorie food gifts for others.
- Cut desserts in half.

5. Be a good guest.

- Pack your favorite lesser-calorie snacks, desserts, special beverage treats, salad dressing, etc.
- Make up a batch of popcorn for your hosts.
- Help prepare a low-calorie meal.

6. Take time out for an attitude check.

- *Maintaining* your weight is more realistic than expecting a great weight loss during the holidays.
- Be picky and selective about what you eat—it's *your* body!
- Enjoy the company, not just the food. People make holidays happy.
- If you do overindulge, don't abandon your pursuit of leanness. Cut back at (don't skip) your next few meals, eat more vegetables and exercise more.

HAPPY HOLIDAYS!

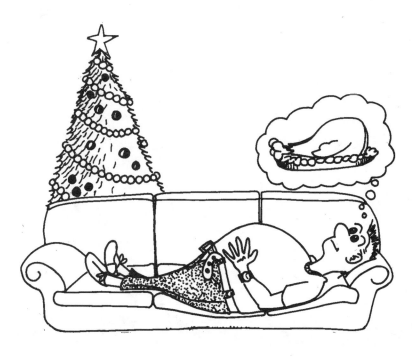

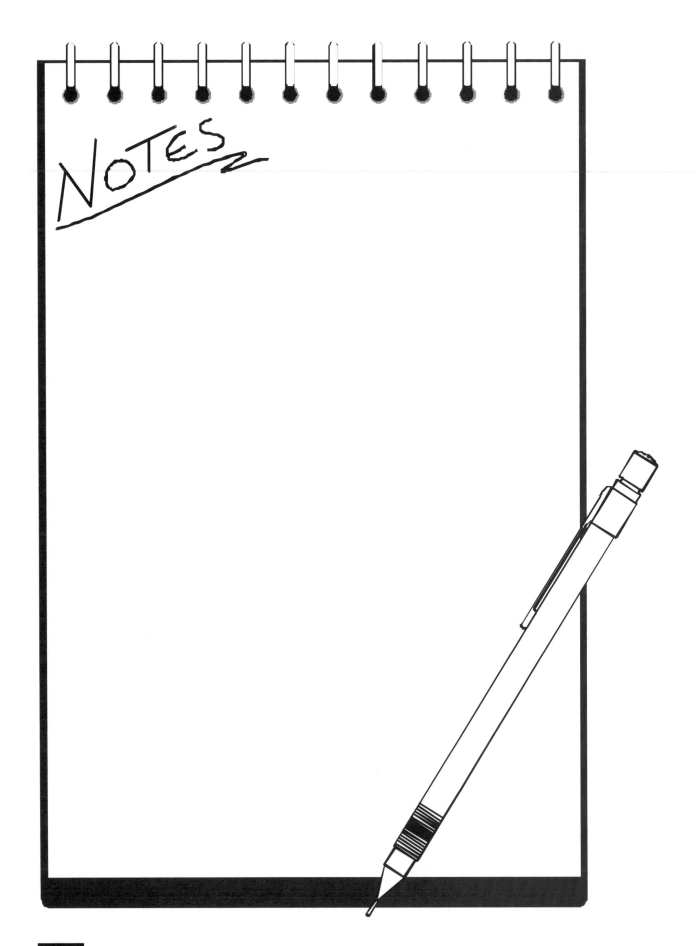

NOTES

Step 8
Watch Your Step -
Do You Eat on Cue?

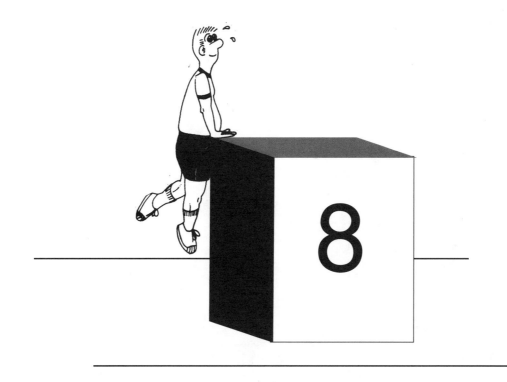

Step 8

What triggers you to eat? Certain places or events? Boredom or stress? In this chapter, I'll introduce you to the types of *food cues* that beckon you to eat—even when you are not hungry. I will explain how to avoid or remove these cues, which will help you gain control of your eating habits. For continued motivation, regularly read my list of "20 Ways to Overcome the Urge to Splurge."

Test your own food cue IQ. If you can reduce the cues, you're one step closer to eating better and losing or managing your weight for life.

Mini-Step 1:
Learn what cues trigger over-eating for you.

Mini-Step 2:
Discover new strategies to help you overcome the "urge to splurge."

ACTION STEPS

①   Identify and remove food cues that trigger eating.
②   Take a few steps to prevent and avoid splurges.

Know Your Food Cues

What triggers you to overeat? **Food cues** signal you to eat…even when you are not hungry. Cues include the following: aromas, vending machines, candy dishes, billboards, bakeries, restaurants, ice cream shops, TV, movies, afternoons, ads, coupons, "special times of day," emotions, stress.

Remember, you can either avoid or remove "cues" or change your response to them.

Make a list of the environmental or emotional cues that are the biggest culprits causing you to eat when you are not hungry.

1. _____   4. _____

2. _____   5. _____

3. _____   6. _____

☑ **Look at how you can easily minimize food contact in the following scenarios. Check the ones you're willing to try.**

STORING FOOD

❑ Store food out of sight and in inconvenient places. As the saying goes, "Out of sight, out of mind." No more candy dishes or cookie jars out at home!

❑ "Hide" problem foods in opaque containers that you cannot see through or in the back of cupboards, the refrigerator or freezer, or refrigerator drawers. If it's a real problem food, don't even purchase it!

❑ Encourage family members to keep problem foods out of sight.

❑ Keep cut-up fruit and veggies in your fridge at eye level.

SERVING FOOD

❑ Serve from the stove; avoid serving dishes on the table. This encourages seconds.

❑ If foods are on the table, place them away from you (such as chips at Mexican restaurants).

CLEANING UP

❑ Clean up immediately. Ask someone else to scrape the dishes and put away leftovers so you won't snack on leftovers.

❑ Freeze or refrigerate leftovers for future lunches or dinners. Store in appropriate portion sizes to avoid overeating.

AFTER-DINNER ACTIVITIES

❑ Leave the table immediately. Involve yourself in activities—preferably physical activity such as walking, biking or gardening.

❑ If you stay at the table and converse, remove the plates and serving dishes. Sip on water, coffee or tea, if anything. Or, change rooms to end eating.

❑ Eat a sugar-free mint or brush your teeth right after a meal to discourage continued eating.

❑ Close the kitchen door and turn off the light. The kitchen is "closed for the night."

WHERE DO YOU EAT?

❑ Eat all meals and snacks in one room and at the table to avoid associating food with different settings at home – TV room, bedroom, etc. Make this place attractive and inviting. Use a placemat and your favorite plates and glassware.

❑ Sit down whenever you eat anything. This helps you control "extra" unconscious eating while lying down or standing to prepare food or grabbing food from the refrigerator.

❑ Avoid places where you tend to overeat, such as all-you-can-eat buffets.

❑ Avoid the kitchen for activities such as using the phone, writing letters, etc.

WHAT DO YOU DO WHILE EATING?

❑ Taste your food, feel the texture and savor each bite.

❑ Don't let reading, writing, watching TV or working make you oblivious to a delicious meal or the company with you. Multitasking will not aid digestion!

❑ Identify emotion-related eating: boredom, fatigue, anger, guilt, stress, loneliness. Alter your response to these circumstances. (Refer to the "Treat Yourself" list on p. 37.)

❑ Make a list of alternative activities to replace overeating: necessities, hobbies, exercise, relaxation, etc.

1. _____   3. _____   5. _____

2. _____   4. _____   6. _____

☑ **Make a list of ways to reduce triggers that encourage you to eat. For example:**

Cue	Strategy
1) Donuts at office	Walk in room with drink in hand and talk, talk, talk.
2) Movie popcorn	Take a healthy snack from home; avoid food area; go straight to your seat. Share small popcorn.
3) Alcohol at parties	Limit to one drink; order water or sugar-free soda.
4) _____	_____
5) _____	_____

© 2009, *The Cooper Clinic Solution to the Diet Revolution* by Georgia G. Kostas, M.P.H., R.D., L.D., Dallas, Texas

20 Ways to Overcome the "Urge to Splurge"

☑ **Select the techniques most effective for you.**

❑ **Remove temptation.** Don't keep "binge" foods such as chocolate, chips or ice cream at home. If they must be there, store and conceal out of sight.

❑ **Buy mini-portions.** Go for smaller, pre-portioned servings (i.e., mini-cereal boxes, snack packets of M&Ms, individually wrapped Fudgesicles, etc.).

❑ **Select lower-calorie versions** such as frozen nonfat yogurt vs. ice cream.

❑ **Be prepared**. Think about vulnerable occasions before they hit…and have some planned strategies.

❑ **Delay a binge.** Get distracted for 10 minutes. In other words, call a friend, play a computer game, take a walk, water your plants, drink a tall glass of water. An impulse will pass.

❑ **Eat slowly**. Savor every bite. Eat with others—not in secrecy.

❑ **Get busy.** Enjoy a new hobby, music, housework, project, computer, walking, shower, manicure, cleaning—or go to sleep!

❑ **Leave the room.** Don't let yourself stay in the kitchen. Motion transforms emotion.

❑ **Identify stop signs.** Does a mint, apple, carrot, glass of milk or water signal "eating is over," and prevent or stop a binge? Find a "stop food" that works for you or a "stop activity," such as exercise or brushing your teeth.

❑ **Stop, Look, Listen.** Before indulging, ask yourself, "What was dissatisfying to me today?" "What can I do about it?" Is eating a "coping mechanism" for emotions and other stressors? Learn to confront and deal with emotions in a constructive way. Be proactive. The urge to binge may disappear. Seek expert assistance for skills.

❑ **After a binge, move!** Do something active and constructive. Do not linger and feel guilty—you will only eat more. Mop, sweep, wash your car, do gardening, wash your hair, run errands. Move, don't mope!

❑ **Regain control.** Write down what you'll eat at your next three meals, and take a walk!

❑ **Stay positive**. Don't let a slip-up make you give up. Look for progress, not perfection.

❑ **Never undercut calories.** You may overeat later.

❑ **Do not deprive yourself of favorite foods**. Deprivation triggers binge-eating. Set "ground rules" to include your favorite foods in appropriate portions.

❑ **Space meals and snacks regularly**. Eat every three to six hours to keep blood sugar levels stable. A drop in blood sugar can trigger a binge. Do not skip or delay meals. Eat on time to let your body adjust to a routine.

❑ **Eat a little fat.** A little fat goes a long way in keeping you "full" and satisfied for hours. Eat at least 5 grams of fat at breakfast and at least 10 grams at lunch and supper. For sustained energy and blood sugar lasting five to six hours, eat with the P-C-F balance (see p. 48).

❑ **Do not overtrain**. Overexercising burns a lot of calories. When blood sugar drops, hunger soars.

❑ **Get centered**. Avoid "all-or-none thinking," "deprivation/bingeing" cycles. Move toward middle ground. Eat moderate portions of all foods.

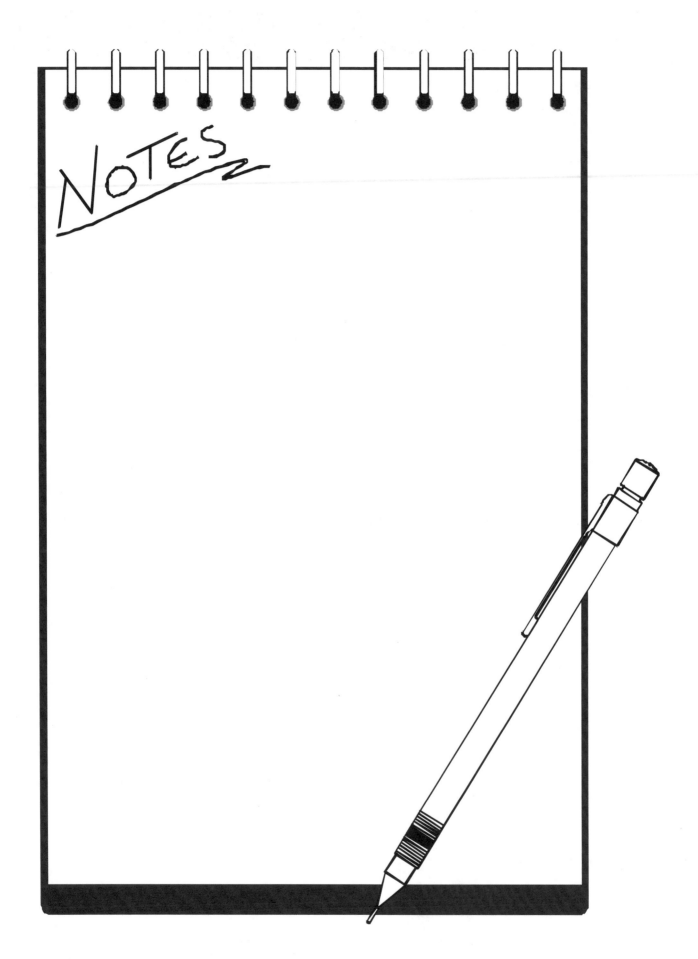

NOTES

Step 9
Mind Your P's and Cues

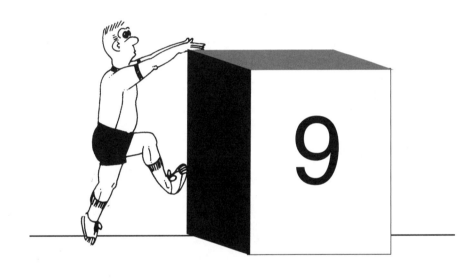

Step 9

Mini-Step 1:
Plan ahead.
Think before you eat.

Mini-Step 2:
Size up your portions
to down-size your size.

Mini-Step 3:
Slow down your pace to eat
less and win the weight race.

If you've ever ordered a pasta dish at an Italian restaurant, chances are you've received several servings—not just one. Over the years, the American plate has gotten larger, and many diners hold fast to the "bigger is better" mentality. The truth is, your body doesn't need as much as it's usually fed. I will show you in this chapter how to develop an eye for size. I'll cover three important P's: planning, portions and pace. These three healthy habits will help keep you on track.

P - "Plan" ahead to prevent impulse eating and poor choices.

P - "Portion" your food - control portions to control weight.

P - "Pace" yourself. Slow down to eat less!

If you can mange your P's and Cues, you're four steps closer to managing your weight with more ease.

ACTION STEPS

① Plan ahead by writing down meals **before** eating. This helps you "think before you eat".

② If you get hungry for a "problem" food, wait 10 minutes before eating. The impulse may disappear.

③ Learn what a true "healthy portion" is. Reserve 1/4th of your plate for protein and 3/4th of the rest of it for vegetables, wholegrains and fruit.

④ Slow down! Allow 20 - 30 minutes per meal and savor every bite.

Planning

"To fail to plan is to plan to fail!" Prior thought helps you avoid impulse eating and provides a lifetime of weight control. Planning prevents the day's circumstances, your moods, your environment, etc., from interfering with your good intentions. It also keeps you aware of your eating and prevents automatic or unconscious eating that may lead to compulsive eating. When it comes to preparing meals and trying to avoid problem foods, think about the situation beforehand so you won't make a bad last-minute decision. In addition, creating "ground rules" helps you keep portions and calories in check...especially when eating favorite foods.

☑ What strategies will you try?

MEALS

- ❏ **Pre-think** meals and snacks to free you from "thinking food" all day.
- ❏ **Write down** what you'll eat before eating. At one meal, pre-think the next.
- ❏ **Pack** a lunch. Now you are in control of this meal!
- ❏ **Vary** breakfast and lunch menus. Keep these meals inviting!

FOOD PREPARATION

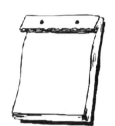

- ❏ **Modify recipes,** using lower-calorie ingredients.
- ❏ **Do not sample** as you cook or clean up. Those extra calories add up! Instead, sip on a low-calorie beverage or munch on a raw carrot.

PROBLEM FOODS

- ❏ **Don't buy them!**

  My problem foods are: _____

- ❏ **Conceal** and store them properly if they are in the house.
- ❏ Buy satisfying, low-calorie **food substitutes** for problem foods.
- ❏ Try **alternative activities** to do in place of snacking: music, reading, needlework, sewing, sports, walking, sleeping, relaxation, carpentry, house projects, phone calls, bills, letters, etc.
- ❏ **Eat one small serving** if this food is impossible to avoid.
- ❏ **Delay** eating this food for 10 minutes. Chances are, you won't want it.

MEAL PLANS

- ❏ Predict and pre-plan meals for the week by writing them down (see forms on p. 199-200).
- ❏ **Add a vegetarian** meal for each meal out at restaurants.

GROUND RULES

- ❏ **All foods fit in** . . . just set your own **ground rules** to eat within reason. (See ideas on the next page.)

Ground Rules

WANT TO LOSE OR MAINTAIN WEIGHT WHILE ENJOYING YOUR FAVORITE FOODS?

Avoid "all-or-none" thinking and "off-and-on" dieting! Set your own "ground rules" with specific foods to enjoy "freedom with boundaries"—eating all foods in set amounts.

Ground Rules

Sandwiches	❑ No mayonnaise (use fat-free mayonnaise or mustard); 1 slice of cheese at most ❑ Ask for fruit, soup, beans, slaw or tomato slices to replace chips and fries ❑ Ask for "double" tomatoes, "double" lettuce
Burgers	❑ ¼ lb. meat; no mayo; no bacon; double tomato/double lettuce ❑ Order meat off bun and pat grease with a paper towel before placing on bun
Steaks	❑ Choose a tenderloin or filet or top sirloin cut; 4-6 oz. only
Baked Potato	❑ 1/2 restaurant size (=100 calories) ❑ Top with salsa (0 calories) or 1 Tbsp. sour cream (30 calories)
Chips/Fries/Peanuts	❑ Eat 10-12 (100-120 calories) at most
Entrees	❑ Split in half (the usual portion is 6 to 8 oz.)
Desserts	❑ Split in half at least
Ice Cream/Frozen Yogurt	❑ 1 scoop (junior or small size) in a dish; no toppings
Salad	❑ Dressing on the side; no bacon, egg or croutons on top; ❑ 1-2 Tbsp. regular dressing or 3 Tbsp. light dressing
Sauces/Toppings/ Dressings/Gravies, etc.	❑ On the side only; add sparingly
Eggs	❑ 3 a week at most; make omelets with 1 egg and 3 egg whites
Cookies	❑ 3 small or 1 big one at a time
Bread with meals	❑ 1 slice or 1 roll
Oils/Fats	❑ 1/2 - 1 Tbsp. per meal
Added butter	❑ 1 pat (1 1/2 tsp.) per meal (1/2 on bread and 1/2 on potato, for example)
Pizza	❑ 2 slices only and add a big salad ❑ Think of salad as the entrée; pizza as the "bread" with a topping
Meat	❑ Think of meat as a flavoring agent or side dish – not the main course
Pasta	❑ 1 cup at most as side dish; 2 cups as entree
Mexican Chips	❑ Take 5-10; break each one into 5-6 pieces; eat slowly; ❑ Replace chips with soft corn tortillas with salsa; 8 chips=200 cal., 3 tortillas=200 cal.
Appetizer	❑ Fruit; salad; 1 cup soup; hot tea; shrimp cocktail; steamed soy beans; sliced tomatoes
Finger Foods	❑ Eat one piece at a time – grapes, dry cereal (such as oat squares), popcorn, carrot sticks, pretzels, raisins, vegetables (string bean, carrot slice, etc.)

MEAL PLANS

_____ MILK _____ VEGETABLE _____ FRUIT
_____ STARCH _____ MEAT _____ FAT

Shopping List

	Monday (sample)	Tuesday	Wednesday	Thursday	Friday	Saturday	Sunday
BREAKFAST Milk	1 C. skim milk						
Veg.							
Fruit	1 orange						
Starch	2 English muffin halves						
Meat							
Fat	1 tsp. margarine						
Free							
LUNCH Milk							
Veg.							
Fruit	1 apple						
Starch	2 wholewheat bread slices						
Meat	2 oz. turkey						
Fat	1 tsp. mayon.						
Free	1 tsp. mustard, lettuce, tomato						
SUPPER Milk							
Veg.	salad, 1/2 C. carrots						
Fruit	1/2 C. broccoli						
Starch	1/2 C. brown rice, 1 roll						
Meat	3 oz. chicken, broiled						
Fat	1 T. Ranch drg						
Free							
SNACKS	8 oz. fat-free yogurt, 1 C. grapes						
TOTAL DAILY	Milk ☒☒☐ Fruit ☒☒☒ Veg. ☒☐ Starch ☒☒☒☒☒ Meat ☒☒☒ Fat ☒☒☐						

© 2009, _The Cooper Clinic Solution to the Diet Revolution_ by Georgia G. Kostas, M.P.H., R.D., L.D., Dallas, Texas

MEAL PLANS

| | MILK | VEGETABLE | FRUIT |
| | STARCH | MEAT | FAT |

Shopping List

	Monday (sample)	Tuesday	Wednesday	Thursday	Friday	Saturday	Sunday
BREAKFAST Milk / Veg. / Fruit / Starch / Meat / Fat / Free							
LUNCH Milk / Veg. / Fruit / Starch / Meat / Fat / Free							
SUPPER Milk / Veg. / Fruit / Starch / Meat / Fat / Free							
SNACKS							
TOTAL DAILY Milk / Fruit / Veg. / Starch / Meat / Fat							

200 Step 9
© 2009, *The Cooper Clinic Solution to the Diet Revolution* by Georgia G. Kostas, M.P.H., R.D., L.D., Dallas, Texas

Portions Count

The key to losing weight and keeping it off is portions! Many people eat nutritiously, but without portion control, too much of even the right food can make you gain weight. Try these portion control ideas:

1. **Measure portions** before eating. Use measuring cups and spoons, and scales to weigh meats/cheeses. 3 oz. 🥄 = 🎲

2. **Avoid seconds**. Relax and think. Let 20 minutes pass before going for the second helping. Chances are, you won't want seconds!

3. **Use smaller dinner plates** or bowls to satisfy your psychological need to see a **full** plate. Spread food to cover the plate. Use a small dish for cereal.

4. **Leave some behind**. Break away from the "clean plate syndrome," the compulsion to eat everything on the plate. Take 1/2 home for tomorrow's lunch.

5. **Eat baby-bites**. Cut food into smaller pieces and eat one bite at a time. You chew more and the meal lasts longer.

6. **Measure easy-to-overdo foods**:
   - Cheese, 1 oz.
   - Meat, 3 oz.
   - Salad dressing, mayonnaise, margarine, and peanutbutter, 1 Tbsp.
   - Starches, 1/2 to 1 c.
   - Nuts, 1-2 Tbsp.
   - Juice, 4-6 oz. (1/2 to 3/4 c.)

7. **Measure your glass sizes at home**. Is your juice glass 4 oz., 6 oz., or 8 oz.?

8. **Use the "plate" rule**. Reserve 1/4th of the plate for the protein or entrée, and 3/4th of the plate for plant foods (vegetables, grains, fruit).

9. **Don't measure forever**. As time goes on, you'll become a good judge. "Spot check" yourself now and then.

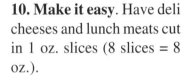

10. **Make it easy**. Have deli cheeses and lunch meats cut in 1 oz. slices (8 slices = 8 oz.).

11. **Buy portioned sizes**.
   - 3 oz. boneless, skinless chicken breasts, etc.
   - Cheese slice "singles"
   - Frozen dessert bars
   - 4 oz. steaks (ask the butcher)

12. **Split** an entrée when eating out. Most are 6-8 oz., and you need only 3-4 oz.

13. **Always slice fresh fruit**. Slices are more filling than one whole fruit.

14. **Don't worry about vegetable portions**. Eat as much as you like.

15. **Use your fist or a tennis ball as a measure** of 1 cup of pasta, rice, vegetables, fruit, etc.

TIP

Eat 2 fists of vegetables per 1 fist of starchy food.

 =  OR

© 2009, *The Cooper Clinic Solution to the Diet Revolution* by Georgia G. Kostas, M.P.H., R.D., L.D., Dallas, Texas

Pace Yourself

Are you a fast eater? Slow down! Slow eaters tend to eat less. I'm convinced that the following practices will not only help slow you down, but also will make the meal more enjoyable! Which will you try?

1. **Use the "20-minute rule."** It takes about 20 minutes after eating to feel full. Eating fast, without pausing or slowing down, leads to excessive eating.

2. **Eat and chew slowly,** taking 20-30 minutes for meals and 10 minutes for snacks.

3. **Be the last one** to finish eating at the table.

4. **Lay down your utensil** between bites. **Sip** on a beverage between bites.

5. **Complete each bite** before taking the next bite.

6. **Take smaller bites**—like a 2- to 3-year-old—one popcorn kernel at a time.

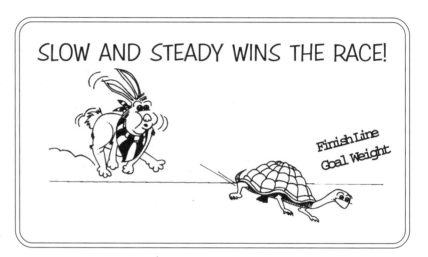

7. **Pause** during the meal to sip water or talk with people at the table or enjoy the atmosphere. Put your hands in your lap.

8. **Serve food in courses**—salad before entree or vice-versa. Courses slow you down!

9. **Eat "slow" foods**—foods with **"crunch"** such as popcorn, pretzels, hard rolls, fresh fruit, raw vegetables, toasted bread for sandwiches, baked potatoes (not mashed), corn-on-the-cob, etc. Try **hot liquids** such as soup, broth, hot tea, low-calorie hot cocoa. These are "filling" and slow you down...both pluses for weight management.

10. **Enjoy** your eating environment. Serve food attractively. Play soft music. Keep surroundings relaxed, pleasant and attractive. No loud TV!

11. **Converse** with each person at the table. Talking will slow you down!

12. **Savor** every bite—the flavors, aroma, texture, color. Involve your senses. Appreciate each bite. Eat mindfully.

13. **Use a baby spoon** to take smaller bites. (Try using the "sample spoon" at Baskin Robbins for your ice cream scoop! I personally use colorful little gelato spoons!)

Step 10
Lighten Your Load by Lightening Up Your Cooking

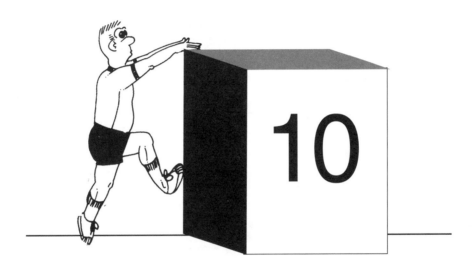

Step 10

Mini-Step 1:

Try some new "Cooking Tips" and "Fun Foods."

Mini-Step 2:

Find creative ways to eat more veggies!

Mini-Step 3:

Try a new low-calorie recipe (Appendix D or your own).

Becoming a wiser "chef" and shopper doesn't require going to cooking school. In this step, I provide practical cooking tips that just about anybody can put to good use. For example, I've taken a lasagna recipe (375 calories with 30 fat grams) and modified the ingredients to create a lower-fat entrée that's irresistible (190 calories with 9 fat grams). Check out my chocolate cake makeover, as well. You won't believe recipes that taste this good can be so healthy!

Do you enjoy fun foods? Learn how to make them healthier and delicious. Use the list of "Low-fat Cooking Substitutes" to shave dozens of calories off some of your favorite recipes.

Are you bored with vegetables? Look at the 30+ simple ways you can prepare and enjoy them and eat more. Note which five vegetables contain the most nutrients.

ACTION STEPS

① Prepare foods in a healthy way with more vegetables and fewer calories, fat, sugar and salt.

② Try 3 new ways to prepare and season vegetables this week. Make meals revolve around veggies.

③ Enjoy thinking about how particular foods add quality to your life. Enjoy the tastes of eating well.

Cooking Tips

Here are some step-by-step ways to add flavor and nutrition while reducing calories, fats, sugar and salt.

STEP 1: **CHOOSE LEAN**

- Select fish, poultry and lean cuts of meat (see meat cuts p. 64).

- Trim excess fats from meats before cooking. Remove skin from poultry before or after cooking.

- Use water-packed tuna and salmon.

STEP 2: **COOK LEAN**

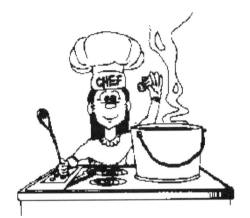

- Bake, broil, grill, poach, stir-fry, microwave, steam or boil rather than deep-fry. (Frying can add 200 calories.)

- Use cooking sprays and non-stick pans to replace oil for sautéing or stir-frying.

- Chill soups and stews and lift off congealed fat, or use a strainer to pour off fat.

- Make gravies with fat-free broth, skim milk and cornstarch.

- Serve foods simply, without added sauces.

STEP 3: **SEASON LEAN**

- Cook onions, green pepper and other vegetables in a little broth or use bouillon cubes instead of sautéing them in fat. Add garlic powder and onion powder to enhance flavor.

- Season vegetables with herbs and spices and unsalted chicken or beef broth or bouillon cubes rather than bacon, butter, ham hocks or salt pork.

- In cheese sauces, use fat-free milk and nonfat or low-fat cheese instead of whole milk, regular cheese and butter (see list of cheeses p. 124-125). Also, use evaporated skim milk for thicker sauces, replacing whole milk or cream.

- To season foods, use reduced-fat soft margarine or margarine pump sprays or fat-free butter-flavored granules (sprinkles), such as Molly McButter.

- Add sharp, strong flavors to recipes: red bell pepper, red onion, sundried tomatoes, cilantro, garlic, salsa, pico de gallo, cumin, red pepper flakes, soy sauce, Worcestershire sauce, barbecue sauce, Tabasco, balsamic vinegar, poblano or chili peppers, jalapenos, liquid smoke, flavored tomato and spaghetti sauces, catsup, fresh lime or lemon, fruit juices, capers, mustard, feta cheese, sliced Kalamata olives, etc. Sharp, tantalizing flavors are so satisfying, they help us eat less!

STEP 4: **THINK LEAN**

- Plan color at each meal.

- Keep portions appropriate: Twice the veggies as the amount of starches/grains.

- "Lighten up" your own favorite recipes, or buy a low-fat cookbook for new recipe ideas.

STEP 5: **SUBSTITUTE LEAN**

- See the recipe makeovers in this section for lasagna and chocolate cake.

- Instead of sour cream or vegetable dips, use light sour cream or plain nonfat yogurt blended with non-fat cottage cheese and seasonings, or plain nonfat yogurt mixed with a ranch dressing packet. Also, use on baked potatoes, salads and sandwiches.

- Use non-fat cottage cheese (blended) in place of cream cheese or sour cream in recipes. Or, use fat-free or light sour cream and cream cheese products.

- Replace oil in cake, brownie and muffin recipes, or packaged mixes with an equal portion of applesauce or strained fruit (baby food), pureed prunes, non-fat yogurt or low-fat buttermilk.

- Reduce sugar in recipes by 1/4 to 1/3 without affecting the final product; reduce fat by 1/2.

- Use naturally sweet flavors instead of excess sugar (i.e., vanilla, cinnamon, almond and cherry extracts, raisins, banana or concentrated apple juice.

- Select fresh fruits as sweet desserts.

Low-Fat Cooking Substitutes

Recipe calls for:	Substitute:
1 whole egg	1/4 c. egg substitute or 2 egg whites
1 c. shortening or butter (baking)	3/4 c. liquid oil or 1 c. margarine (2 sticks)
1 Tbsp. oil/butter (sautéing)	2 Tbsp. broth or wine, or 1 tsp. oil with vegetable cooking spray and nonstick pan, or light margarine
1 Tbsp. shortening or butter	2 tsp. liquid oil or 1 Tbsp. margarine or 1 Tbsp. light margarine
1 Tbsp. butter (seasoning)	1 Tbsp. light margarine or fat-free butter-flavored pump spray or granules (i.e., Molly McButter)
1 square chocolate (1 oz.)	3 Tbsp. dry cocoa powder + 1/2 Tbsp. liquid oil
1 c. whole milk or cream	1 c. fat-free milk or 1 c. fat-free evaporated milk
1 c. sour cream	1 c. nonfat yogurt or fat-free or low-fat cottage cheese (in blender) or 1 c. nonfat sour cream
1 oz. cream cheese	1 oz. low-fat cottage cheese (in blender) or 1 oz. fat-free or low-fat cream cheese
1/4 c. oil (in baking cake mixes, brownies, muffins, pancakes)	2 Tbsp. oil + 2 Tbsp. nonfat yogurt (or 1/4 c. applesauce, mashed banana, strained fruit (baby food), pureed or strained prunes, or nonfat yogurt)
1 egg + 3 Tbsp. oil (in brownie mix)	1/2 c. nonfat plain yogurt or 1/4 c. finely ground flaxseeds
1 Tbsp. mayonnaise	1 Tbsp. fat-free or light mayonnaise, or 2 Tbsp. nonfat yogurt (in tuna or potato salad, etc.)
1 c. cream soup	1 c. light cream soup (i.e., Campbell's Healthy Request Cream Soup)
1 oz. cheese (American, cheddar, etc.)	1 oz. of reduced-fat or fat-free cheese, or 3/4 oz. regular cheese (or grate cheese to use less)
1/2 c. nuts	1/2 c. Grape-Nuts or omit completely

Recipe Makeover: Lasagna

Thought chocolate cake and lasagna were off-limits? Think again. With a few recipe modifications, you can create foods you can enjoy just as much as the "real thing". Try these two recipes, and see what I mean!

New Makeover suggestions

Omit oil, spray bottom of pan with non-stick vegetable oil or thin layer of tomato sauce

- Omit and add vegetables (spinach, zucchini, etc.) instead.
- Use less meat (1 lb. lean beef and no pork, or ½ lb. lean beef and ½ lb. pork). Brown and drain fat from meat before adding to tomato sauce.
- Change type of meat (for example, ½ lean beef and ½ ground turkey/chicken or use chicken in place of meat.

Replace regular ricotta cheese with fat-free or part-skim ricotta cheese or fat-free or low-fat cottage cheese. Note comparison.

Use part-skim mozzarella or reduced-fat mozzarella (1 oz. mozzarella = 8 g fat vs. 1 oz. reduced-fat mozzarella = 6 g fat) or…use less cheese (4 oz. instead of 6 oz.)

Use less parmesan (4 oz. instead of 8 oz.).

Omit eggs or use 2 egg whites or ¼ c. liquid egg substitute

Original Recipe Lasagna *(Yield: 16 servings)*

	Calories	Fat (g)
2 Tbsp. olive oil	238	27
2 cloves garlic	8	0
2 lb. lean ground beef	1725	117
½ lb. ground pork	381	22
4 c. canned tomatoes	200	2
1 c. beef broth or stock	16	0
3 tsp. salt	0	0
½ tsp. pepper	2	0
1 c. mushrooms, fresh	20	1
¼ c. oregano	72	1
1 ½ c. (12 oz.) ricotta cheese	593	44
1/3 lb. (5 oz.) mozzarella cheese	1045	38
2 c. (8 oz.) parmesan cheese	80	68
1 egg	80	6
12 oz. noodles	1190	5

Nutrient analysis per serving:
375 calories, 30 g fat, 75 mg cholesterol

Note:

	Ricotta Cheese			Cottage Cheese	
	Calories	Fat (g)		Calories	Fat (g)
Regular, 1/2 c.	215	16	⇒	120	5
Low-fat, 1/2 c.	170	10	⇒	80	1
Fat-free, 1/2 c.	80	0	⇒	70	0

 Lighter version nutrient analysis per serving:
190 calories, 9 g fat, 33 mg cholesterol

Recipe Make-over: Chocolate Cake

New
Makeover suggestions

Original Recipe

Replace 2 oz. chocolate (28 g fat) with 6 Tbsp. cocoa (0 g fat) plus 4 Tbsp. sugar (0 g fat).

Replace 1 stick butter with ½ stick margarine (0 g cholesterol) and ¼ c. strained prunes (baby food) or replace butter with ½ c. strained baby food or ½ c. applesauce.

Replace 4 eggs with 8 egg whites (0 g fat) or 1 c. egg substitute (0 g fat).

Replace 3 oz. chocolate (42 g fat) with 6 Tbsp. cocoa (0 g fat) + 3 Tbsp. margarine (30 g fat).

Replace 3 Tbsp. butter with 3 Tbsp. margarine (0 g cholesterol).

Add 6 Tbsp. skim milk to liquefy frosting further.

** Alternative Frosting Option:
Replace frosting with fat-free chocolate syrup (35 cal/Tbsp.)

Chocolate Cake with Frosting
(Yield: 12 servings)

CAKE	Calories	Fat (g)
1 ¾ c. flour	735	2
3 Tbsp. baking powder	12	0
¼ tsp. salt	0	0
1 tsp. cinnamon	6	0
2 oz. bitter chocolate	265	26
½ c. (1 stick) butter	840	97
1 ½ c. sugar	1080	0
4 eggs	260	22
½ c. milk	75	4
1 tsp. vanilla extract	15	0
FROSTING**		
3 oz. bitter chocolate	397	43
3 Tbsp. butter	315	37
¼ c. coffee	1	0
1/8 tsp. salt	0	0
2 c. (1 lb.) powdered sugar	992	0
1 tsp. vanilla extract	15	0

Nutrient analysis per serving:
415 calories, 19 g fat, 100 mg cholesterol

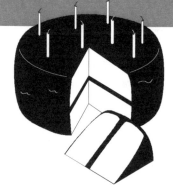

Lighter version nutrient analysis per serving:
350 calories, 7 g fat, 2 mg cholesterol

Step 10

Fun Foods Made Healthy

You can eat nutritious foods and still enjoy yourself. Try some of the ideas I've provided below. Create some of your own concoctions—using healthy ingredients, of course!

CRUNCHY SNACKS

- **Veggies and Dip:** 1 c. raw vegetables + 1/2 c. yogurt-based dip, fat-free dip or dip made with light sour cream or light cream cheese; or use light ranch dressing as dip
- **Nachos:** 1 corn tortilla (quartered and toasted) + 1 oz. grated nonfat or low-fat cheese + jalapeno pepper slices and optional salsa
- **Tortilla or pita chips:** Cut tortillas or pitas into eighths and bake at 400 degrees until crisp
- **Tostitos:** Toast corn tortilla, break into chips.
- **Wholewheat crackers:** Toast Shredded Wheat cereal
- **Blend a commercial Chex mix** with your favorite unbuttered Chex cereals for a great treat

CHEESE

- **Cheese toast:** 1 slice reduced-calorie bread + 1 oz. (3 Tbsp.) mozzarella cheese
- **Celery and cheese:** 3 celery sticks + 1 oz. skim ricotta cheese filling

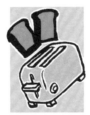

POPCORN

- **Cheesy popcorn:** 2 c. air-popped popcorn + 2 Tbsp. Parmesan cheese
- **Buttered popcorn:** 2 c. air-popped popcorn + butter-flavored pump spray
- **Herbed popcorn:** Combine 1/2 tsp. (each) marjoram, oregano, basil, onion powder and garlic powder; shake on popcorn
- **Nacho popcorn:** Shake nacho or taco seasoning mix on popcorn

Tip: *To make seasonings stick to air-popped popcorn, place popped popcorn on cookie sheet; spray with nonfat cooking spray and add seasonings. Place in oven for 10-15 minutes.*

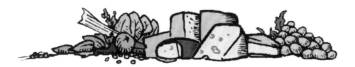

POTATO TOPPINGS

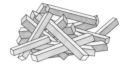

- **Cheesy potato:** 1 small baked potato + 1 oz. (3 Tbsp.) nonfat or low-fat cheese
- **French fries:** Broil red potato slices on each side. Sprinkle with Parmesan cheese
- **American potato:** 1 small baked potato + butter-flavored pump spray + 1 Tbsp. fat-free sour cream + 1 Tbsp. cheese
- **Mexican potato:** 1 small baked potato + picante sauce
- **Chinese potato:** 1 small baked potato + "lite" (low-sodium) soy sauce
- **Italian potato:** 1 small baked potato + 3 Tbsp. spaghetti sauce
- **Greek potato:** 1 small baked potato + 1 Tbsp. crumbled feta cheese + 1 Tbsp. nonfat yogurt
- **Yogurt potato:** 1 small baked potato + low-fat yogurt + low-fat mozzarella cheese

MINI-MEALS

- **Mini pizza:** 1 tortilla or English muffin half + 2 Tbsp. tomato sauce + 1 Tbsp. grated cheese + 2 Tbsp. green pepper
- **Lasagna:** Use chicken or make a vegetarian lasagna.
- **Stir-fry vegetables** in fat-free broth, water or wine instead of oil until crisp-tender
- **Cereal and milk:** 1/2 c. cereal + 1/2 c. nonfat milk

COLD DAIRY TREATS

- **Fruit and yogurt:** 1/2 c. mixed fruit topped with 1/2 c. plain nonfat yogurt
- **Milk shakes:** Blend 1 c. fat-free milk + fresh fruit (frozen) + flavor extract + cinnamon + ice (A refreshing dessert without excess sugar and fat calories.)
- **Smoothies:** Blend nonfat yogurt with 1 banana (frozen, sliced) and 1/2 c. frozen strawberries
- **Chocolate treat:** 1/2 c. plain nonfat yogurt + 1/2 packet sugar-free cocoa drink mix
- **Freeze fruit juice** using popsicle sticks to make low-calorie popsicles
- **Freeze grapes and sliced bananas** for a refreshing treat

How to Make Great-Tasting Veggies

Are you eating three vegetables every day? To improve your record, try these cooking methods that add flavor and pizzazz! (See Step 2 for the many benefits of a veggie-filled diet.)

VARY COOKING METHODS

Grill vegetables outdoors or roast or broil in oven with a touch of olive oil. Eat as a side dish or as tortilla or fajita fillings. Try red new potatoes, sweet potatoes, eggplant, zucchini, yellow squash, red bell pepper, carrots, celery.

Stir-fry vegetables...in nonstick skillets (add broth, if needed); or cook mushrooms first and use their "juice" for stir-frying. Add as many vegetables as possible: red bell pepper, red onion, celery, carrots, broccoli, cauliflower, green beans, snow peas, cabbage, asparagus, etc.

Sauté spinach in a little olive oil and garlic. Try also with zucchini, broccoli, asparagus, green beans and yellow squash.

Season vegetables by topping with melted low-fat cheese or parmesan, fat-free butter granules or "butter flavored" pump spray. Or, add Knorr bouillon cube(s) dissolved in hot water to vegetables as they cook.

Mash carrots or cauliflower into mashed potatoes. Mash butternut squash.

Start any dinner with sautéed carrots, celery, onion, garlic. Add this combo to navy beans, any stir-fried dish, green beans, chicken, seafood, squash.

Add sharp flavors to any vegetable: red bell pepper, cilantro, red onion, chili peppers, sun-dried tomatoes, red pepper flakes, chili powder, cumin, Italian or Greek seasoning blends.

Steam or microwave acorn squash. Top with a teaspoon of brown sugar or honey and lemon juice and spray butter.

Buy frozen bags of mixed vegetables; thaw and stir-fry with chicken or lean ground beef or soy crumbles, plus sliced onion in a little olive oil and cooking spray.

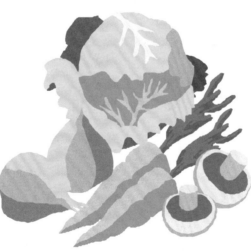

Microwave an ear of corn, sweet potato or red new potato or edamame beans for a snack!

Add green peas, carrots, celery, onion, green pepper and mushrooms to casseroles, mixed dishes and stews for color and flavor.

Add to rice, pasta and corn: colorful veggies such as minced carrots, parsley, celery, onion, green peas, red bell pepper, broccoli, tomatoes...whatever you like best. Serve hot one day, and the next day chill and add light Italian dressing for a cold salad.

MAKE YOUR MEAL REVOLVE AROUND VEGGIES

 Top a baked potato with:

- spinach + mozzarella cheese + cottage cheese and/or nonfat yogurt
- broccoli + mushrooms + low-fat or nonfat cheddar cheese
- picante sauce (and/or cottage cheese)
- spaghetti sauce + low-fat or nonfat cottage cheese, ricotta or parmesan cheese
- low-fat or fat-free cottage cheese or fat-free sour cream and picante sauce
- baked beans, diced tomatoes and onions

 Stuff vegetables, such as stuffed squash, tomatoes, peppers. For stuffing, use rice and ground turkey or tuna salad, or beans/rice mixture.

 Make spinach or broccoli dips, using nonfat yogurt or cottage cheese as a base.

 Stuff a pita pocket with mixed vegetables or salad.

 Make stews with 1 part lean meat, 10 parts vegetables. Or, make "vegetable stew" (tomatoes, onion, celery, beans, corn, green peas, carrots, green beans, squash, red cabbage, etc.).

Bake zucchini or carrot muffins and breads.

 Make a shish-ka-bob of vegetables and/or add more vegetables than meat shish-ka-bobs.

 Fill tortillas with spinach, cottage cheese, parmesan cheese and heat.

 Layer vegetables in a casserole pan as follows (bottom to top): onions, yellow squash, zucchini, tomato (all sliced in "rounds"): drizzle a little olive oil on top, then bread crumbs (4-5 Tbsp.) and parmesan cheese (4-5 Tbsp.). Bake at 350 for 30-40 minutes.

 Make a vegetarian pizza with lots of tomato, zucchini, green or red pepper, onion, mushroom, olives and carrots.

 Eat more beans: black beans, navy beans, kidney beans, soy (edamame) beans, etc. Add to rice, spaghetti sauces, pizza, chili, tortillas, tacos, soups, salads. Blend beans with picante sauce for bean spread, or try hummus spread. If you're feeling adventurous, try boiled soybeans. They are sweet and delicious! (Beans are rich in all vegetable nutrients.) Try cold bean salads (corn/blackbean; lentil/rice; blackeye pea, etc.)

EAT MORE FRESH RAW VEGGIES:

Buy baby carrots, already washed, peeled and ready to eat; snack on cherry tomatoes, fresh sugar snap peas, crisp celery, red bell pepper slices, steamed edamames.

Make a big colorful salad every night with dark-green lettuce, red bell pepper, red onion, tomato, cucumber, celery, carrots, etc. The more veggies, the better.

Add shredded broccoli, cabbage or carrots (available in bags at grocery stores) to sandwiches, wraps, soups, salads, pizza, spaghetti sauce, dips, spreads, humus.

Drink tomato or carrot juice for beverages. Or, try new fresh squeezed vegetable juice blends.

Add raw vegetables to:
- cold green bean or three-bean salads
- carrot-raisin salad
- Waldorf salad (apples, celery, cheese, nuts, green pepper)
- fruit salads (sliced carrots and celery)
- Jell-O salad (grated carrots in place of fruit)
- spinach salads with oranges, red bell pepper, pears
- coleslaws with fruit (pineapple, raisin, apple)
- marinated vegetable mix (carrots, celery, broccoli, cherry tomatoes, yellow squash, etc.)
- pickled vegetables (okra, carrots, corn, etc.) in salads

REMEMBER: GO FOR COLOR!

■ Make veggies the focus of a meal. Add meat, fish and poultry as "side dishes."

■ The five most nutrient-rich vegetables are broccoli, beans, carrots, tomatoes and potatoes.

■ The most antioxidant-rich vegetables have deep colors: **Romaine lettuce (not iceberg), spinach, broccoli, greens, tomatoes, carrots, sweet potatoes, red bell pepper, corn, red onion, beets, red cabbage, acorn squash, etc.**

■ The most phytochemical-rich vegetables **are beans, deep-colored vegetables, garlic, onion and soybeans (and soy products).**

■ These "cruciferous" vegetables help prevent cancer: **cabbage/coleslaw, broccoli, cauliflower, Brussels sprouts, bok choy, broccoli sprouts. Eat these at least four times a week.**

Quick Meal Ideas

CROCKPOT IDEAS

ITALIAN SPAGHETTI: Add chicken pieces or strips and favorite jar spaghetti sauce. (Optional: add sliced carrots, onions, celery.) Slow cook 6-8 hrs. Serve over pasta or rice.

STEW: Add beef stew chunks, quartered new potatoes, baby carrots (1 bag), 1 huge onion (chopped), yellow and zucchini squash (sliced), 1 can or thawed-out frozen green beans, 1 small can tomato sauce, 2 Knorr bouillon cubes, Italian seasonings. Slow cook 6-8 hrs. Can also simmer on stove top for 45-50 minutes.

CHILI: Brown/drain fat off ground beef. Put beef, onions, canned beans in pot and cook 4-5 hrs. (If you like, add tomatoes, carrots). Add chili powder.

MISCELLANEOUS

- **TURKEY ROLL-UPS**: Surround broccoli spear with 1 cheese slice and 1 turkey slice (or 1 ham slice). Heat and eat.
- **MINI-PIZZAS**: Use English muffin or tortilla as crust. Add pizza sauce, cheese, toppings.
- **BLACK BEANS** (canned): heat in microwave with chopped baby carrots and onions. Remove. Stir in salsa to taste. Fill tortillas. Sprinkle on cheese (Kraft 2% fat). Can add chopped tomato, lettuce.
- **BEANS** (canned): add to rice or bean soup for a great dinner. Add a salad.
- Take advantage of "**CREATE-A-MEAL**" frozen vegetable meals. Add chicken, ham, beef. Stir-fry.
- **CHICKEN**: Buy whole-roasted at the grocery store (or restaurants such as Boston Market); remove the skin; slice and add to vegetables, rice or soup meals at home.

> ➢ **See recipes in Appendix D.**

COOK AHEAD & BUILD MULTI-MEAL IDEAS

CHICKEN BREASTS: Cook (bake/broil/grill) 14 skinless breasts one weekend. Freeze. Use as needed.

Day 1- Serve fresh cooked with rice, green peas, baby carrots, salad.
Day 2- Serve sliced in stir-fry (frozen or fresh vegetables).
Day 3- Serve sliced, sauteed with onions and green peppers and fill tortillas (fajitas or soft tacos). Add lettuce, tomato, grated cheese, pico de gallo.
Day 4- Dice and add to macaroni and cheese for kids, with side salad or green vegetables.
Day 5- Reheat with spaghetti sauce and top pasta or baked potato.
Day 6- Thaw chunks and add to leftover pasta with thawed frozen vegetables for pasta salad.

GROUND BEEF: Brown 2 lbs. of lean ground beef; drain; divide and freeze in baggies. Thaw & use as needed.

Day 1- Reheat with spaghetti sauce for pasta.
Day 2- Reheat with taco seasoning mix for soft tacos.
Day 3- Reheat with tomato sauce and seasonings as "Sloppy Joes" for kids.
Day 4- Add to macaroni and cheese (boxed).
Day 5- Add to soups to make heartier.
Day 6- Make homemade pizza - split loaf of french bread; top with ground beef, grated cheese, spaghetti sauce, onions, peppers.

SALADS: Buy ready-to-serve bags. Top with:

1. Pre-cooked chicken breast
2. Shrimp (purchase boiled)
3. Turkey ham
4. Beans and grated cheese (taco salad)
5. Cooked lean ground beef
6. Cottage cheese

© 2009, *The Cooper Clinic Solution to the Diet Revolution* by Georgia G. Kostas, M.P.H., R.D., L.D., Dallas, Texas

Easy Ways to Add Nutrients to Family Favorite Meals

One-dish Meals: Plants + Protein = Flavor + Nutrition

- **Fajitas** - use flank steak, sirloin or chicken strips, or shrimp. Add grilled onion, red/green bell pepper, zucchini, mushrooms. Choose wholewheat or corn tortillas. Add as sides: beans, pico de gallo (lots) or salsa; tomato; lettuce.

- **Spaghetti, pizza or tomato sauces** - add 85-95% lean ground beef, soy crumbles or 85% lean ground turkey; grated carrots, onions, extra tomatoes (fresh or canned), bell pepper, garlic, mushrooms, celery and leftover veggies, etc.

  Fast steps: start with sauce from a can or jar; blend veggies in a blender or chop fine.

- **Pizza toppings** - add 85-95% lean ground beef, ham, chicken or soy pepperoni circles; grilled onion, red/green bell pepper, mushrooms, chopped broccoli or spinach, olives, grated carrots; regular or soy cheese and extra tomato sauce.

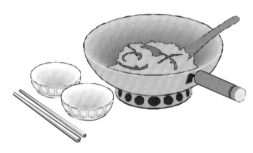

- **Stir-fries** - add to round steak strips, chicken or shrimp: at least 5 colorful veggies, snow peas, carrots, yellow squash, Chinese cabbage, garlic, edamames, nuts, red bell pepper, etc. Serve over brown rice.

- **Stew or pot roast** - add to lean chuck or round roast: carrots, onions, red potatoes w/skin, green beans, tomato sauce, wine, soy sauce. Slow-cook in crockpot.

- **Sandwiches, pitas or wraps** - use leftover beef or chicken, steak strips, deli roast beef/ham/turkey; add extra tomatoes, cucumber, fresh or roasted bell pepper, grated carrots, red onion, grated cabbage, hummus, etc.

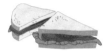

- **Tacos or tortillas** - add to 85-95% lean ground beef: onion, beans, salsa or pico de gallo, tomato, lettuce.

- **Chili or soup** - add to 85-95% lean ground beef: onion, red/green bell pepper, celery, carrots, mushrooms, tomatoes, beans, leftover veggies.

- **Salads** - add dark red/green lettuce, tomatoes, cucumber, red onion, red/green bell pepper, celery, any beans (garbanzo, black, kidney, pinto, etc.), edamames, grated red cabbage, carrots, artichokes, olives, mandarin oranges, leftover cooked veggies (broccoli, green beans, cauliflower, etc.), beets, nuts, seeds, ground flaxseed. Top with lean protein: meat, poultry, tuna, salmon, shrimp or tofu for one-dish meals.
  Salad dressing: add 1/2 c. canned cranberry (sauce or whole) to 1/2 c. olive oil/vinegar dressing or to your favorite light Italian dressing or vinaigrette. The cranberries cut the calories per Tbsp. of dressing in half and add antioxidants. You may also blend 1 tsp. flaxseed + 2 tsp. olive oil for every Tbsp. oil needed.

- **Stuffed vegetables** - fill bell peppers, cabbage rolls or eggplant with ground beef, brown rice, diced tomatoes, celery, onion, carrots, tomato sauce as filling.

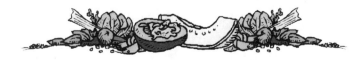

Delicious Veggies: Phyto-Nutrients "Phyte" for Your Health

Use as side dishes or pair with lean protein as one-dish meals:

❈ **Broccoli** - saute w/red bell pepper in olive oil. Eat cherry tomatoes on the side.

❈ **Broccoli, carrots, cauliflower, onion** - steam and season w/olive oil and fresh lemon juice blend.

❈ **Spinach, onion, garlic** - Saute together in olive oil; may stir in brown rice and lemon juice (or serve rice as a side dish); add tomatoes on the side. *Greens go great with red meat - they complement each others' flavors and nutrition.*

❈ **Roasted veggies** - slice and marinate at least five veggies together (broccoli, yellow squash, red bell peppers, red onions, carrots, green beans, asparagus, etc.)

❈ **Navy or cannelloni beans** - saute w/ olive oil and dices carrots, celery, onion.

❈ **Beans and rice** - black or red beans + brown rice.

❈ **Rice with onions** - season brown or wild rice with sauted yellow onions and tumeric.

❈ **Rice medley** - combine brown rice w/ pintos, soybeans or lentils, onion, raisins, nuts, carrots; may add drained, pre-cooked ground beef for flavor and nutrition; serve hot; add a salad for a complete meal.

❈ **Sweet potatoes** - broil potato rounds after spritzing each side with olive oil. Or microwave potato.

❈ **Mash potatoes** with cauliflower or carrots.

❈ **Guacamole + tomato** - add chopped tomatoes or pico de gallo or salsa to guacamole for flavor and maximizing nutrient value; also add avocado and tomato to salads, sandwiches, hamburgers, tacos.

❈ **Spice up dishes** with cilantro, rosemary, oregano, cumin, tumeric, hot peppers, jalapenos, cinnamon.

Breakfast Ideas - Begin each day with a healthy start!

Studies show breakfast eaters do better academically, miss fewer days from school or work and are more likely to be a healthy weight. Start each day with protein, grains and fruit.

Oatmeal or hot wholegrain cereals - top with fresh, frozen (thawed) or dried berries, ground flaxseed, prunes, almonds, walnuts, dried tart cherries or cranberries, raisins, cinnamon, bananas; cook in soy or lowfat milk.

Dry cereals - add to Kashi or any wholegrain cereal: walnuts, ground flaxseed, fresh or dried fruit (raisins, cranberries, blueberries); add lowfat or soy milk.

Quesadillas or toasted grilled cheese sandwiches - just add fruit and milk!

Frozen multi-berry packages - heat with a little sugar and use as topping for oatmeal, pancakes, Kashi waffles, yogurt; or add to smoothies with yogurt, soy or lowfat milk.

Eggs - cook any way. (Scrambled with cheese helps keep energy up longer!) Add wholewheat toast, sliced fruit or orange juice, and milk.

Sandwich or wrap - filled with ham and cheese or peanutbutter and banana.

Healthy Homemade Snacks

❈ **Snack mix** - add wholegrain chex cereals, corn chex, rice chex, Cheerios, raisins, soynuts, nuts. Eat as a snack or top salads and yogurt (substitute for chips).

❈ **Peanutbutter** or almondbutter on wholewheat bread, crackers or celery.

❈ **Edamames (in pods)** - steam and eat; these are great party appetizers or snacks.

❈ **Cheese** - with apple slices, wholewheat crackers (Triscuits) or grilled cheese sandwich

❈ **Salsas** - make mango or peach salsa or chutney; use with Triscuits or baked chips, or use as a side with chicken or main dishes.

❈ **Pico de gallo** - serve as a side to seafood, poultry or meat dishes. Great with snacks.

❈ **Fruit** - any type, hot or cold. Serve as a snack, appetizer or dessert. Or make a salad with grapes, apples, blueberries and oranges to maximize antioxidants.

❈ **Chocolate and fruit** - dip fresh strawberries or bananas, dried apricots, in melted chocolate.

❈ **Sundae** - top fat-free yogurt with fresh peaches, blueberries or seasonal fruit; sprinkle nuts or crunchy dry cereal on top.

❈ **Smoothies** - blend berries, a banana, favorite fruit and fat-free yogurt or milk with ice.

❈ **Raw veggies with hummus or Ranch dip** - carrots, broccoli, celery, cherry tomatoes, cucumbers.

❈ **Pizza** - especially homemade!

❈ **Chocolate milk or homemade hot cocoa.**

Step 11
Food: It's What's Inside That Counts

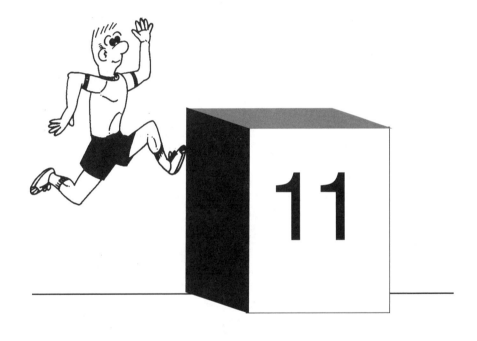

Step 11

Mini-Step 1:

Get to know food . . . sources of calcium, fiber, sugar, sodium and caffeine.

Mini-Step 2:

Value the benefits of water and whole foods.

Foods are a treasure chest of vital nutrients for our best health. By emphasizing top-quality foods daily, we feed our bodies with "high-octane" fuel and feel our best. Don't take a "shortcut" to weight management by selecting primarily low-calorie, low-nutrient processed foods . . . Go for quality, wholesome, nutrient-dense foods!

Simple Steps you can take daily:

- add more fiber, calcium, water daily and
- eat less sugar, sodium, caffeine, processed foods

The menus throughout this book incorporate these guidelines.

Are you consuming enough *calcium* for strong bones? See how to get enough calcium from food.

Do you eat enough *fiber* each day? Fiber promotes weight control and helps prevent numerous health problems. Soluble fiber reduces cholesterol levels. Refer to the chart on p. 221 to make sure you're getting the suggested 20-35 g each day.

And what about *sugar*? Too much of it leads to weight gain. How much do you eat, unaware? Same goes for *sodium*—it's everywhere. Take a look at p. 229. It goes without saying that foods are best in their natural state.

How much *caffeine* do you consume daily, and how much is considered "safe"? *Water* is the beverage of choice (see p. 230), but you coffee lovers will be happy to know that a little of your favorite drink is OK. Moderation is the key.

What's the scoop on **additives**? Review the Food and Drug Administration's approved list of food additives. Cut back on processed foods and choose whole foods whenever possible. Remember, by *minimizing* processed foods, you can *maximize* nutrients!

ACTION STEPS

① Each day eat at least three fruits, three vegetables, three wholegrains (with one serving of bran cereal or beans) to get 20-35 g fiber. Avoid processed foods. Focus on fresh and "whole foods."

② Take inventory of how much calcium you consume each day. How can you consume more?

③ Read labels to look for hidden sources of sugar and salt.

④ Determine how many milligrams of caffeine you drink each day. Limit it to 200 mg.

⑤ Drink 6 - 8 glasses of water a day.

Bone Up on Calcium

At all ages, men and women need calcium for strong bones, teeth and exercising muscles. In particular, women need extra calcium after age 30 to prevent osteoporosis, or "softening of the bones", which manifests itself in women after age 50. (See p. 150 for exercise diagrams to help prevent osteoporosis.) Below is a chart to determine if you eat enough calcium, followed by other tips that will motivate you to do all you can, while you can, to meet your body's calcium needs.

Daily Calcium & Vitamin D Needed:				
Adults	Ages	Amount (mg)	Number of 300 mg Calcium Equivalent Foods*	Vitamin D
Men	19-65	1000	2-3 servings	800 - 1000 IU
	65+	1500	3-4 servings	800 - 1000 IU
Women	19-50	1200-1500	3-4 servings	800 - 1000 IU
	50+	1500	3-4 servings	800 - 1000 IU
With low bone density	all ages	1500	3-4 servings	800 - 1000 IU

* 1 cup milk = 300 mg calcium

Factors to Promote Strong Bones

- Adequate calcium daily and a balanced, healthy diet
- Regular weight-bearing exercise such as walking (not biking or swimming), at least five times a week
- Strength training with light weights, 2-3 times a week
- Sunlight exposure, 10-15 minutes a day, to stimulate vitamin D production in skin, which aids calcium absorption. Most Americans need more Vitamin D. Consult with your physician about lab work and supplements.
- Estrogen replacement or medications as directed by your physician
- Therapeutic high dosages of prescription Vitamin D may help (10,000 - 50,000 IU Vitamin D3 for 6-8 wks.)
- Not smoking
- Limited soft drinks, caffeine (one cup coffee/day), and sodium to reduce blocking calcium's absorption
- Isoflavones in soy products, estrogen-like compounds that increase bone density
- Potassium and magnesium—in greens, beans, wholegrains, vegetables, fruit
- Vitamin K daily from greens (lettuce, spinach, broccoli, cabbage, etc.)
- Omega-3 fats in seafood (especially salmon, mackerel, sardines).

Calcium Supplements: Which Are Best?

Use Foods First; Supplements Next!
- **Calcium citrate** (found in Citracal and citrus juices with added calcium citrate maleate) is absorbed best.
- **Calcium carbonate** is found in Tums, Caltrate, Viactiv, etc. Take with food.
- **Calcium phosphate**, **calcium lactate** and **calcium gluconate** *are not* absorbed as well.
- Avoid bone meal and dolomite due to potential lead contamination.
- Never exceed 2000 mg of calcium daily from food & supplements combined.

Ways to Boost Calcium Supplement Absorption

- Take calcium supplements with food (stomach acidity aids absorption), or with a dairy product (lactose and vitamin D aid absorption), or with orange juice or tomato juice (vitamin C boosts calcium absorption).
- Never take supplements with caffeine-containing beverages such as tea, coffee and cola or high-fiber foods (caffeine and fiber impair calcium absorption).
- Take supplements with vitamin D, especially if you are without daily sunlight exposure (see amounts above).
- Space calcium supplements at 5 - 6 hour intervals. Smaller amounts, (up to 500 mg) are absorbed better.

Beyond bone-building: Calcium helps lower blood pressure, prevent colon cancer and lose weight.

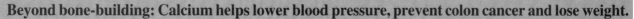

Boost your calcium intake!

Calcium Food Sources

500 mg Calcium
Lactaid 100 Milk, calcium-fortified, fat-free, 1 c.
General Mills Total whole grain cereal or Total Raisin Bran, 1/2 c.
Quaker Instant Oatmeal Nutrition for Women, 1 pkt.
Frulatte Smoothies - 6 flavors, 10.5 oz.
Nestles Carnation Instant Breakfast drink, 1 carton
GeniSoy Ultra XT Protein Powder (3 flavors), 1 scoop
Silk Soy Milk calcium fortified, 1 c.
Blue Bell sugar-free low fat ice cream, 1/2 c.

450 mg Calcium
Lucerne fat-free plain yogurt, 1 c.
Stoney Field Farm non-fat yogurt, 1 c.
Edy's/Dreyer's fat-free frozen yogurt, 1/2 c.

400 mg Calcium
Yogurt, nonfat or low-fat, 1 c. (350-400 mg)
Kraft 2% Milk Cheese w/added calcium, 1/4 c.

350 mg Calcium
Borden Plus Kid Builder 1% low-fat milk, 1 c.
Hood Carb Countdown Milk, fat-free - reg or choc, 1 c.
Bordens Plus fat-free milk, 1 c.
Tropicana, Minute Maid m Minute Maid Lite or Florida's Natural Orange Juice **w/calcium + Vitamin D** , 1 c.
Lucerne or Columbo Light fat-free yogurt, 1 c.
Clift Lima Bars, all flavors, 1 bar
Café Latte, fat-free, 12 oz.
Ronzoni Smart Taste Pasta w/Calcium & fiber, 2 oz.

300 mg Calcium = calcium in 1 cup milk
Milk, fat-free, 1%, 2%, whole, 1 c.
Soy or rice milk, calcium-fortified, 1 c.
Borden fat-free or 2% cheese slices, 1 slice
Tofu, Azumaya Lite, 2.8 oz.
Galaxy Veggie Soy slices, 1-1/2 slices
Lucerne 2% cottage cheese, calcium fortified, 1/2 c.
Parmesan & Romano, (3 Tbsp. or 1/4 c.) 1 oz.
Kraft finely shredded Parmesan cheese, (1/4 c.) 1 oz.

Mootown Twirls string cheese, 1 piece
Nonfat dry milk, 5 Tbsp.
Nestle or Swiss Miss fat-free calcium-fortified hot cocoa, 1 packet
V-8 Juice with Calcium, 1 c.
Yoplait Nouriche Light Smoothie, 11 oz.
Pria Power Bar, 1 bar
Power Bar Performance, 1 bar
Macaroni and cheese, 3/4 c.
12" Cheese pizza, 2 slices
Krusteaz muffin mix, 1 muffin
Eggo Homestyle frozen waffles, 2 pieces
Special K Plus Cereal, 1/2 c.
Iron Kids Bread (Rainbow), 2 slices
Earthgrains Heart Healthy Plus bread w/ added calcium & fiber, 2 slices
Weight Watchers Yogurt, 6 oz.

250 mg Calcium
Swiss cheese, 1 oz.
Kraft 2% Milk American or Swiss singles, 1 oz.
Kraft snackable cubes, 1 oz.
Kraft free Shredded Cheese, 1 oz., 1/4 c.
Dannon Light 'n Fit Yogurt, 6 oz.
Blue Bell Light Ice Cream, 1/2 c.
Precious Ricotta Cheese, fat-free, 1/4 c.
Precious Mozzarella Sticks Plus, 1 oz.
Edamame Beans, 1 c.

200 mg Calcium
Cabot 50% or 75% less fat cheeses, 1 oz.
Cheddar cheese, 1 oz.
Lowfat Healthy Choice String Cheese, 1 piece
Part-Skim Mozzarella cheese sticks, 1 stick
Soy/tofu Singles ("veggy"), 1 slice
Yoplait Light fat-free yogurt, 6 oz.
Kellogg's Nutrigrain Cereal Bar, 1 bar
Sesame seeds, 2 Tbsp.
Propel Calcium Fitness Water, all flavors, 16 oz.
Wheatena, 1/3 cup (dry)

175 mg Calcium
American cheese, 1 oz.
Oysters, 3/4 c. (170 mg)
Salmon, canned with bones, 3 oz. (170 mg)

150 mg Calcium
Kraft fat-free singles, 1 slice
Velveeta light, 1 oz.
Mini Babybel Cheese, 1 oz., (1 round)
Kraft String-Ums, 2% milk string cheese, 1 stick
Cottage Cheese 1% fat, 1/2 c.
Dannon Light 'n Fit yogurt smoothie, 7 oz.
Fiber One or All-Bran cereals, 1/2 c., (100-150 mg)
Earthgrains Calcium-fortified Bread, 1 slice (100-150 mg)
Custard pudding, 1/2 c.
Broccoli, 1 c.
Collard greens; most greens, 1/2 c.

100 & under mg Calcium
Spinach or mustard greens cooked, 1/2 c.
Ice cream or ice milk, 1/2 c.
Instant oatmeal, 1 packet
Yoplait GoGurt yogurt, 1 tube
Calcium-fortified margarines (Shedd's, I Can't Believe It's Not Butter, etc.), 1 Tbsp.
Almonds, 1/4 c. (90 mg)
Beans, cooked, 1 c. (90 mg)
Cottage cheese, 2% (low-fat), 1/2 c. (80-100 mg)
Kale, cooked, 1/2 c. (75 mg)
Broccoli, cooked, 1/2 c. (70 mg)
Orange, 1 medium, (55 mg)

Calcium Alternatives
Ensure Plus w/calcium added, 1 packet (300 mg) + 1 c. fat-free milk, (600 mg total)
Viactiv calcium chocolate chews, 1 piece (500 mg)
Bayer Women's aspirin 81 mg, 1 tablet (300 mg)
Tums chews, 1 piece (500 mg)
Knox gelatin, 1 scoop (300 mg)
Calcium supplements, 1 tablet (300 - 600 mg)

How to Get 1500 Mg of Calcium Daily

Basic Daily Plan:

2 c. milk or yogurt	600 mg	
1 c. orange juice with calcium	300 mg	**Totals**
1-2 calcium-rich foods or supplements	300 mg	**1500 mg**
Overall diet	300 mg	

Sample High-Calorie, Low-Calorie Menu:

	Calcium (mg)	Calories	Fat (g)
2 c. skim milk	600	200	Trace
2 slices Kraft 2% cheese (singles)	500	100	6
1/2 c. spinach, cooked	100	25	0
1 orange, medium	50	50	0
1 apple, large	10	80	0
3 slices bread	75	210	3
3 oz. chicken, baked	12	150	6
Tossed salad w/ 1 Tbsp. Parmesan	130	50	2
1 baked potato, medium	15	140	0
1 carrot	25	25	0
TOTALS	**1517 mg**	**1030 cal**	**17 g**

Tips to Increase Calcium

1. **Select calcium-fortified foods** (see above) and add new ones that come out often.

2. **Add nonfat dry powdered milk to:**

mashed potatoes	oatmeal
cornbread or muffins	casseroles
high-calcium Alba cocoa	liquid milk
macaroni & cheese	spaghetti sauce
homemade yogurt made from skim milk	pizza sauce
homemade milk & fruit shakes/smoothies	pancakes
	soup

3. **Add grated cheese** to salads, baked potatoes, vegetables, soup, toast and grits.

4. **Choose cheeses with more calcium:** Swiss, Parmesan, Romano, Ricotta; 2% milk cheeses.

5. **Read calcium labels!** A food labeled with a Daily Value for calcium of 20% means 200 mg calcium.

Fiber Facts

Like fruits and veggies, **fiber** is an important part of healthy eating. Unfortunately, studies have shown that most Americans eat half the recommended amount—**20-35** grams per day—and, as a result, we are putting ourselves at risk for possible health problems such as colon cancer.

Fiber is essentially the "bulk" or "roughage" in your diet that pushes food through the digestive tract more smoothly, aiding digestion and elimination. The **key sources** are wholegrain breads and cereals, wheat bran, fresh fruits and vegetables, peas, beans, nuts, seeds, oats, psyllium, popcorn, barley and brown rice. Further, there are two types of fiber with different health benefits:

- **Insoluble:** found in plant coatings, peels, seeds, kernels, bran, strings. Sources include wholegrains, apple or fruit peels, nuts, beans, seeds (berries, tomatoes, grapes), bran kernels, popcorn, oranges, pear, celery or melon strings, potato peels.

- **Soluble:** found in the water-soluble complex carbohydrate content of food and characterized by "stickiness" after cooking. Key sources include apples, oats, beans, peas, psyllium, bananas, citrus fruit, Brussels sprouts, carrots, eggplant.

10 Ways to Eat More Fiber

How can you be sure to consume 20-35 grams of fiber each day?

☐ 1. **Eat eight or nine fiber-rich plant foods daily** (3 fruit, 3 vegetables, 3 wholegrains, 1 serving beans or bran cereal).

☐ 2. **Eat beans or foods with bran (wheat or oat) every day.** By eating 1/2 c. to 1 c. bran cereal (i.e., Fiber One) or beans daily, you consume 50% of the fiber you need. Add bran or bran cereal to other cereals, muffins, cookies, pancakes, bread recipes, meat loaf; or add as a topping on tossed or fruit salads, or on yogurt.

☐ 3. **Eat 1/2 c. cooked oat bran cereal** or 1 1/2 c. cooked oatmeal daily to lower cholesterol.

☐ 4. **Add unprocessed bran to foods, gradually increasing the amount—up to 3 Tbsp. a day.** Excessive amounts may lead to impaired absorption of some nutrients. Drink more water as you add bran.

☐ 5. **Eat vegetables raw or slightly cooked.** Do not overcook!

☐ 6. **Eat fresh fruit** instead of canned, peeled or pureed fruit or juices.

☐ 7. **Choose breads and cereals labeled "wholewheat" or "wholegrain" as the first ingredient.** Avoid brown-colored breads labeled "wheat flour" with "caramel" coloring. Look for "100% wholewheat flour."

☐ 8. **Eat hot oat bran, oatmeal and wholegrain cereals** instead of refined cereals such as Cream of Wheat and Cream of Rice, etc.

☐ 9. **Eat a variety of fiber-rich foods**, since different foods contain varied types of fiber with different benefits.

☐ 10. **Read and compare food labels.** Did you know 7 reduced-fat wholewheat Triscuits contain 3 grams of fiber?

Reasons to Eat More Fiber

Enjoy these wonderful benefits of a fiber-rich diet:

1. **It promotes weight control.** Fiber-rich foods take longer to eat and create a feeling of fullness and satiety; a very high-fiber intake (55-60 g/day) may help block fat absorption and promote fat excretion.
2. **It enhances good digestion and elimination.**
3. **It acts as a "natural laxative"** to reduce constipation and promote regular elimination.
4. **It decreases the risk of colon cancer and perhaps other cancers.**
5. **It helps prevent and treat diverticulosis.**
6. **It prevents and treats spastic colon, hemorrhoids and other digestive problems.**
7. **Soluble fiber from any food reduces cholesterol levels.**
   - **3 grams oat fiber daily (in 1 1/2 c. cooked oatmeal or 1/2 c. cooked oat bran)**
   - **7 grams psyllium fiber daily (in 1 Tbsp. sugar-free Metamucil or in a few breakfast cereals)**
8. **Soluble fiber stabilizes blood sugar levels,** which helps control appetite and lowers insulin requirements in people with diabetes.

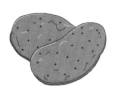

Tips to Improve Digestion and Elimination:

- Consume more **fiber and water.**
- **Eat slowly** in a relaxed environment and chew food well.
- **Eat regular meals, exercise daily and get adequate rest.**
- **Eat at least 8 to 9 high-fiber foods daily.** (Refer to list on next page.)

Important Note:

When increasing fiber, drink 10-12 glasses of fluids per day, at least half of which is water. Fiber absorbs liquid to form larger and softer stools that are easier to pass. Too little fluid may cause dehydration and constipation.

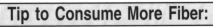

Tip to Consume More Fiber:

Eat daily at least:
    3 fruit (6 g fiber)
    3 vegetables (6 g fiber)
    3 starches, especially wholegrains (6 g fiber)
    1 serving bran cereal or beans (5 - 10 g fiber)
Total: 20 - 35 g of fiber!

Eat wholegrains
for
maximum fiber!

Fiber Content of Foods

GRAINS (1/2 c. unless otherwise noted)

	Fiber (g)
Fiber One Original (General Mills)	14.0
Fiber One Honey Clusters (1 c.)	13.0
* All-Bran with Extra Fiber (Kellogg)	13.0
All Bran Buds (Kellogg) (1/3 c.)	13.0
Kashi Good Friends (1 c.)	12.0
Gnu Bar, Cinnamon Raisin	12.0
Nature's Path Flax Plus Raisin Bran (3/4 c.)	11.0
* 100% Bran (Nabisco) (1/3 c.)	10.0
Kashi Go Lean (1 c.)	10.0
Fiber One Chewy Bar	9.0
Earthgrains Extra Fiber 100% Wholewheat bread (2 slices)	9.0
Flat Out Wrap - Light Sundried Tomato	9.0
Kashi Go Lean Crunch (1 c.)	8.0
Thomas Light Multigrain English Muffin	8.0
Nature's Own Double Fiber Bread (1 slice)	8.0
Orowheat Double Fiber Bread (1 slice)	8.0
Ry Krisp Light Crackers (5)	7.0
Nature's Path & Grain Synergy (2/3 c.)	6.0
Barbara's Puffins Cinnamon (3/4 c.)	6.0
Wasa Fiber Rye & Multigrain Crispbread (3 slices)	6.0
Quaker Oat Bran (1/3 c. dry - cooks to 2/3 c.)	6.0
Corn Bran (Quaker)	6.0
Light 100% wholewheat bread (2 slices) (read labels)	6.0
Instant Oatmeal, Weight Control (Quaker)	6.0
Bran Chex (Post)	5.0
Kashi Heart to Heart (3/4 c.)	5.0
Nature's Path Multigrain Oat Bran (2/3 c.)	5.0
Natural Bran Flakes (Post) (3/4 c.)	5.0
Fiber One Yogurt	5.0
All Bran Multi-Grain Crackers (18)	5.0
40% Bran Flakes (all brands)	4.5
Kashi Granola Bars	4.0
Smart Balance Light Butter Popcorn	4.0
Raisin Bran (Kellogg, Post, General Mills)	4.0
Multi-Bran Chex (General Mills)	4.0
* Wheat germ (1/4 c.)	4.0
Complete Bran Flakes	4.0
Shredded Wheat n Bran (Nabisco) (2/3 c.)	4.0
Wheatena (Uhlmann)	4.0
Barley, cooked	4.0
Low-fat flour tortilla, soft (Tia Rosa) (1)	4.0
Shredded Wheat (Nabisco)	3.3
Instant oatmeal (Ralston, Quaker)	3.0
Popcorn, air-popped (3 c.)	3.0
Reduced-fat or Low Sodium Triscuit crackers (6)	3.0
Fruit 'n Fiber (Post)	3.0
Frosted Mini-Wheats (Kellogg)	3.0
Grape-Nuts (Post) (1/3 c.)	3.0
100% Wholegrain Wheat Chex (Ralston)	3.0
Low-fat granola (Kellogg)	3.0
Wholewheat spaghetti, cooked	3.0

	Fiber (g)
Graham crackers (2 squares)	2.8
Brown rice, cooked	2.1
Nutri-Grain (Kellogg)	2.1
Total (General Mills)	2.0
Wheaties or Cheerios (General Mills)	1.5
Wholewheat bread, 1 slice (read label)	2-3
Special K or Corn Flakes (1 c.)	1.0
Rye bread (1 slice) (read label)	0-2
Mission Carb Balance Wholewheat Tortilla, fajita size (1)	8.0
La Tortilla Factory Wholewheat 10 Carb tortilla, small (1)	7.0
Corn tortilla, soft (1) (read label)	2-3
Flour tortilla, soft (1)	1.0
Kashi Heart to Heart waffles (2)	5.0
Aunt Jemima Buckwheat Pancake Mix 4" pancakes (2)	1.0

VEGETABLES (1/2 c. cooked)

Sweet potato (1 large); Green peas (1/2 c.)	5.0
Brussels sprouts; Corn	4.0
Potato, baked with skin (1 medium)	4.0
Hominy	3.0
Carrots (1 raw or 1/2 c. cooked); Broccoli	3.0
Spinach, collard greens; Acorn or butternut squash	3.0
Asparagus; Green beans; Okra; Turnips	2.0
Bean sprouts	1.5
Mushrooms, raw; Zucchini; 1/2 Tomato	1.0
Lettuce (1 c.); Celery (3 stalks)	1.0

FRUITS (raw)

Strawberries; Blueberries (1 c.)	4.3
Blackberries; raspberries (1/2 c.)	4.0
Apple or pear with skin (1 medium)	4.0
Prunes, dried (5) or prune juice (1 c.)	3.5
Orange (medium); Banana (large)	3.0
Grapefruit (1/2 large); Peach (large)	2.0
Cantaloupe (1/4 small); Watermelon (1 c.)	1.0
Grapes (15); Raisins (2 Tbsp.)	1.0

LEGUMES/BEANS/NUTS/SEEDS

Psyllium seeds (5 Tbsp., 1 oz.)	20.0
Black bean soup (1 c.)	10.0
Kidney beans, lentils, pinto beans, chickpeas, cooked (1/2 c.)	7.0
Flax seeds (3 Tbsp., 1 oz.)	7.0
Split peas; White, black or lima beans, cooked (1/2 c.)	5.0
Nuts/Seeds (1/4 c., 1 oz.)	3.0

EXTRA FIBER SOURCES

Metamucil Wafers (2)	6.0
* Unprocessed bran flakes (such as Millers Bran) (2 Tbsp.)	5.4
Metamucil, 1 Tbsp.	3.0

NO FIBER

Milk, cheese, yogurt, poultry, fish, meat, margarine, oils, dressings

➤ See cereal list, p. 225

Add to soups, beverages, cooked or dry cereals, spaghetti sauce, stews, casseroles, meat loaf, muffins, bread, rolls, pancakes, salads, yogurt.

Sugar

Excessive sugar inevitably leads to weight gain and poor health and fitness. One teaspoon of sugar (all forms) equals 15 calories. These are "empty" calories that do not provide vitamins, minerals or fiber. It's easy to eat too much sugar, even unaware. Once again, "knowledge is power."

What is Sugar?

Sucrose, the technical term for **sugar**, occurs naturally in sugar cane or sugar beets. A "simple carbohydrate," it is easily absorbed by the body. Sugar is the most popular food additive. It adds taste, texture, appearance, color, thickening and firmness while acting as a preservative.

Refined sugar (simple carbohydrates) increase blood sugar levels within 15 minutes, resulting in "quick energy." This lasts only a few minutes because insulin reacts immediately to lower blood sugar. This rapid drop may make you feel less energetic and crave more sugar. On the other hand, complex carbohydrates such as fruits, vegetables, starches and wholegrains are broken down slowly by your body, allowing a more constant blood sugar level that gives longer, lasting energy. Eat more complex carbohydrates, especially those with fiber, and you'll find you want less sugar. Plus, you'll have more energy and control over your "sweet tooth" and appetite.

FORMS OF SUGAR	
Some forms of sugar are indicated by words ending in:	
"-ose"	**Other forms include:**
Dextrose	Brown sugar
Fructose	Corn syrup
Galactose	Dextrin
Glucose	Honey
Lactose	Maple syrup
Maltose	Molasses
Mannose	Sorghum
Sucrose	Table sugar
	Sugar alcohols (sorbitol, mannitol, dulcitol, zylitol)

What is the Glycemic Index?

This is a rating system that indicates how fast the natural or added sugar in food is absorbed into your bloodstream. When you eat several foods together (mixing proteins-carbohydrates-fats), the Glycemic Index is low (desirable), sustaining your blood sugar and energy, controlling appetite.

Where Is Sugar?

Sugar is added to a great variety of foods, prepared commercially and at home:

cakes, pies	fruit yogurt	peanutbutter
canned fruit	ice cream	pudding
cereal	jam, jelly	salad dressing
cookies, candy	ketchup	soups
soft drinks	non-dairy coffee creamers	spaghetti sauce

Read labels when you shop, and look for "sugar" and its other names. Remember that ingredients on the label are listed from greatest quantity to least. Thus, if some form of sugar is one of the first three ingredients—or if various forms of sugar are listed separately throughout the ingredient list—then the product is most likely high in sugar content. Find a lower-sugar product if possible. Or, choose a very small portion of the sugar-rich food. Ask yourself if this food is really worth its calories. If not, move on.

Why Limit Sugar?

Excess sugar may lead to these health problems:

❏ **Tooth Decay:** Bacteria thrive on sugar and destroy tooth enamel, causing cavities.

❏ **Extra pounds:** Sweets compact a lot of calories into a small amount of food. Excess sweets lead to excess calories that are stored as body fat.

❏ **Diabetes or Pre-diabetes:** Excess sugar calories may lead to excess weight, which requires more insulin than the body can supply; diabetes may result. Check your blood sugar levels regularly.

❏ **Hypoglycemia:** Although sugar does not cause hypoglycemia, people with hypoglycemia should avoid sugar to prevent unpleasant symptoms such as shakiness, headaches, weakness, fatigue, confusion and to help maintain constant blood sugar levels.

❏ **Heart Disease:** Excess sugar promotes insulin production, converting blood glucose to fatty acids and triglycerides, which may deposit in arteries and lead to atherosclerosis.

❏ **Triglycerides:** Excess sugar may elevate triglycerides (fats) in the blood, increasing one's risk of heart disease.

How Can I Learn to Eat Less Sugar?

Below are 15 ways to eat less sugar. Which ones will you implement?

❏ **Cut back**. The less sugar you eat, the less sugar you want. The more you eat, the more you want. Sugar can trigger a craving for more sweets or more food. If sugar leads to compulsive overeating or bingeing, avoid it. Otherwise, eat it with limits.

❏ **Choose sugar-free products**. Substitute unsweetened fruit juice or plain water for regular soft drinks, punches and fruit drinks containing large amounts of sugar.

❏ **Buy unsweetened cereals** such as shredded wheat, puffed wheat or puffed rice.

❏ **Eat fewer and smaller desserts**.

❏ **Reduce sugar in recipes**. Use concentrated fruit juice, cinnamon, nutmeg or flavor extracts such as vanilla and almond for added flavor. Replace 1/4 cup of sugar with a mashed banana in cookies.

❏ Make it a habit not to buy simple carbohydrates. Instead, buy and **eat fresh fruits**.

❏ **Don't use sweets as rewards**. Buy a new CD, tape or video…or call a friend.

❏ Drink coffee or tea without sugar. Drink flavored, **unsweetened coffees or teas**.

❏ **Sweeten cereal by adding fruit**, raisins, vanilla extract or cinnamon instead of sugar.

❏ **Read labels for "sugars."** Know what you are eating.

❏ **Eat sugar-free, nonfat frozen yogurt** as a treat.

❏ **Split a dessert** with two to four other people if you really want it. Eat it slowly and enjoy!

❏ **Learn fun alternatives for sweets**. For example, choose a bagel instead of a donut. Or add a teaspoon of jam (15 calories) to bread as a sweet snack.

❏ Rather than buy a candy bar, select miniature **"fun size" candy portions** (about 75 calories).

❏ **Set a limit**: 100 to 150 "sweet calories" daily (i.e., a small yogurt or 12 oz. soda). **READ LABELS!**

Hidden Sugars

Food Item	Amount	Sugar (tsp)
BEVERAGES		
colas	12 oz.	10
gingerale	12 oz.	7
orange-ade	12 oz.	9
root beer	12 oz.	6
7-Up	12 oz.	9
sweet cider	12 oz.	7
canned fruit juices (sweetened)	1/2 c.	2
CANDIES		
chocolate milk bar	3 oz.	5
chewing gum	1 stick	½
fudge	1 oz. square	4 ½
gum drop	1	2
hard candy	4 oz.	20
Lifesavers	1	½
peanut brittle	1 oz.	3 ½
marshmallow	1	1 ½
CAKES AND COOKIES		
angel food cake	1 (4 oz. piece)	7
banana cake	1 (2 oz. piece)	2
cheesecake	1 (4 oz. piece)	2
chocolate cake (no icing)	1 (4 oz. piece)	6
chocolate cake (iced)	1 (4 oz. piece)	10
coffee cake	1	4 ½
cup cake (iced)	1	6
fruit cake	1 (4 oz. piece)	5
jelly roll	1 (2 oz. piece)	2 ½
pound cake	1 (4 oz. piece)	5
sponge cake	1 (1 oz. piece)	2
strawberry shortcake	1 serving	4
brownies (unfrosted)	3/4 oz. square	3
chocolate cookies	1	1 ½
fig newtons	1	5
ginger snaps	1	3
nut cookies	1	1 ½
oatmeal cookies	1	2
sugar cookies	1	1 ½
chocolate eclair	1	7
cream puff	1	2
donut (plain)	1	3
donut (glazed)	1	6

Food Item	Amount	Sugar (tsp)
DAIRY PRODUCTS		
ice cream (1/3 pint)	(3 ½ oz.)	3 ½
ice cream bar	1 (depending on size)	1-7
ice cream cone	1	5 ½
eggnog, all milk	8 oz.	4 ½
ice cream soda	1	5
cocoa, all milk	1 c. (8 oz.)	4
ice cream sundae	1	7
chocolate, all milk	1 c. (5 oz. milk)	6
malted milk shake	10 oz.	5
sherbet	1/2 c. (1 scoop)	9
DESSERTS		
apple cobbler	1/2 c.	3
custard	1/2 c.	2
French pastry	1 (4 oz. piece)	5
Jell-O	1/2 c.	5
apple pie	1 slice (average)	7
cherry pie	1 slice	10
cream pie	1 slice	4
custard pie	1 slice	10
coconut pie	1 slice	10
lemon pie	1 slice	7
peach pie	1 slice	7
pumpkin pie	1 slice	5
banana pudding	1/2 c.	2
bread pudding	1/2 c.	1 ½
chocolate pudding	1/2 c.	4
rice pudding	1/2 c.	5
tapioca pudding	1/2 c.	3

Add it up:

Based on the these charts, how much hidden sugar do you eat daily?

Approximately _____ teaspoons.

A 12 oz. soda contains 9-10 tsp. of sugar!!

Cereals: Top Choices

Choose those with more wholegrains & fiber, less sugar:

- at least 3 grams of fiber
- no more than 8 grams sugar added
- 2 grams fat or less
- 300 mg sodium or less
- wholegrains as the 1st ingredient listed

Most of the following cereals meet these criteria. Note popular cereal comparisons.

Cereals	Serving Size (1 ounce)	Calories	Sugar (g)	Fiber (g)	Fat (g)	Sodium (mg)
100% Bran *(Post)*	1/2 c.	80	7	10	1	150
All-Bran *(Kellogg)*	1/2 c.	80	6	10	1	285
All-Bran w/ Extra Fiber *(Kelloggs)*	1/2 c.	50	0	14	0	110
All-Bran Bran Buds *(Kelloggs)*	1/3 c.	70	8	13	1	200
Alpen	1/4 c.	110	5	3	2	60
Complete Wheat Bran Flakes *(Kelloggs)*	3/4 c.	90	5	5	0	220
Cheerios *(General Mills)*	1 c.	100	1	3	2	280
Multigrain Cheerios Plus *(General Mills)*	1 c.	110	6	3	1	200
Crunchy Corn Bran *(Quaker)*	3/4 c.	90	6	5	1	250
Fiber One *(General Mills)*	1/2 c.	60	0	13	1	125
Fiber One Honey Clusters *(General Mills)*	3/4 c.	120	4.5	10	2	210
Grape Nuts *(Post)* (2 oz.)	1/2 c.	200	5	7	1	300
Kashi Go LEAN (1.4 oz.)	3/4 c.	120	7	10	1	35
Kashi Go LEAN Crunch (1.9 oz.)	1 c.	200	13	8	3	95
Kashi Good Friends (1.9 oz.)	1 c.	170	9	12	2	130
Kashi Heart to Heart (1.2 oz.)	3/4 c.	110	5	5	1	90
Kashi Mountain Medley Granola (w/ .3 g Omega-3 ALA)	1/2 c.	220	12	6	7	110
Mini-wheats, unfrosted *(Kelloggs)*	15 biscuits	100	.5	3	1	5
Multi-Bran Chex *(General Mills)*	1/2 c.	90	6	4	1	120
Nature's Path Flax Plus Raisin Bran	3/4 c.	180	16	11	5	280
Nature's Path Optimum Slim (1.9 oz.)	1 c.	180	10	11	2	250
Puffed Kashi	1 c.	70	0	2	0	0
Raisin Bran *(Kellogg)*	1/2 c.	90	10	4	1	175
Raisin Bran Total *(General Mills)*	1/2 c.	85	10	3	0	120
Shredded Wheat *(Nabisco)*	1 lg. biscuit	80	0	3	0	0
Shredded Wheat (spoon size) *(Post)*	1/2 c.	100	0	4	0	0
Shredded Wheat 'n Bran *(Post)*	1/2 c.	100	0	4	1	0
Total Wholegrain *(General Mills)*	3/4 c.	100	5	3	1	200
Uncle Sam Cereal (with flax seed)	1/2 c.	110	0	7	1	65
Wheaties *(General Mills)*	1 c.	100	4	4	1	200
Whole Grain Wheat Chex *(General Mills)*	2/3 c.	100	3	3	1	230

approximately ½-oz. serving

Diet and Dental Health

Dental disease is the most prevalent disease known to man; yet it is *preventable*. Our best defenses against dental decay and periodontal disease, which weakens teeth and gums, are **proper nutrition** and **dental care**. These two defenses go hand-in-hand: Poor dental health interferes with good nutrition; and poor nutrition interferes with good dental health. You can strengthen your teeth and gums and resist dental decay. Here's how:

Proper Dental Care:

- Brush teeth thoroughly after meals or after eating a "sugar-rich" food.
- Floss once a day.
- Brush tongue and gums.
- Do not open bottles or packages with your teeth.
- Schedule dental check-ups twice a year, and request fluoride treatments as needed.
- Rinse your mouth after meals and snacks. Drink a glass of water.

> **Note:**
>
> *Steps 1, 2 and 3 remove or reduce oral bacteria, which produce acids from food sugar that decay (demineralize) tooth enamel. Plaque formation can lead to gum disease.*

Proper Nutritional Care:

1. Eat a **well-balanced**, healthy diet.
2. Avoid **simple sugars** in sodas and sweets (see p.222.)
3. **Read food labels**.
4. If you must eat sweetened foods, eat them **with** meals, not between meals.
5. **Avoid frequent snacking** of sugar-containing foods or beverages.
6. **Choose unsweetened between-meal snacks**: fresh fruits and vegetables, milk, cheese, sugar-free yogurt, bagels, peanutbutter, whole grain breads and crackers, cooked or dry cereal, popcorn, nuts, seeds, sugarless drinks and chewing gum.
7. **Chew high-fiber foods** for healthy gums, teeth and jaw muscles (i.e., bran cereals, nuts, apples, carrots, celery, seeds, popcorn, bagels).
8. **Avoid "sticky" sweets** including caramels, peanut butter, candy bars and raisins.
9. **Include calcium** for strong bones and teeth. Dairy products such as fat-free milk, cottage cheese, low-fat cheese or low-fat yogurt, as well as tuna, salmon and green leafy vegetables, are the best sources of calcium.
10. **Never chew on ice**. This breaks down the enamel.
11. Include a source of **vitamin C** daily for healthy gums: citrus fruit and juices, tomatoes, broccoli, potatoes, green leafy vegetables, strawberries and melon.
12. **Never eat extremely hot or extremely cold** beverages and foods. Thermal irritation can crack teeth.
13. **Avoid** comforting a baby with a **bedtime milk or juice bottle** as the child goes to sleep. The result is "nursing bottle mouth," where teeth are destroyed by decay.
14. It's not just the **amount** of sugar you eat that is important. Other factors that contribute to cavities (tooth enamel decay) are:

- **Frequency**—the more often you eat sugar-rich foods, the more often acids form on teeth and erode tooth enamel.
- **Length of time**—the longer sugar is in your mouth (from cough drops, Lifesavers, candies, etc.), the longer acid attack continues.
- **Physical form**—soft, sticky sweets such as caramels, toffees, mints, peanutbutter cracker sandwiches, candied apples, etc., are difficult to clean from teeth.

> ### It is up to you!
> Only you can prevent dental decay and disease.
> Take care of your teeth and gums, and they will last a lifetime.

© 2009, *The Cooper Clinic Solution to the Diet Revolution* by Georgia G. Kostas, M.P.H., R.D., L.D., Dallas, Texas

Limit Your Sodium

Sodium is a mineral that occurs in almost everything you eat. Even is you never added salt (NaCl) to your food, your sodium (Na) intake would exceed what you need. Excess sodium is linked to high blood pressure, which affects 1 in 3 American adults. Sodium also increases heart disease risk by stiffening arteries. That is why it is so important to limit sodium intake, even if your blood pressure is normal. The American Heart Association recommends consuming no more than 2300 mg of sodium daily (in 1 teaspoon of salt). Most Americans consume 5000 mg daily! To lower blood pressure: lose weight, exercise, eat the DASH way (below) and limit alcohol and sodium.

How to Sensibly Cut Back on Sodium:

☑ Do not add salt, salt seasonings, bouillon or broth to food during cooking.

☑ Add a little salt (if you must) at the table. Try sea salt or kosher salt. Both contain as much sodium as table salt, but you'll add less of these tasty, larger crystals!

☑ Try salt-free seasonings or salt substitutes in place of salt. Examples:

	Sodium in 1/4 Tsp
Mrs. Dash; "Salt-free" McCormick or Kroger's seasonings	0 mg
McCormick Seasonings (all types)	240 mg
Morton Lite Salt	290 mg
Lawry's Seasoned Salt or meat tenderizers	380 mg
Morton's "Nature's Seasons" seasoning blend	380 mg
Compare to Table Salt or Sea Salt	**600 mg**

☑ Eat wholesome foods - the more natural and less processed or "instant", the better.

☑ Check your medicines. Some contain sodium (2 tablets Alka-Seltzer = 1134 mg sodium).

☑ Replace high-sodium foods with lower-sodium options. See ideas next page.

☑ Follow the DASH Diet (Dietary Approach to Stop Hypertension). The high potassium, magnesium, calcium and plant nutrient content of this plan lowers high blood pressure, even when your sodium intake exceeds 2300 mg. Low sodium eating lowers blood pressure further.

DASH Diet	**Sodium (mg)**	**Calories**
2-3 large fruit + 2-3 cups vegetables	0	400
3 wholegrains (3 bread slices) *	450	300
3 other starchy foods (potato, etc)	0	250
3 c. nonfat milk yogurt (or lowfat cheese)	375	300
6 oz. lean meat, fish, poultry	300	300
2 Tbsp. unsalted nuts or 1/2 c. beans/peas **	0	100
3 tsp. healthy oils, unsalted margarine	0	150
TOTALS	**1125 mg**	**1800 calories**

* breakfast cereals add 300-500 mg/serving; oatmeal, brown rice or pasta adds 0 sodium

** cooked at home without salt: canned = 900 mg Na; unsalted canned beans/peas = 500 mg Na

These foods lower Blood Pressure, Cholesterol and Weight

Seasoning With Herbs and Spices

Herbs and spices can add pizzazz to any meal, without salt. Try these ideas:

FOOD	SEASON WITH ...	See "Cooking Tips" p. 105-106 for more ideas.
Beef	allspice, bay leaf, caraway seed, garlic, marjoram, dry mustard, nutmeg, onion, pepper, green pepper, thyme	
Fish	bay leaf, curry, marjoram, dry mustard, lemon, parsley, margarine, lemon juice, green pepper, tomatoes	
Poultry	basil, curry, garlic powder, mint, rosemary, thyme	
Veal	bay leaf, curry, ginger, marjoram, oregano, rosemary, thyme	
Eggs	curry, dry mustard, onion, paprika, parsley, thyme, green pepper, tomatoes	
Asparagus	caraway seed, lemon juice, mustard seed, sesame seed, tarragon	
Beans	basil, dill seed, unsalted French dressing, lemon juice, marjoram, mint, mustard seed, nutmeg, oregano, sage, savory, tarragon, thyme	
Broccoli	caraway seed, dill seed, mustard seed, oregano, tarragon; lemon juice and oil	
Cabbage	caraway seed, dill seed, mint, mustard seed, dry mustard, nutmeg, poppy seed, savory, thyme, vinegar	
Cauliflower	caraway seed, chives, dill seed, lemon juice, mace, nutmeg, parsley, rosemary, tarragon	
Corn	curry, green peppers	
Cucumbers	basil, dill seed, lemon juice, mint, tarragon, nutmeg	
Eggplant	chives, grated onion or garlic, marjoram, oregano, chopped parsley, tarragon	
Lettuce salad	basil, caraway seed, chives, dill, garlic, lemon, onion, tarragon, thyme, vinegar	
Onions	caraway seed, mustard seed, nutmeg, oregano, pepper, sage, thyme	
Peas	basil, dill, marjoram, mint, oregano, lemon, parsley, green pepper, poppy seed, rosemary, sage, savory, thyme	
Potatoes	basil, bay leaves, caraway seed, chives, dill seed, mace, mustard seed, onion, oregano, paprika, parsley, green pepper, poppy seed, rosemary, thyme	
Spinach	basil, garlic, mace, marjoram, nutmeg, oregano; lemon juice and oil	
Squash	allspice, basil, cinnamon, chives, cloves, fennel, ginger, mace, mustard seed, nutmeg, onion, rosemary	
Sweet potatoes	allspice, cardamom, cinnamon, cloves, nutmeg	
Tomatoes	allspice, basil, bay leaf, curry, marjoram, onion, sage, thyme	

LOWER SODIUM OPTIONS

Instead of these:	TRY THESE ...
Deli meats, ham, bacon, cold cuts, hot dogs, sausage, salt pork	Fresh or frozen meat, poultry and fish, low-sodium deli meats
Canned and smoked fish: anchovies, caviar, herring, sardines	Tuna packed in water (reduced sodium brands), 50% less sodium Light Tuna
Processed cheese and cheese products	Natural Swiss, low-sodium Swiss, cheddar, mozzarella
Boullion cubes, canned or dried soups	Homemade soups, frozen soups (Tabatchnick), Swanson low-sodium broths, Healthy Choice, Amy's, Campbell's Healthy Request, Progresso's 50% less sodium soups
Canned vegetables, tomato juice, sauerkraut, pork and beans	Fresh or frozen vegetables, low sodium canned varieties, bagged beans
Chips, dips, pretzels, salted nuts or popcorn	Melba rounds, Wasa Light Rye, low-sodium Saltines and Wheat Thins
Bottled salad dressings, olives, pickles, relishes, horseradish	Wishbone Salad Spritzers, homemade oil and vinegar dressings, low-sodium bottled brands
Bottled sauces: BBQ, chili, steak, soy, tomato, tartar, Worcestershire, mustard, ketchup, spaghetti sauce	Heinz No Salt Added ketchup, Tabasco, lite soy sauce, Kitchen Bouquet, no-salt added canned tomato sauce, Prego Heart Smart spaghetti sauce
Salts and spices containing salt or MSG, lemon pepper, meat tenderizers; garlic salt; onion salt	Sodium-free seasonings, salt substitutes, herbs and spices, fresh lemon, a pinch of sugar; garlic powder; onion powder
Most breakfast cereals, instant oatmeal packets, cereal bars	Oatmeal, Kashi, shredded/puffed wheat, puffed rice, Wheaties, low-sod Rice Krispies
Frozen dinners, pizza, fast foods	Entrees with less than 800 mg of sodium

Even small reductions in your sodium intake help your overall health!

Sodium Comparisons

Notice how sodium content increases in foods as food processing increases. You are better off eating as many foods as possible in their natural, unprocessed state.

AS FOODS	Sodium (mg)	ARE PROCESSED...	Sodium (mg)	SODIUM INCREASES	Sodium (mg)
Apple 1 medium	1	Applesauce 1 c.	6	Apple Pie 1/8, frozen	482
Bread 1 slice	130	Homemade Biscuit 1 biscuit	175	Canned Biscuit 1 biscuit	270
Butter or Margarine, unsalted 1 Tbsp.	3	Trans-free Tub Margarine 1 Tbsp., unsalted	85	Butter or Margarine, regular 1 Tbsp., salted	80-150
Cabbage 1 c.	22	Cole Slaw 1 c.	150	Sauerkraut 1 c., canned	1,760
Chicken 3 oz., baked	86	Fast Food Chicken 3 oz., fried	500	Chicken Pie 1 frozen pie	863
Corn 1 ear	1	Corn Flakes 1 c.	325	Canned Kernels 1 c.	400
Soup, canned 1 cup	800-1200	Soup, canned, Lower Salt 1 c. (Amy's Healthy Choice, Progresso)	500	Frozen Soups 1 pouch (Tabatchnick)	420
Lemon 1 lemon	3	Soy Sauce 1 Tbsp.	1,330	Salt 1 tsp.	2,300
Peanuts (No Salt) 1 oz. (30 nuts)	1	Peanuts, salted 1 oz. (30 nuts)	115	Peanutbutter 2 Tbsp.	250
Cheese, Natural 1 oz.	95-150	Cheese Spread 1 oz. (2 Tbsp.)	490	Cheese Soup 1 c., canned	1,020
Potato - Baked 1 oz.	5	French Fries 1/2 c. (18 fries)	120	Potato Chips 1/2 c. (10 chips)	200
Tomato 1 medium	4	Tomato Juice 1 c. (Campbell's)	680	Tomato Soup 1 c. (Campbell's)	1,420
Tomato Paste 1 c. (Contadina)	160	Tomato Sauce 1 c. (Contadina)	1,120	Spaghetti Sauce 1 c. (Prego)	1,160
Tuna in Water 3 oz.	345	Tuna in Oil 3 oz.	375	Tuna Noodle Casserole 1 c.	845
Water, tap 12 oz.	4	Soft Drink 12 oz.	50	Club Soda 12 oz.	90

Even if foods are labeled "low sodium" or reduced sodium", read the fine print. Choose products with less than 150 mg sodium per serving.

Water

...Good to the Last Drop!

Did you know that your body can survive only three to five days without water? I can't overemphasize the need for Mother Nature's best and most basic beverage. Our bodies thrive on water. In fact, water makes up about 80% of our muscle mass, 60% of our red blood cells and more than 90% of our blood plasma.

Why Water?

1. Regulates every living cell's processes and chemical reactions.
2. Aids digestion and absorption of foods and nutrients.
3. Transports nutrients and oxygen.
4. Excretes waste products.
5. Helps to maintain normal bowel habits and prevent constipation.
6. Assists new tissue development.
7. Lubricates joints in your body, providing a protective cushion for tissues.
8. Maintains normal body temperature. Loss of water through perspiration cools the body and prevents it from building up internal heat (dehydration).
9. Contributes to the proper concentrations of blood electrolytes (electrolyte balance).
10. Prevents/delays fatigue from dehydration.

Replenish Often

➢ **Drink at least eight glasses of fluids each day, half of which are water.** Don't count caffeinated drinks! Teas, colas and alcohol have a dehydrating effect, which means they decrease body fluids. Why so much water? You need it to replenish that which is lost through perspiration (skin), lungs, body functions, urine, stool and air travel. A 2-5% loss of body water causes you to become weak; 15 to 20% is fatal. That means a loss of 7 pounds for a 150-pound person = 5% loss.

➢ During the hot summer months, increase your fluids. And if you are adding fiber to your diet, drink more water to prevent constipation.

➢ If you have any friends who are athletes, you may note that they drink water constantly. Why? Water loss, more than salt or sodium loss, impairs an athlete's performance. Water helps them gain the edge they need to perform.

> **NOTE:** *For every hour of air travel, you lose 1 cup of water. Drink ample water to prevent fatigue. Driving for hours, golf, yard work, home chores can be dehydrating.*

Tips to increase water intake daily:

- Add lemon, lime or orange slices to a glass of water.
- Keep a clear pitcher of water (2 qt.) on your desk or work area.
- Carry a squeeze bottle filled with water — in your car, at meetings, etc. Drink two 32 oz. bottles a day.
- Drink 16 oz. water at each of three meals a day, 8 oz. upon rising and 8 oz. before bedtime.

Caffeine

We've been talking about nutrients your body needs. Caffeine is actually a drug that reduces your absorption of some vitamins and minerals. *Caffeine* belongs to a family of chemical compounds called *xanthines*. Other substances in this group are *theophylline* (in tea) and *theobromine* (in chocolate and cocoa). Several studies on caffeine have produced conflicting results. However, one very credible report showed that more than 200 milligrams of caffeine a day (2 cups brewed coffee) led to the development of unpleasant symptoms—nervousness, anxiety, irritability, insomnia, gastrointestinal problems, irregular heart beat, etc. Thus, my advice: *Drink up to 2 cups or 1 mug coffee daily, not to exceed 200 mg caffeine.*

How Caffeine Affects Your Body

Wondering why you should limit caffeine? Let me explain its effects. Caffeine:

- may cause rapid heartbeats or skipped heartbeats
- may lead to a rise in blood pressure and body temperature
- promotes acid secretion in the stomach (not advisable for persons with ulcers or gastric irritation; avoid decaffeinated coffee also since it has the same effect)
- relaxes your muscles or respiratory system, digestive tract and kidneys, causing increased urinary output — a dehydrating effect
- can cause diarrhea
- can lead to central nervous system disturbances including nervousness, insomnia, irritability, anxiety, headaches, twitching muscles, difficulty sleeping, etc.
- in pregnant women, may interfere with normal fetal development because it readily crosses the placenta
- may lead to or aggravate fibrocystic breast disease in some women
- interferes with calcium and iron absorption

How Much Is *Too* Much?

Remember: Caffeine is a *drug*. Drinking three to four cups of caffeine-containing beverages (300-400 mg of caffeine) per day may make you psychologically and physically dependent. Gradually break the habit—especially if you have heart disease, gastrointestinal problems, hypertension, emotional problems, ulcers, gastritis, diverticulosis, spastic colon, indigestion, hypoglycemia or diabetes. Just to prepare you for the reactions: caffeine withdrawal may result in headaches, nervousness, depression, drowsiness and irritability...for 2-3 days only.

Alternatives to Caffeine

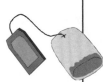

- Decaffeinated coffee, tea and colas contain only a minute amount of caffeine. However, they may still stimulate stomach acid and produce heartburn.
- Choose steam-decaffeinated coffee to avoid chemical solvents.
- Drink water, juice, herb teas—all naturally caffeine-free.
- Try grain-based beverages as alternatives to caffeine: Postum, Cafix, Pero. (Postum is made from bran, wheat and molasses.)
- See next page . . .

Sources of Caffeine

	Mg Per Serving	
Coffee	**6 oz.***	**10 oz.***
Brewed, drip method	115	190
Percolated	110	185
Instant	60	100
Flavored (Café Francais, Vienna, etc.)	30	50
Grain blends (Mellow Roast, Sunrise, Luzianne-chicory)	15-40	25-35
Espresso (2 oz.)	70	
Decaffeinated	3	5
Tea		
Regular, 1 bag	45	45
Regular, loose	40	65
Instant	30	50
Decaffeinated	0	0

Cola Beverages — **12 oz. serving**

Coca-Cola	50
Diet Coke	40
Dr Pepper, regular and diet	40
Pepsi Cola – regular and diet	35
Tab	45

Non-Cola Beverages

Mountain Dew	55
Sunkist Orange soda	45
Barq's Root Beer	20
Diet Sunkist, Fanta drinks, Shasta drinks	0
Sprite, regular and diet; 7-Up, regular and diet	0
Root Beer (Hires, A&W, Diet Barq's Root Beer)	0
Nehi (orange, strawberry, peach)	0
Nehi Red	5

*Note:

Small coffee cup = 5-6 oz.
Your mug may be 10-12 oz.

Caffeine in Starbucks Coffees:
6 oz. coffee = 150 mg
18 oz. coffee = 250 mg
2 oz. espresso = 180 mg

Chocolate

Baker's, 1 oz.	25
Milk chocolate candy, 1 oz.	6
Chocolate milk, 8-oz. cup	5
Hot cocoa, 6-oz. cup	5

Other

Starbucks coffee ice cream, 1 c.	50
Dannon coffee yogurt, c.	45

Drugs: per pill

Aspirin, Midol, Anacin, Dristan, Sinarest, etc.	30
Excedrin	60
No Doz, Vivarin	100-200

What's the Scoop on Additives?

Food additives serve a multitude of purposes. They are used as stabilizers, thickening agents, flavor enhancers (i.e., sugar and salt), emulsifiers, acidic or alkaline or neutralizing agents, preservatives, antioxidants (to protect fats from becoming rancid during storage), nutritional supplements and food colors.

Benefits and Risks Involved With Their Use:

➢ **Benefits**: prolonged shelf life, spoilage prevention, enhanced food appearance of flavor or texture and added nutrients.

➢ **Risks**: related to the quantity and choice of additives used and their known and unknown potential dangers. *All* foods, as well as additives, are essentially chemical compounds. Therefore, additives are not "unnatural," nor are they automatically harmful.

The Food and Drug Administration has compiled a "Generally Recognized as Safe" (GRAS) list of 415 additives tested and approved as safe at specified levels. This list, first started in 1958, is updated on a regular basis. According to the last assessment, the vast majority of additives are considered safe at levels currently used. Their benefits of longer food shelf life, convenience, a greater food supply and variety, added nutrients and food appeal seem to outweigh their risks. Further, the human body is able to handle minute levels of almost any substance without serious health consequences. Some experts believe the decline in stomach cancer in America since the 1930s is related to the use of additives. On the other hand, most authorities agree that excessive amounts of any substance can be potentially dangerous. *My take on it: The less, the better.*

How to Avoid Excessive Levels of Additives

The most sensible suggestion is grandmother's long-standing advice: Eat a well-balanced diet, with a variety of foods, in moderation. The more varied our diets, the more healthful nutrients we are likely to consume…and the less likely we are to eat excessive levels of potentially dangerous substances. Eat fresh foods and "whole" (unprocessed) foods to maximize nutrients and minimize additives.

The following page lists common additives.

Common Additives

CLASSIFICATION	TYPES	PURPOSE	USED IN
Antioxidants	BHT, BHA, vitamin E, ascorbic acid (vitamin C), citric acid, EDTA	prevent oxidation that leads to rancidity of fats and discoloration of fruits; extend shelf life	breakfast cereals, baked products, margarine, sauces, salad dressings, processed fruit, snack foods, fats, oil, shortening
Preservatives	benzoic acid, sodium benzoate, calcium propionate, citric acid, lactic acid, propionic acid, potassium sorbate, sulfur dioxide, sodium nitrate, salt, sugar, paraben, sulfites	inhibit growth of bacteria, yeast and mold; extend shelf life	pastries, baked goods, dried fruit, canned fruit, vegetables, meats and soups; acidic foods; cured meats, bacon; olives; cheese; salad dressing
Emulsifiers	monoglycerides, diglycerides, lecithin, propylene glycol mono stearate, polysorbate, carrageenan	blend liquids together for more uniform consistency, texture and stability	mayonnaise, salad dressings, margarine, chocolate, whipped toppings, gelatin, pudding, ice cream
Stabilizers and Thickeners	agar, cellulose, guar gum, gelatin, pectin, dextrin, alginate compounds, propylene glycol, fat substitutes	maintain uniform color, flavor and smooth texture	mayonnaise, salad dressings, ice cream, dessert dairy products, jam, jelly
Coloring Agents	*Natural:* chlorophyll (green), beet or tomato powder (red), caramelized sugar (brown), carotene (yellow). *Synthetic:* Red No. 3 and No. 40, yellow No. 5	enhance color	canned fruit and vegetables, bakery products, desserts
Flavoring Agents	*Natural:* vanilla, cocoa, lemon, orange, spices, sweeteners, sugar, lactose, mannitol. *Synthetic:* fruit flavors, monosodium glutamate (MSG), hydrolyzed vegetable protein (HVP—another name for MSG), saccharin, aspartame	enhance flavor or modify original taste and/or aromas	beverages, baked goods, cereals, dessert mixes, candy, sauces, many canned foods, soup, stews, oriental foods, hot dogs, sauce mixes, dietary products, etc.

Note:

Limit MSG, HVP, sodium nitrate and nitrite, sulfites and saccharin. Some people react to these additives.

New Foods - How Safe?

Genetically engineered foods: Foods modified to be more pesticide-resistant, spoilage-resistant, sweeter, deeper in color, etc. We've been consuming them for decades. They appear safe.

Irradiated foods: Foods treated with radiation to kill bacteria contaminants. No evidence has proven them harmful. Astronauts have eaten irradiated foods without harm since 1973.

Functional foods: Foods with nutrients or components added in ample amounts for additional health benefits. For example, orange juice fortified with calcium.

Organic foods: As labeled "USDA-certified organic", these foods are grown without synthetic pesticides or fertilizers, hormones, antibiotics or genetic engineering.

- They may not be safer than conventionally grown foods since bacteria can be found on all produce. Wash everything!
- Some reports indicate organic foods contain higher levels of some nutrients, particularly antioxidants.
- Since organic foods are more expensive, "go organic" for those foods you most frequently consume, which are most likely to have more pesticide residue. The top 12, in descending order, are:

Peaches	Spinach	Pears	Strawberries
Celery	Apples	Lettuce	Grapes (imported)
Cherries	Nectarines	Bell peppers	Potatoes

Natural foods: As labeled on meat and poultry *only*, USDA defines "natural" as no added artificial flavors or colors, chemical preservatives or ingredients added. USDA does not require "natural" to mean "no hormone or antibiotic" exposure of animals. "Natural" has no official definition for non-meat products.

Free-Range foods: No official definition exists. It means animal/poultry has *access* to the outdoors, but no guarantee of *going outdoors*.

Grass-fed meat: "Grass-fed" and "grass-finished" have the same meaning; the last 6 months of life, the cow is fed grass (a finishing diet), rather than grain (usually corn). For the first 12 months, all cows are 100% grass fed. Grains promote marbling, which produces a more tender meat. With correct cooking methods, leaner meat cuts can be tender as well.

Hormone-free: Not a legal claim since all animals produce their own hormones.

Sources: USDA National Organic Program: www.ams.usda.gov/nop/; Environmental Working Group: www.foodnews.org; Organic Trade Assn: www.ota.com

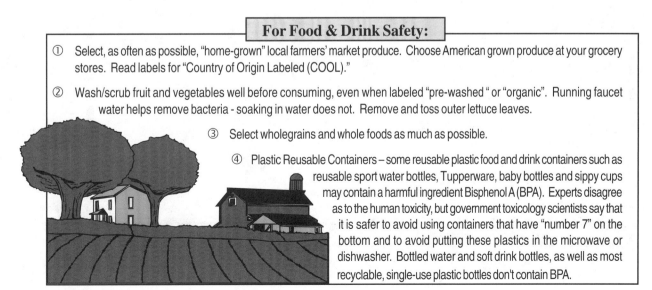

For Food & Drink Safety:

① Select, as often as possible, "home-grown" local farmers' market produce. Choose American grown produce at your grocery stores. Read labels for "Country of Origin Labeled (COOL)."

② Wash/scrub fruit and vegetables well before consuming, even when labeled "pre-washed " or "organic". Running faucet water helps remove bacteria - soaking in water does not. Remove and toss outer lettuce leaves.

③ Select wholegrains and whole foods as much as possible.

④ Plastic Reusable Containers – some reusable plastic food and drink containers such as reusable sport water bottles, Tupperware, baby bottles and sippy cups may contain a harmful ingredient Bisphenol A (BPA). Experts disagree as to the human toxicity, but government toxicology scientists say that it is safer to avoid using containers that have "number 7" on the bottom and to avoid putting these plastics in the microwave or dishwasher. Bottled water and soft drink bottles, as well as most recyclable, single-use plastic bottles don't contain BPA.

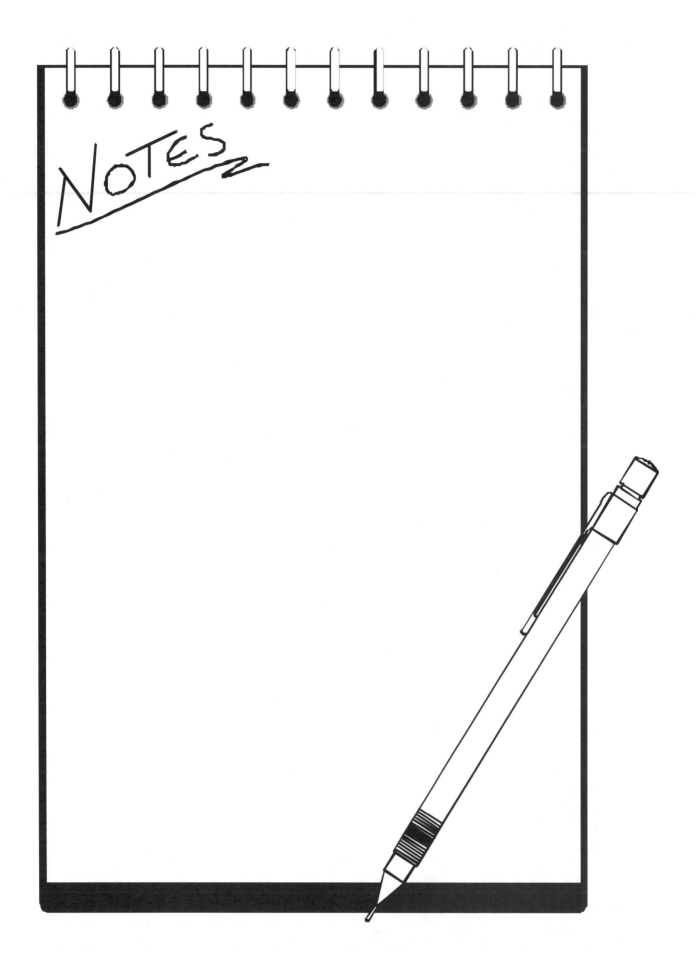

NOTES

Step 12
Lessen Stress for
More Success

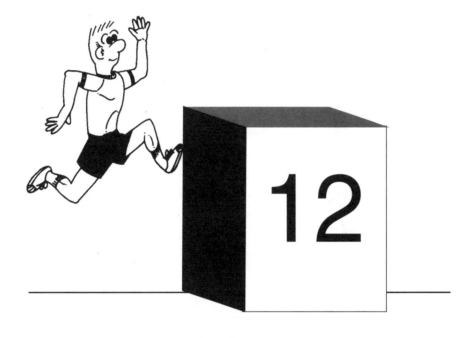

Step 12

Mini-Step 1:
Tune into yourself.
Nourish your inner psyche.

Mini-Step 2:
Lessen stress.

Mini-Step 3:
Practice relaxation techniques.

Struggling with mastering new eating and exercise patterns? Look within. Inner disharmony from stress and/or emotional struggles often disrupt the best intentions. To achieve a balanced lifestyle, one must focus on those spiritual, mental and emotional aspects of inner well-being that sometimes get neglected. In this step, we'll talk about some of those areas:

- how to tune into yourself
- how to lessen the symptoms of stress
- how to overcome job-related stress
- effective relaxation techniques
- eating/exercise tips to give you energy

A changed inner person can inspire outer changes in behaviors. Likewise, changed eating and exercise (outer) patterns can motivate changes within. What a great opportunity for personal growth, a renewed spirit, successful lifestyle changes, and peace with food and one's self.

ACTION STEPS

① Identify and reduce stressors.

② Practice relaxation techniques. Relax without food.

③ Eat regular, healthy, balanced meals for less stress and more energy.

Inner Psyche

How Well Are You Taking Care of Your Inner Self?

Inner psyche refers to your spiritual, mental and emotional self. These areas contribute to the "balance" you're trying to achieve on your road to total well-being. Your "inner" health affects your self-attitude and life-attitudes. It motivates you to take care of yourself and promotes confidence to do so. Lack of inner contentment can disrupt any worthy goals and plans for weight control, healthy eating and exercise...because it zaps energy and enthusiasm.

Nourish and exercise your inner self with appropriate reading, family time and communication, fellowship with others (individually and in groups), challenges and opportunities for growth. Self-reflect. Spend time with God. Love and serve others. Try to "make it someone else's day." Your inner person will be enriched, and you'll be able to meet your goals.

> *"It is the most beautiful of compensations of this life that no man can try to help another without helping himself."*
>
> **--Albert Schweitzer**

When you are content and fulfilled by your choices and activities, food becomes less of a focus in life.

Nourish Yourself

- Develop your special gifts and talents.
- Wear flattering clothes.
- Enjoy varied activities and learning new skills.
- Seek personal growth.
- Expand your interests and friendships.
- Appreciate yourself and your own attractiveness.
- Remind yourself of qualities you like in yourself and in your appearance.

Tune Into Yourself

Do you eat for emotional reasons or for unmet needs? *Emotional eating* often results from unresolved conflict, anger, fatigue, boredom, stress, loneliness. Do you need more attention, more social activities, better relationships, more job fulfillment, more fun and recreation, more recognition or a greater meaning in life? Food is a poor substitute.

The counsel of a professional therapist, trusted friend, pastor or religious leader may direct you to solutions.

To feel you are in control of your weight and your life, accept responsibility for the choices you make. Learn assertiveness skills, do things you enjoy, accept yourself and pursue your own interests and enrichment times. You'll find new fulfillment and less hunger.

Seek Moderation

In place of an "all or none" attitude toward eating and a chronic "losing weight"/"gaining weight" lifestyle, try a new approach of *moderation*. Set your own boundaries or "ground rules" for foods to limit. Enjoy the freedom of eating anything within your chosen guidelines.

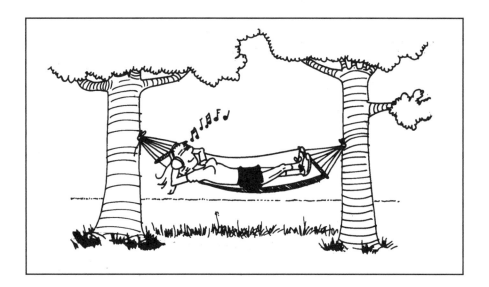

Take charge of your life!

It's the only one you've got!

Stress and Relaxation

What Is Stress?

Almost everyone encounters stressful periods—from a specific crisis (death, marriage, relationships, divorce, change in jobs, etc.) or from day-to-day hassles (traffic, losing keys, missing the bus, uncertainties, etc.). Stress can be positive, stimulating your best efforts.

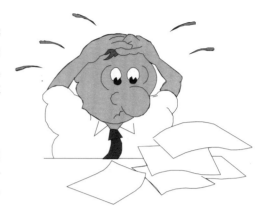

On the other hand, prolonged stress can lead to organic disease; or to excessive eating, smoking, drinking, sleep difficulties, anxiety, depression, irritability and susceptibility to cancer, ulcers, headache, hypertension and heart problems.

How Do You Handle It?

Learn to cope with stress so it does not work against you.
- Learn how to experience less stress.
- Prevent excessive or chronic stress.
- Identify events that trigger stress for you (rush-hour traffic, too many phone calls during the day, finances, lack of time, etc.)

1. _____   5. _____

2. _____   6. _____

3. _____   7. _____

4. _____   8. _____

How Does Your Body Respond to Stress?

_____ rapid heart beat; chest pains   _____ tense back, neck/shoulder

_____ headaches   _____ migraine headache

_____ jaw tension aches   _____ allergies or skin rashes

_____ high blood pressure   _____ diarrhea

_____ constipation   _____ fatigue

_____ stomach ache, heartburn   _____ anxiety

_____ overeating or bingeing   _____ withdrawal, isolation

_____ eating less/undereating   _____ more infections/colds

_____ depression/burnout   _____ insomnia

_____ tenseness/irritability   _____ compulsiveness

5 Simple Ways to Lessen Stress

Be aware of the people, places and things that cause you stress. Learn to respond in ways that lessen your stress.

 1. Predict/Strategize.

- Identify the causes of stress and work toward solutions.

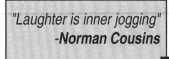

"Laughter is inner jogging"
-Norman Cousins

 2. Communicate.

- Talk to someone you can trust. Communicate your feelings.

 3. Have realistic expectations. Limit activities.

- Don't take on more than you can accomplish. Set limits and say *no* to excessive demands. Be assertive.
- Set priorities. Plan ahead. List your necessary tasks in order of importance and tackle one at a time. Solve difficult tasks when you are energetic and simple tasks later in the day.
- Organize your time. Pace yourself. Identify your most productive time and allow for rest periods. Avoid too many appointments, deadlines and unnecessary obligations.
- Don't try to be perfect. Work to the best of your efforts and ability. Avoid criticism for not achieving an "impossible" task. Take deserved credit for a task well-done.
- Plan for a change. Coping with the unexpected is a great stressor. Try to avoid too many big changes at the same time, and accept and prepare for change.

 4. Take time out.

- Escape and pursue pleasures. Read a book, go to a movie, listen to music, take a walk, walk your dog, enjoy a hobby. *Avoid* escaping to food, smoking, alcohol, etc.
- Slow down. Practice walking slower, eating slower, driving slower and talking slower. Really listen to someone talking with you. Look at their faces.
- Avoid situations and places that are noisy and crowded. Take the back streets, eat in quiet restaurants and shop in smaller stores.
- Make time for yourself and have fun! Get involved in a hobby or something that helps you to forget stressors of the day. Learn to relax mentally and physically. Pamper your body with a massage, facial, pedicure or bath.
- Work at your friendships. Help others. Practice complimenting others several times a day. Seek social support.

5. Make self-nourishing a habit.

- Build a positive self-image. Realistically accept your special gifts and limitations. Do a good job. Be dependable. Develop a life purpose. Stay close to your support system of friends.
- Balance your life with work and play, seriousness and laughter, etc.
- Take care of yourself. *Eat right and exercise regularly.* Take a nap. A healthy, well-nourished and well-exercised body handles stress better than a weak, poorly nourished one. Limit caffeine in coffee, tea, colas and chocolate. Avoid salt and refined sugars. Eat breakfast and avoid late-night snacks. Eat three meals daily at regular times. Eat slowly.

- Hug someone. Touching gives us a sense of well-being, comfort and security.
- Smile! Positive emotions help fight stress. Don't hold grudges. Learn to forgive.
- Listen to quiet, soothing music. Sounds of rain or waves at the seashore are relaxing. Wind chimes and a bird feeder in the backyard can be a source of relaxation. Enjoy beautiful pictures or photographs.
- Avoid self-medication. Alcohol and drugs only reduce your resistance and cover up your problems.
- Meditate or pray.
- Breathe deeply.
- Use the power of imagery and "get away" (see p. 245).
- Think positive thoughts. Notice the better outcomes.
- Utilize the "**Big 3**" coping solutions:
    1. *Commitment:* to self, family, friends, values, meaningful work
    2. *Control:* sense personal control over your life
    3. *Challenge:* see change as an opportunity

PURSUE HAPPINESS FROM:

H appy thoughts

A ltruism; service

P urpose in life

P laytime

I ntimacy

N ever retiring

E xercising regularly

S pirituality

S mile

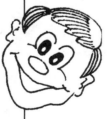

"One thing I know: The only ones among you who will be really happy are those who will have sought and found how to serve."

-*Albert Schweitzer*

Simplify Your Life!

Ten Ways to Overcome Job Stress

☑ 1. **Maximize your productivity and efficiency.**
   - Plan ahead.
   - Know your responsibilities, deadlines, expectations.
   - Organize your day.
   - Write down everything to "unburden" your memory.
   - Reduce interruptions. Answer e-mail and phone calls at specific times daily.

☑ 2. **Keep your office area and desk neat.** Create a pleasant working environment around you.

☑ 3. **Seek out positive co-workers who offer encouragement.** Avoid negative people and office gossip.

☑ 4. **Set aside time for play.**
   - Take a creative lunch break at an antique shop, cafe, park (picnic), walking paths, bench (to read).
   - Exercise with a co-worker.

☑ 5. **Get enough sleep.** Trade TV for sleep.

☑ 6. **Change your scenery.**
   - Go to another room.
   - Walk down the hall.
   - Go outside.
   - Take a day off to de-stress.

☑ 7. **Change your routine.**
   - Go out to breakfast on occasion.
   - Meet a co-worker for lunch or a walk.

☑ 8. **Do not take work home every night.** Come in earlier or stay a little later. Never stay more than one hour past regular leaving time.

☑ 9. **Slow down.** Tune into your physical and emotional self. Live in the "now." Don't worry about tomorrow.

☑ 10. **Find ways to slow down your pace** at regular intervals in the day to help you enjoy your life and change your awareness of time.

Relaxation Techniques

for Office or Home

If you have problems relaxing, try some of the following techniques below. It will make a difference!

1. **Learn to breathe deeply.** This increases oxygen in your blood, strengthens abdominal and intestinal muscles, and releases tension.

   - Think of your lungs in 3 parts.
   - Breathe in and fill up the bottom part, lifting your diaphragm and keeping your chest still.
   - Fill the middle area of your lungs, and feel your chest expand.
   - Fill the upper portion, and feel your shoulders rise slightly.
   - Set a regular time each day for deep, slow breathing. Do 10 breaths, four times a day.

2. **Practice these muscle relaxing exercises.** Breathe deeply throughout the exercises, and feel tension leave your body.

   - **Clench each fist** and hold 10 seconds. Relax. Repeat five times.
   - **Rigidly straighten** both arms and hold for 10 seconds. Relax. Repeat twice.
   - **Shoulder rotation**: Stand with arms to side, rotate shoulders forward 10 times and then backward 10 times.
   - **Neck rotation**: Take a full deep breath and exhale. Drop head to chest and rotate to right, then to left 8 times.
   - **Shrug your shoulders**, bringing them up to your ears. Hold 10 seconds and pull back down. Repeat 5 times.
   - **Arm rotation**: Stand up and extend arms outward by your sides. Rotate arms, making 10 small circles in one direction. Increase the size of your circles and repeat 10 times. Repeat in opposite direction.
   - **Overhead stretches**: Reach up with right arm 8 times and then with left arm 8 times.

3. **Practice Imagery Techniques.**

   - Be relaxed. Find a quiet place to be alone, away from other people, noise, activity and the phone.
   - Tensions block the success of visual suggestions.
   - Sit in a comfortable chair in comfortable clothing. Turn down the lights and close your eyes.
   - Take a deep, full breath and exhale fully and completely.
   - Keep your eyes shut, and drift away to a time or special place that you found to be calm, relaxing and peaceful (i.e., the beach, a hike in a wooded area, a walk in the fields, vacation spot, etc.).
   - Let your imagination go, and put yourself completely into this environment—the smells, the cool or warm feeling, the sounds, the feelings that made it peaceful. Stay with this scene until you feel completely relaxed. Enjoy for about 5 minutes—or longer, if you have time.
   - When relaxed, open your eyes and move your arms and legs. *Feel the calm.*
   - Practice at least once a day to "get away from it all!"

© 2009, *The Cooper Clinic Solution to the Diet Revolution* by Georgia G. Kostas, M.P.H., R.D., L.D., Dallas, Texas

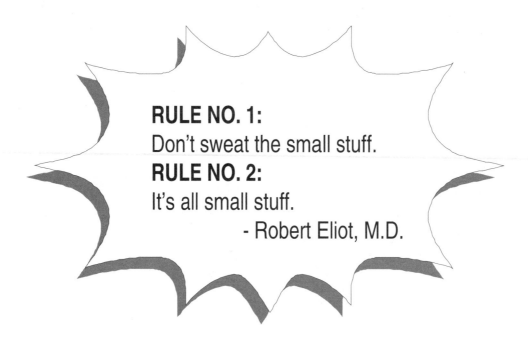

RULE NO. 1:
Don't sweat the small stuff.
RULE NO. 2:
It's all small stuff.
                    - Robert Eliot, M.D.

"If you can't fight and you can't flee, learn to flow."
                                        - Robert Eliot, M.D.

"Most folks are about as happy as they make up their minds to be."
                                        - Abraham Lincoln

"To err is human, to forgive divine."
                                        - Alexander Pope

"Other people are not in the world to live up to your expectations."
                                        - Fritz Perls

"I can't give you the formula for success, but I can sure give you the formula for failure: Try to please everybody."
                                        - Abraham Lincoln

"People can alter their lives by altering their attitudes."
                                        - William James

"Better keep yourself clean and bright; you are the window through which you must see the world."
                                        - George Bernard Shaw

Relaxation Checklists
for Office or Home

☑ **Check/add specific activities you can use to relax:**

_____ A long walk

_____ Exercise (vigorous, moderate or recreational)

_____ Movies, TV, videos

_____ Concerts, plays, performing arts

_____ Hobbies, interests

_____ Music, listening or performing

_____ Rhythmic motion (i.e., dancing; sitting in a rocking chair; watching a water fountain, blowing trees, rain or swimming fish)

_____ Sing

_____ Escape with your headphones

_____ Communicate (in person, phone, letter, e-mail)

_____ Use journal to transfer thoughts and frustration

_____ Take a shower or long bath

_____ Meditate/Pray

_____ Think and analyze problems

_____ Emphasize leisure

_____ Read a good book

_____ Sleep/nap/rest

_____ Daydream

_____ Socialize (attend meetings, programs w/others)

_____ Review picture albums of pleasant events and times

_____ Touch, hug

_____ Laugh, cry (express feelings)

_____ other: _____

_____ _____

_____ _____

Use Your Hands:

_____ Carpentry

_____ Painting

_____ Sewing

_____ Gardening

_____ Needlepoint

_____ Gifts

_____ Knitting

_____ Car work

_____ Picture albums

_____ Artwork

_____ Musical instruments

Take Mini-Vacations:

_____ Smell/pick flowers

_____ Note nature: a sunrise or sunset, moon, stars

_____ Enjoy a piece of art

_____ Feel the warmth of the sun

_____ Sense a cool breeze

_____ Enjoy a rainbow

_____ Listen to birds or trees swaying

_____ Have a picnic

_____ Eat by candlelight

_____ Change your scenery

_____ Change your pace

_____ "Connect" with someone

_____ Help someone

Eating and Exercise Tips
to Energize You and Reduce Stress

The relaxation strategies I've suggested will be much more effective if you put into place the eating and exercise tips mentioned throughout the pages of this book. Here is a summary of the eating/exercise steps you can take to feel like a new person!

1. **Eat sensibly.** Choose healthy, low-fat, high-fiber foods.

2. **Eat regularly**—every three to six hours. Snack as needed. Do not skip or delay meals. Eat breakfast. And, of course, eat P-C-F (see p. 47-48) to keep energy up and stress down.

3. **Eat easily digested foods**...simple foods with fiber.
   - Focus on fruit, vegetables, grains, starches.
   - Skip fried, greasy, spicy, rich foods.

4. **Minimize caffeine, nicotine, alcohol.**

5. **Limit salt, sugar, fat, cholesterol.**

6. **Drink lots of water**—eight glasses per day. Dehydration causes fatigue.

7. **Reach a healthy weight in a healthy way.** Do not "crash diet."

8. **Exercise every day for 30 minutes.** Break it into two 15-minute sessions if necessary. Go longer when you can.

9. **Seek balance in your exercise routine:** Go for aerobic endurance, flexibility and strength.

10. **Get fit, and stay there.** Fitness, endurance and strength reduce stress. Moving works wonders!

Step 13
Build a Support System

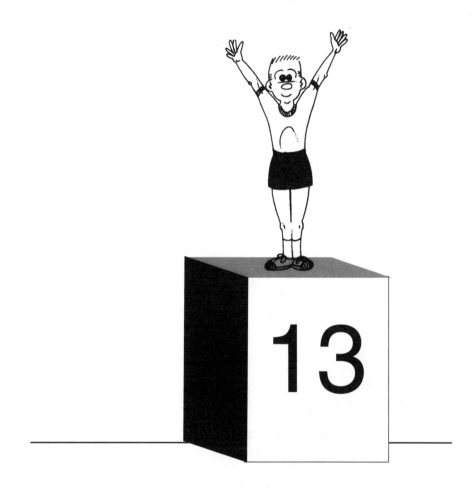

Step 13

Mini-Step 1:
Surround yourself with support - people, places, activities, skills and thoughts.

Mini-Step 2:
Be your own best supporter - practice positive thinking.

Studies have shown that support groups help people make lifestyle changes. If you can team up with a friend and implement the steps outlined in this book, you are sure to experience success—and it will be more fun. Having a person or team supporting you keeps you accountable and encouraged. You'll think twice before helping yourself to seconds or skipping exercise! Join a bike club, YMCA, dance club or low-fat cooking class, for example, and surround yourself with others to reinforce your interests.

It's possible that some of your closest friends and family members won't be supportive of your new lifestyle. How do you handle that? See my tips on p. 251-252. Practice positive self-talk, monitor your progress with records and follow the other guidelines recommended for "self-support" on p. 255.

Remember that at any given time, someone else is making the same types of changes you are and has faced similar struggles. Others *already* have crossed the finish line and, like them, "*You can do it!*"

ACTION STEPS

① Identify the people and factors that encourage or positively influence you . . . they are your support team. Give them specifics on *how* they can support you and what kind of feedback they can give you.

② Learn to cope with non-supportive behaviors.

③ Join clubs and classes that reinforce your new interests and goals.

④ Be your own best friend. Practice positive self-talk; be optimistic about your successes. Reward yourself for behaviors you've changed (see ideas on p. 37).

Your Support Team

When trying to lose weight, have you ever felt that...

- No one cares or is interested? Others are overly interested?

- You are teased even though you are changing and losing weight?

- Your friends and/or family are pessimistic or non-supportive?

- You are being sabotaged—given high-calorie foods? Given food as a sign of affection? Told that you are becoming too skinny?

- People insist that you eat dessert, seconds, etc.?

The people in your environment play a very important and influential role in your program and in your life. People can be a source of reinforcement and rewards—noticing changes, complementing you, giving you feedback and encouragement. Let them know!

Take Control

Be vocal! No one can read your mind. Be explicit about what you need and want.

1. Ask for daily support and encouragement. Be specific. Tell others *how* to support you.

2. Ask for feedback. What type of feedback do you desire? When?

3. Ask for praise.

4. Ask for cooperation and assistance. Tell others *how* to assist.

5. Ask for participation in exercise, shopping, cooking, counseling, education, pre-planning, cue elimination, etc.

6. Entertain with low-calorie, attractive, fun foods.

7. Do not use food for sharing and affection. Request that love be expressed in other ways. Ask for flowers, books, music, etc.

8. Let others know that you do not want food offered to you.

9. Minimize conversations about food.

10. Exercise with your family and friends or with a class.

11. Ask close friends and family not to continue eating tempting foods around you.

12. Get involved in activities that take you outside of yourself—ceramics, sewing, gift-making, bowling, team sports, painting, carpentry, yard work, church groups, charities, etc.

13. Plan family gatherings to include activities, not just food.

14. Thank others for their support and encouragement.

How Do You Handle Non-Supportive People?

People have different ways of reacting to someone losing weight. Be sensitive to the factors that may cause negative responses, conscious or unconscious, from others:

- They may feel threatened by your self-discipline and self-control—and pressured to match your accomplishments.
- Your improved appearance may create new, uncertain feelings within others. With a "new look," will you want a new type of relationship? Will your personality change?

Keeping these factors in mind, remember not to let others control you. You must control your own life. Ask yourself these questions:

1 Are your expectations of others unrealistic?

2 How do you reinforce others' supportive behaviors?

3 How can you positively cope? Respond?

4 How can you let others get involved?

5 How can you ask for the support you want? Others may not know how to help you, so be specific.

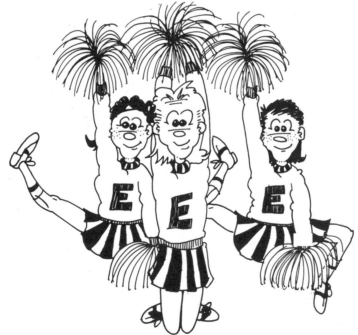

Remember: Your program and the education you give others may benefit them! *You can make a difference!*

Social and Community Support

There's tremendous value in surrounding yourself with ongoing support. Try to focus on the following types of people and activities:

❶ Associate and socialize with others of similar values, motives, goals and "coping skills" to acquire stronger behavioral skills and easier social adjustment skills.

❷ Join clubs or groups that reinforce your interests: spas, gyms, low-fat cooking classes, bike club, dance group, etc.

❸ Join self-help groups. Their benefits:

- social outlet/peer support
- role models (participants) representing obtainable goals
- motivation and self-confidence
- problem-solving practice
- self-responsibility

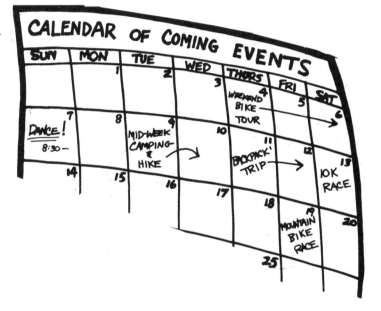

❹ Participate in self-help activities:

- lead the class
- check buddy's food records or exercise log
- write newsletter
- contribute recipes
- develop phone check system

❺ Take classes that motivate your desired behaviors and knowledge:

- The discipline of regular meetings will reinforce and commit your behaviors.
- Enriched skills make tasks easier and more desirable.
- A camaraderie of class friends provide support and encouragement.

❻ Find a "partner" with whom you can communicate and work. Commit to a common goal and action plan.

❼ Develop communication skills and interpersonal relationship skills.

Environmental Support

How do your surroundings impact your decisions? Motivate yourself to stay fit and eat well by…

❶ …participating in active events.

- walks, races, swim meets, tennis tournaments, etc.
- hiking trips, ski trips, bike trips
- intramural sports
- treadmill test
- active vacations
- children's activities
- charity bike-a-thons or similar events

❷ …going to the right places.

- gyms and exercise facilities—a healthier after-work activity than bars
- nonfood environments—socialize with a friend outdoors, not in front of the television or at a food counter
- church, charity groups—activities that put others first
- home and work—keep your surroundings free of "food cues"

❸ …managing your time well. Don't use food as a:

- procrastinator
- transition
- time-filler, such as when waiting for a bus or plane
- coffee break
- leisure or recreational activity or pastime
- reward
- comfort

❹ …knowing your reaction to media.

- Enjoy health, fitness, weight control magazines and tapes instead of high-fat cooking magazines and food catalogs.

Self-Support

While it's helpful and motivating to have people in your life who are supportive of lifestyle choices, remember that you are your No. 1 cheerleader. Nobody can make the choices for you. You can talk and think yourself into healthier behaviors by following the steps below:

❶ Practice positive self-talk when excuses and discouragement seep in. Write down your positive responses.

NEGATIVE THOUGHTS	POSITIVE THOUGHTS
(a) I overate and feel guilty. I might as well keep eating and forget this program.	It's OK. I enjoyed it. Now it is time to get back on track and keep going.
(b) I shouldn't have eaten that candy. That blows the whole day. I'll start over tomorrow.	I won't procrastinate; I'll start back right now. A small mistake won't hurt.
(c) When I eat out, I have to eat everything on my plate. After all, I paid for it.	I'm eating out because of the company or the convenience. That's what I'm paying for. I'll take half home for tomorrow.
(d) I always blow it on weekends or at parties or after dinner.	I'll plan ahead to avoid undesirable situations; and I'll keep healthy choices at home.
(e) If I don't eat this now, I might never have another chance.	Ridiculous! There are always fun foods to enjoy. I'll enjoy it more when I've lost some weight.

❷ Be your own best friend. Treat yourself to activities that please you as you make progress. Refer to your "Treat Yourself" list on p. 37.

❸ Compliment yourself daily for reorienting your lifestyle and practicing new behaviors, attitudes, self-confidence, etc. (The scales are not the only sign of progress!)

❹ Monitor your progress with records—food, exercise, weight, inches, clothing sizes. View any progress a step in the right direction.

❺ Manage your thinking. Improve your self-attitude by:
- being *assertive*—you must help yourself.
- being *realistic*—allow room for imperfection. Take small steps of change.
- being *optimistic*—feel positive about yourself, your successes and your ability to reach and maintain health goals.
- being *proud*—you are living a healthier lifestyle.

❻ Practice self-imagery:
- Envision yourself being more slender, confident and content.
- Picture yourself living an active lifestyle.
- See yourself managing eating occasions in a positive way.

❼ List your priorities in life. Arrange your commitments to give your health and weight the attention they deserve.

My Support Team

☑ Write it down. To whom do you turn for support of your new lifestyle? Identify people and factors that encourage you. Surround yourself with them! Add to the examples below.

Who / What?	How Are They Supportive?

SOCIAL

☑ best friend Mary — ◆ exercise partner; emotional support
☑ weight control class — ◆ team motivation
☐ _____ — ◆ _____
☐ _____ — ◆ _____
☐ _____ — ◆ _____

ENVIRONMENTAL

☑ join YMCA — ◆ exercise class and participants
☑ charity walk/run — ◆ motivational goal
☐ _____ — ◆ _____
☐ _____ — ◆ _____
☐ _____ — ◆ _____

SELF-SUPPORT

☑ positive self-attitude — ◆ keep thinking of positive steps and ability to reach your goals
☑ encourage self daily — ◆ take one day at a time
☑ be realistic — ◆ lose one pound a week, don't expect perfection
☑ be alert and aware — ◆ keep food + exercise records; weigh weekly
☐ _____ — ◆ _____

NON-SUPPORTIVE BEHAVIORS

☑ family snacking at night — ◆ drink low-calorie beverages; make low-fat popcorn for all, enjoy as a family
☐ _____ — ◆ _____
☐ _____ — ◆ _____
☐ _____ — ◆ _____
☐ _____ — ◆ _____

PSYCHE

☑ positive self-image — ◆ focus on positive qualities – fitness
☑ appearance — ◆ smaller clothing size, feeling good, complements
☑ confidence boosters — ◆ focus on challenges achieved
☐ _____ — ◆ _____
☐ _____ — ◆ _____

Step 13   © 2009, *The Cooper Clinic Solution to the Diet Revolution* by Georgia G. Kostas, M.P.H., R.D., L.D., Dallas, Texas

Step 14
Moving Onward
and Upward

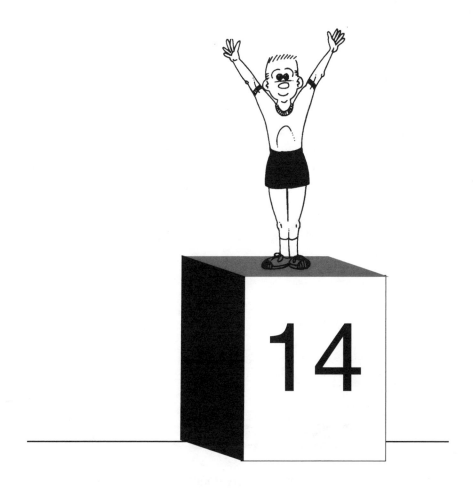

Step 14

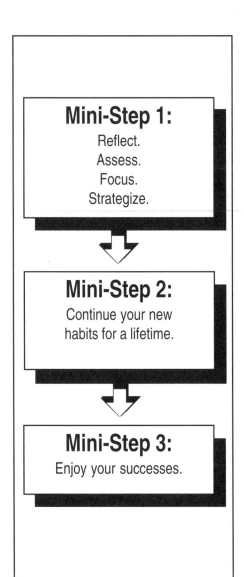

Mini-Step 1:

Reflect.
Assess.
Focus.
Strategize.

Mini-Step 2:

Continue your new
habits for a lifetime.

Mini-Step 3:

Enjoy your successes.

By now, you have crossed some major hurdles in your journey for better health and weight management:

- You've modified your eating habits and taken steps to manage your weight.
- You've made personal decisions regarding appropriate goals and strategies.
- You've taken appropriate actions and enjoyed success and beneficial effects of weight management.

The purpose of this book has been to teach you skills and techniques so you can manage your social, physical and personal environments. *You now have the skills to take charge of your eating behavior and weight.* Continue your efforts to make necessary habit changes and to strengthen changes you have already made. Remember, it takes time and repeated practice to establish permanent new eating patterns. Be patient, persistent and optimistic!

To further your success, you must reassess your progress and problem areas on a regular basis, set small goals, reach these and continue moving forward. Take the self-assessment quiz on p. 259-260 to see where you stand, and review the material (p. 261-263) from time to time to keep each step fresh and alive.

CONGRATULATIONS!

ACTION STEPS

① Make a list of your successful changes. What new weekly goals and strategies will help you maintain a healthy lifestyle?

② Re-read each step in this program for positive reinforcement. Keep going! Small changes add up!

③ Keep focusing on your newly forming lifestyle and the benefits and rewards you are enjoying. Surround yourself with support.

④ MAKE YOUR NEW HABITS LAST A LIFETIME!

Self-Assessment Quiz

It's time to reflect on your successes, goals, trouble spots, etc. Answer the following questions honestly, and use them as a guide.

1 Turn to your **"Assessment of Eating Habits"** form (p.18). Which eating behaviors improved?

Which eating habits do you need to concentrate on improving now?

2 Turn to **"My Overall Game Plan"** (p. 38). Which goals did you achieve?

What areas need work?

3 What new **pleasures** (p. 37) are you enjoying, other than food?

List others you will enjoy:

4 List your priorities in life. Arrange your commitments to give your health and weight the attention they deserve.

5   Identify your greatest challenge in your weight reduction efforts:

- List and test potential solutions:

- My most successful solution(s) are:

6   Where are you in your positive progress toward health and fitness? List areas you need to focus on, and refer to appropriate sections to reinforce your good habits.

7   To keep improving, set weekly eating goals, i.e.:

SOME WEEKLY EATING GOALS:

- Meatless week
- Fish or poultry all lunches
- Meat: 3 times a week
- Vegetarian week
- 2 fruits-a-day week
- No ice cream week
- No nachos week
- No alcohol week
- No soft drinks week
- "3 preplanned meals a day" week
- Slower eating week
- Smart snacks week
- Breakfast daily
- "Brown bag lunch" week

- 5 fish meals week
- "Remove food cues" week
- "All homemade meals" week
- "3 vegetables a day" week
- Sugar-free week
- Measure portions week
- Treat self without food
- Relax without food
- Choose a non-food entertainment
- Exercise if angry or upset
- Eat sitting down only
- Low-fat week
- 2 crunchy foods per meal
- Other:_____

Helpful Strategies: A Review

In the previous Steps, we focused on the strategies listed below. ☑Check the items in column one that need more work. In column two, take note of your "success days." Do you see a pattern?

WHICH NEED FOCUS?		MARK YOUR "SUCCESS" DAYS						

PLANNING AHEAD

		S	M	T	W	TH	F	S
____	Start each day with breakfast.	___	___	___	___	___	___	___
____	Eat three regular, planned meals.	___	___	___	___	___	___	___
____	Choose small, planned snacks.	___	___	___	___	___	___	___
____	Eat lunch daily.	___	___	___	___	___	___	___
____	Eat meals at scheduled times.	___	___	___	___	___	___	___
____	Use a Meal-Menu Planner daily.	___	___	___	___	___	___	___
____	Think before eating. Predict/plan eating-out choices.	___	___	___	___	___	___	___

PROBLEM FOODS

		S	M	T	W	TH	F	S
____	Don't buy problem food: i.e., _____.	___	___	___	___	___	___	___
____	Choose low-cal alternatives: i.e., _____.	___	___	___	___	___	___	___
____	Eat a low-cal instead of a high-cal snack: i.e., _____.	___	___	___	___	___	___	___
____	Chew sugarless gum while cooking.	___	___	___	___	___	___	___
____	Don't sample food when cooking.	___	___	___	___	___	___	___
____	Drink sugar-free drinks.	___	___	___	___	___	___	___

FOOD QUANTITY

		S	M	T	W	TH	F	S
____	Measure portions.	___	___	___	___	___	___	___
____	Leave some food on your plate.	___	___	___	___	___	___	___
____	Take 20 minutes to eat a meal.	___	___	___	___	___	___	___
____	Enjoy one portion; skip seconds.	___	___	___	___	___	___	___
____	Use smaller dishes and utensils.	___	___	___	___	___	___	___
____	Sit down while eating.	___	___	___	___	___	___	___
____	Put utensils down between bites.	___	___	___	___	___	___	___
____	Let someone else scrape dishes.	___	___	___	___	___	___	___
____	Put leftovers away immediately.	___	___	___	___	___	___	___
____	Share servings—particularly an entree, dessert, appetizer or richer food—with a friend.	___	___	___	___	___	___	___

ENVIRONMENTAL CONTROL	S	M	T	W	TH	F	S
____ Keep tempting foods out of sight.	____	____	____	____	____	____	____
____ Take healthy, low-cal snacks and portable food with you.	____	____	____	____	____	____	____
____ Tell fellow peers not to offer you food.	____	____	____	____	____	____	____
____ Avoid places that give you trouble.	____	____	____	____	____	____	____
____ Eat a low-cal snack before eating out to reduce appetite.	____	____	____	____	____	____	____
____ Make special requests in restaurants.	____	____	____	____	____	____	____

COOKING AND ENTERTAINING	S	M	T	W	TH	F	S
____ Fix lower-calorie foods for company.	____	____	____	____	____	____	____
____ Substitute lower-calorie ingredients.	____	____	____	____	____	____	____
____ Try new, low-cal recipes.	____	____	____	____	____	____	____
____ Broil or bake instead of frying.	____	____	____	____	____	____	____

YOUR INDIVIDUAL STRATEGIES	S	M	T	W	TH	F	S
(Write in)_____	____	____	____	____	____	____	____
_____	____	____	____	____	____	____	____
_____	____	____	____	____	____	____	____

FEELINGS/SELF-IMAGE	S	M	T	W	TH	F	S
____ I see myself as slender.	____	____	____	____	____	____	____
____ I see my clothes fitting better.	____	____	____	____	____	____	____
____ I enjoy healthy, balanced meals.	____	____	____	____	____	____	____
____ I feel terrific without food.	____	____	____	____	____	____	____
____ I find comfort in the outdoors, in peace and quiet, with family and friends.	____	____	____	____	____	____	____
____ Activities and exercise make me feel good; food doesn't.	____	____	____	____	____	____	____
____ I have more confidence in myself.	____	____	____	____	____	____	____
____ I enjoy life and people a lot more.	____	____	____	____	____	____	____

EMOTIONS AND THOUGHTS	S	M	T	W	TH	F	S
____ Avoid persons/situations that upset me.	____	____	____	____	____	____	____
____ Interpret events objectively.	____	____	____	____	____	____	____
____ Express feelings objectively.	____	____	____	____	____	____	____
____ Counter excuses and negative thoughts with positive self-talk.	____	____	____	____	____	____	____
____ Use relaxation techniques.	____	____	____	____	____	____	____
____ Go for a walk or talk to someone instead of eating.	____	____	____	____	____	____	____

EATING SITUATIONS		S	M	T	W	TH	F	S
____	Don't eat in the car.	____	____	____	____	____	____	____
____	Let others get their own snacks.	____	____	____	____	____	____	____
____	Do nothing else while eating.	____	____	____	____	____	____	____
____	Remove food cues.	____	____	____	____	____	____	____
____	Eat only at my designated eating place.	____	____	____	____	____	____	____
____	Eat only while sitting down.	____	____	____	____	____	____	____
____	Eat healthy foods, even "on the run."	____	____	____	____	____	____	____

BUYING AND STORING FOODS		S	M	T	W	TH	F	S
____	Shop when not hungry.	____	____	____	____	____	____	____
____	Shop from a list.	____	____	____	____	____	____	____
____	Don't buy "problem foods."	____	____	____	____	____	____	____
____	Avoid tempting aisles.	____	____	____	____	____	____	____
____	Put groceries in trunk on way home.	____	____	____	____	____	____	____
____	Do not open package until ready to use.	____	____	____	____	____	____	____
____	Use opaque instead of clear wrap when storing foods.							

EATING OUT		S	M	T	W	TH	F	S
____	Choose restaurants with varied food selections.	____	____	____	____	____	____	____
____	Order fat-free milk or low-cal drink.	____	____	____	____	____	____	____
____	Eat a low-cal snack before eating out.	____	____	____	____	____	____	____
____	Take own low-cal salad dressing, food or drink.	____	____	____	____	____	____	____
____	Share entrées, desserts and sauces.	____	____	____	____	____	____	____
____	Ask for salad dressing "on the side."	____	____	____	____	____	____	____
____	Order menu items "grilled," "steamed," "without butter," etc.	____	____	____	____	____	____	____
____	Avoid dessert list.	____	____	____	____	____	____	____
____	Call hostess about menu beforehand; plan strategies.	____	____	____	____	____	____	____
____	Make special requests in restaurants.	____	____	____	____	____	____	____

From This Time Forward

As a summary, I've compiled a checklist of helpful hints that I believe will keep your lifestyle in balance and help you enjoy a fuller, more invigorating life. Keep it handy for regular checkups. Be proud of your accomplishments—and enjoy the "new you"!

For Continued Success:

1. **Reassess your problem areas** from time to time.
2. **Continue recordkeeping.**
3. **Reread this manual**, and concentrate on lessons that deal specifically with your eating concerns.
4. **Practice strategies** suggested and devise new ones.
5. **Maintain a supportive environment.**
6. **Be prepared for weight plateaus.** These are normal. Continue your program and the weight will inevitably disappear.
7. **Expect problems** from time to time. **Anticipate ways to cope.**
8. **When you reach your desired weight, gradually add 200 calories per week** until you reach your weight maintenance calorie level.

Maintenance:

1. **Know your weight.** Weight at least once weekly and record.
2. **Keep food records** periodically.
3. **Enjoy your new weight** and rewards associated with it.
4. **Maintain your good eating habits.** Do not eat like a fat person. You know how to eat for your well-being.
5. **Get rid of, or alter, old clothes**. Buy new, flattering outfits. Do not allow yourself an easy road back to your old sizes.
6. **Set a 3-pound weight gain limit for yourself.** As soon as you are over this limit, start immediately to re-establish sound eating habits.
7. **If you need a break, decide to maintain your weight for a week** rather than to lose that week.
8. **Remind yourself of all the work it took to reach your ideal weight.** Do not let it be wasted effort.
9. **Stay active.** Continue to increase daily activity.
10. **Care about yourself.**

My best wishes for your lifelong success!

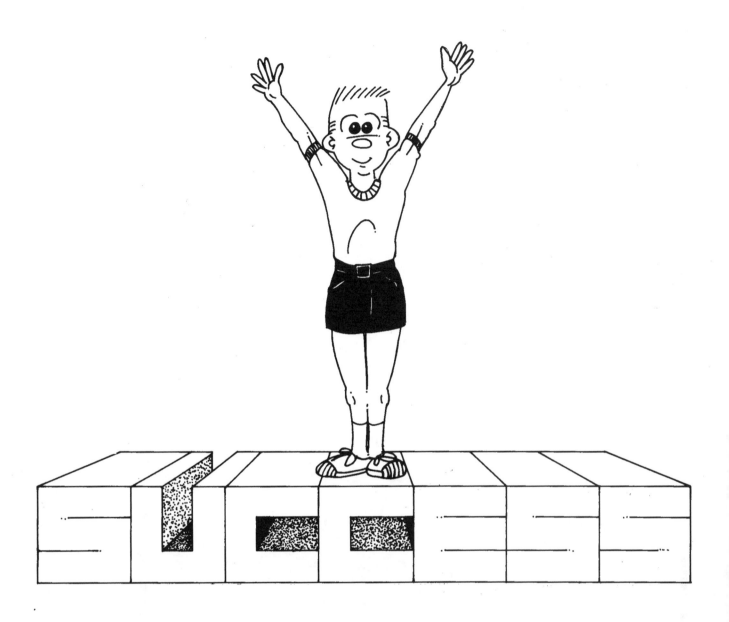

NOTES

Appendix A
RECORDS

- FOOD RECORDS

- EXERCISE LOGS

- WEIGHT GRAPHS

- END-OF-MONTH PROGRESS CHECK

(See Step 1 for examples of completing each record.)

DAILY FOOD RECORD

Date _____

(Write one food on each line.)

Time/ Min. Eating	Place / With Whom	Mood / Activity	Amount	Food - How Prepared	Food Group or Calories	Fat Grams

MONTHLY EXERCISE LOG

Month _____

Goal = 1400 calories a week or 200 a day.

Sunday	Monday	Tuesday	Wednesday	Thursday	Friday	Saturday	Weekly Totals	Cal. Totals*

WEEKLY WEIGHT GRAPHS

Starting Weight _____   Date _____

Desired Weight _____   Date _____

Week No.	Date	Weight	Weight Change	Total Weight Change
0				
1				
2				
3				
4				
5				
6				
7				
8				
8				
9				
10				
11				
12				
13				
14				
15				
16				
17				
18				
19				
20				
21				
22				
23				

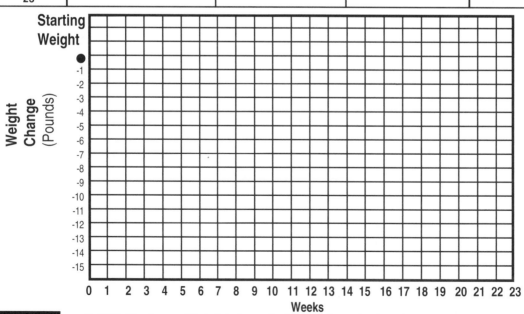

END-OF-MONTH PROGRESS CHECK

Month _____

1. Identify your greatest challenge in your weight reduction efforts: _____

    _____

2. List and test potential solutions: _____

    _____

3. My most successful solutions are: _____

    _____

4. Where are you in your positive progress toward health and fitness? List areas you need to
    focus on and refer to appropriate sections to reinforce your good habits. _____

    _____

Month _____

1. Identify your greatest challenge in your weight reduction efforts: _____

    _____

2. List and test potential solutions: _____

    _____

3. My most successful solutions are: _____

    _____

4. Where are you in your positive progress toward health and fitness? List areas you need to
    focus on and refer to appropriate sections to reinforce your good habits. _____

    _____

Appendix B
Recommended Reading and Resources

- Nutrition
- Weight Control
- Sports Nutrition
- Cookbooks
- Calorie and Nutrient Counters
- Newsletters/Magazines
- Hotlines
- Websites and Internet Sources

RECOMMENDED READING

With the abundance of nutrition and diet books available, it's important to choose nutrition resources that are reliable and factual. Some are based on fads and give erroneous information.

Be sure to scrutinize the author and content before buying the book. It should:

1. **Describe a credible author** including -
   · degrees and background (distinguish between "nutritionist" and R.D., or registered dietitian, and "doctor" and M.D.)
   · work experience

2. **Describe a credible diet** including -
   · emphasis on a variety of foods and not just a single food and/or beverage
   · a realistic, livable approach
   · a healthy balance of protein, carbohydrate and fat intake

I recommend the following books:

NUTRITION

Brody, J. *Jane Brody's Nutrition Book: A Lifetime Guide to Good Eating for Better Health and Weight Control*. Bantam, 1988.
Carpenter, R. and C. Finley. *Healthy Eating Every Day.* Human Kinetics, 2005.
Cooper, K. *The Aerobics Program for Total Well-Being.* M. Evans and Co., 1983.
Cooper, K. *Advanced Nutritional Therapies.* Thomas Nelson Publishers, 1996.
Calvert-Finn, S. *The American Dietetic Association's Guide to Women's Nutrition for Healthy Living.* Perigree/Berkley, 1997.
Duyff, R.L. *The American Dietetic Association's Complete Food and Nutrition Guide.* Wiley, 1998.
Gershoff, S. *The Tufts University Guide to Total Nutrition.* Harper Perennial, 1996.
Herbert, V. *The Mt. Sinai School of Medicine Complete Book of Nutrition.* St. Martin's Press, 1999.
Tribole, E. *Eating on the Run.* Leisure Press, 1992.
Ayoab, K. *The Uncle Sam Diet.* St. Martin's Paperbacks, 2005.

WEIGHT CONTROL

Cooper, K. *The Aerobics Program for Total Well-Being.* M. Evans and Co., 1983.
Bailey, C. *The New Fit or Fat.* Houghton Mifflin Co., 1991.
Blair, S., R. Carpenter, et al. *Active Living Every Day.* Human Kinetics, 2001
Brownell, K. *The Learn Program.* American Health Publishing Co., 1999.
Carpenter, R. and C. Finley. *Healthy Eating Every Day.* Human Kinetics, 2005.
Ferguson, J. *Habits, Not Diets.* Bull Publishing Co., 1997.
Katahn, M. *The T-Factor Diet.* W. W. Norton and Co., 1994.
Kirby, J. *Dieting for Dummies.* IDG Books, 1999.
Kirschenbaum, D. *The Nine Truths about Weight Loss.* Henry Holt and Co., 2000.
Kostas, G. *The Cooper Clinic Solution to the Diet Revolution.* Good Health Press, 2006.
Nash and Long, R.D. *Managing Your Weight and Well-Being.* Bull Publishing Co., 1978.

SPORTS NUTRITION

Berning, J. and Steen, S. *Nutrition in Sports and Exercise.* Aspen Publications, 1998.

Clark, N. *Nancy Clark's Sports Nutrition Guidebook.* Human Kinetics, 2002.

Coleman, E. and Steen, S. *The Ultimate Sports Nutrition Handbook.* Bull Publishing, 1996.

Coleman, E. *Eating for Endurance.* Bull Printing Co., 1997.

Kleiner, S.M. and Greenwood, Robinson, M. *Power Eating.* Human Kinetics Publishers, Inc., 1998.

McArdle, W., Katch and Katch, *Sports and Exercise Nutrition.* Lippincott, Williams and Wolkins, 1999.

Manore, M. *Sports Nutrition for Health and Performance.* Human Kinetics Publishers, Inc., 2000.

Neiman, D. *The Fitness Handbook.* Bull Publishing Co., 1986.

Williams, M. *Nutritional Aspects of Human Physical and Athletic Performance.* Charles C. Thomas, 1991.

Wood, E. *Let's Keep Moving!* Bellaire Wellness Club, PO Box 555, Bellaire, TX 77482, 1999.

COOKBOOKS

(See also "Lowfat Recipes/Cooking" Web Sites)

ADA Family Cookbook. The American Dietetic Association and American Diabetic Association. Englewood Cliffs, NJ: Prentice-Hall, 1991.

The American Heart Association's Cookbook. Times Books, 1999.

The American Heart Association's Meals in Minutes. Clarkson Potler Publishers, 2000.

The American Cancer Society's Healthy Eating Cookbook, 1999. Call 800-ACS-2345.

Brody, J. *Jane Brody's Good Food Book.* Bantam, 1987.

Brody, J. *Jane Brody's Good Food Gourmet.* Bantam, 1992.

Cookery Classics. Cooper Wellness Program. 12300 Preston Rd., Dallas, TX 75230.

Cooper Clinic's *What's Cooking at the Cooper Clinic.* Call 800-444-5764.

DeBakey, M., et.al. *The New Living Heart Diet.* Raven Press/Simon & Schuster, 1999.

Hachfeld, L. and Eykyn, B. *Cooking a la Heart.* Appletree Press, 1991.

Jones, J. *Cook It Light Classics.* MacMilliam, 1992.

McDonald, H.B. *Eat Well, Live Well.* Canada: Macmillan, 1990.

McIntosh, S. *Cooking Light.* Oxmoor House, Birmingham, 1991.

Piscatella, J. *Don't Eat Your Heart Out Cookbook.* Workman Publishing, 1987.

Piscatella, J. *Controlling Your Fat Tooth.* Workman Publishing, 1991.

Ponichtera, B. *Quick and Healthy Recipes and Ideas, Volume I and II,* 1991. 1519 Hermits Way, The Dalles, OR 97058.

Robertson, L. and Flinder, C. *Laurel's Kitchen: A Handbook for Vegetarian Cookery and Nutrition.* B. Ruppenthal's, 1987.

Weight Watchers Cookbook. Weight Watchers International, 1995.

CALORIE AND NUTRIENT COUNTERS

Borushek, Allan. *The Calorie King Pocket Calorie, Fat and Carbohydrate Counter.* Family Health Publications, 2009.

Natow, A. and Heslin, J. *Eating Out Food Counter.* Family Health Publications, 1999.

Netzer, C. *The Complete Book of Food Counts.* Dell Publishing, 1994.

Nutritive Value of Foods, Agricultural Handbook No. 456. U.S. Department of Agriculture. Superintendent of Documents, U.S. Government Printing Office, 1981, Washington, D.C. 20402.

Pennington, J. and Church, H. *Bowles and Church's Food Values of Portions Commonly Used. 16th Ed.,* Perennial Library, 1998.

Pope-Cordle, J. and Katahn, M. *The T-Factor Fat Gram Counter.* W. W. Norton, 1994.

Roth, Harriet. *Fat Counter.* Signet Publishing Co., 1992.

NEWSLETTERS AND MAGAZINES

Supermarket Scoop Newsletter *(New Products)*
and Brand-New/Brand-Name Shopping List
Supermarket Savvy
11102 Lakeside Forest Lane
Houston, TX 77042
(888) 577-2889

Environmental Nutrition
PO Box 420235
Palm Coast, FL 32142
(800) 829-5384
www.environmentalnutrition.com

Tufts University Health & Nutrition Letter
PO Box 57857
Boulder, CO 80322
(800) 274-7581
www.healthletter.tufts.edu

Intelihealth.com
960C Harvest Drive
Blue Bell, PA
(215) 775-5155
www.intelihealth.com

Consumer Reports on Health
PO Box 52148
Boulder, CO 80322
(800) 234-2188

University of California, Berkeley Wellness
Newsletter
Health Letter Associates
PO Box 420235
Palm Coast, FL 32142
(800) 829-9080

Nutrition Action Healthletter
Center for Science in the Public Interest
1875 Connecticut Ave., NW, Suite 300
Washington, D.C. 20009-5728
(202) 332-9110
www.espinet.org

Vitality Magazine
Vitality Inc.
780 Township Line Rd.
Yardley, PA 19067
www.vitality.com

Wellness Lifeline
Health Education Materials
234 Cass Street
Port Townsend, WA 98368
(800) 294-9801
www.winfocat.com

HOTLINES

Toll-Free American Dietetic Association
National Referral Service
Call for Registered Dietitians in your area.
(800) 366-1655
www.eatright.org

Toll-Free Department of Agriculture, Meat
and Poultry Hotline
Call for safe preparation and storage of meat
and poultry.
(800) 535-4555

American Anorexia & Bulemia Association
(212) 575-6200
www.something-fishy.org/ed.htm

National Association of Anorexia Nervosa &
Associated Disorders
(708) 831-3138 or (847) 831-3438

Toll-Free Consumer Nutrition Hotline
Call for educational materials or questions regarding
nutrition.
(800) 366-1655

Toll-Free National Osteoporosis Foundation
Call for educational materials.
(800) 223-9994
www.nof.org

WEBSITES AND INTERNET RESOURCES

NUTRITION/WEIGHT CONTROL

1. **Cooper Clinic/Cooper Aerobics Center:** www.cooperwellness.com & www.cooperaerobics.com
2. **The Cooper Institute for Aerobics Research:** www.cooperinst.org
3. **American Dietetic Association:** www.eatright.org
4. **Ask the Dietitian:** www.dietitian.com
5. **Sports, Cardiovascular and Wellness Dietitians (SCAN) of the American Dietetic Association:** www.nutrifit.org
6. **California Dairy Council:** www.dairycouncilofca.org
7. **Washington State Dairy Council:** www.eatsmart.org
8. **Mayo Health Oasis** (of the Mayo Clinic): www.mayohealth.org
9. **John Hopkins Health Information:** www.intelihealth.com/ih/ihtlh
10. **Tufts University - Nutrition Navigator:** www.navigator.tufts.edu
11. **Columbia University Health Service:** www.goaskalice.columbia.edu
12. **E-diets** *(tips, menus, recipes, chat rooms)*: www.ediets.com
13. **Weight Watchers:** www.weightwatchers.com
14. **Weight Control Information Network:** www.niddk.nih.gov/health/nutrit.html
15. **Fit Day** *(calculates daily calorie intake)*: www.fitday.com
16. **Winninghabits.com** (interactive weight loss coaching)
17. **Center for Science in the Public Interest:** www.cspinet.org
18. **Dole Food Company** (fruits, vegetables): www.dole5aday.com
19. **Diet Site** (general nutrition information): www.dietsite.com
20. **5 a Day for Better Health Company:** www.dcpc.nci.nih.gov/5aday
21. **Vitality:** www.vitality.com
22. **American Cancer Society:** www.cancer.org
23. **American Heart Association:** www.americanheart.org and www.women.americanheart.org
24. **American Council on Exercise:** www.acefitness.org/index.html
25. **Association for Worksite Health Promotion:** www.awhp.org
26. **Centers for Disease Control and Prevention:** www.cdc.gov
27. **Consumer Information Center:** www.pueblo.gsa.gov
28. **Fitness Partner Connection Jumpsite:** www.healingdoc.com
29. **Gatorade Sports Science Institute:** www.gssiweb.com/
30. **U.S. Dept. of Health and Human Services:** www.os.dhhs.gov
31. **U.S. Dept. of Health and Human Services:** www.healthfinder.gov
32. **U.S. Dept. of Agriculture's Food/Nutrition Center:** www.hall.usda.gov/fnic
33. **Web M.D.** *(medical & nutrition information)*: www.webmd.com
34. **MedScape Daily News:** www.medscape.com
35. **Medicine Net** *(practicing doctors' info)*: www.medicinenet.com
36. **CNN Health Online:** www.cnn.com/health
37. **Medline (***National Library of Medicine***):** www.nih.gov/databases/freemedl.html
38. **American Botanical Council** *(reliable herb/medicine info)*: www.herbalgram.org
39. **Health Fraud and Quakery:** www.quackwatch.com
40. **Supplement.com** *(medical info about supplements)*: www.supplementwatch.com
41. **Harvard School of Public Health:** www.hsph.Harvard.edu/nutritionsource/index.html

NUTRITION/DIET ANALYSIS

1. **Nutrient Analysis Tool, University of Illinois:** www.spectre.ag.uinc.edu/~food-lab/nat/ (provides custom analysis of your diet)
2. **Fast Food Facts/Interactive food finder:** www.chowbaby.com and www.calorieking.com (provides comprehensive nutritional data on fast-food menu items) (see p. 283 for more sites)
3. **Diet Analysis and Food & Activity Tracking:** www.nutribalance.com, www.foodworks.com, www.fitday.com, www.personalhealthanddietmanager.com (by Two Peaks Software), www.calorie-count.com, www.calorieking.com, www.eDiets.com, www.myfooddiary.com, www.nutrawatch.com, www.weightwatchers.com, www.dietpower.com, www.nutridiary.com, www.MyPyramidTracker.com
4. **Nutribase by Cybersoft, Inc.:** www.nutribase.com
5. **Cyberdiet:** www.cyberdiet.com
6. **Balance Log by Healthetech:** www.healthetech.com
7. **Diet Watch:** www.dietwatch.com (diet buddy)
8. **DietSite:** www.dietsite.com
9. **Food databases:** www.calorieking.com, www.nutridata.com, www.nal.usda.gov/fnic/foodcomp/data, www.caloriescount.com
10. **Recipe analysis:** www.per-serving.org/links.asp, www.NutritionData.com
11. **For Pocket PC's, PDA's and mobile phones:** www.calorieking.com, www.hangango.com, www.nutrihand.com, www.fitday.com, www.ars.usda.gov/Main/site_main.htm?modecode=12-35-45-00, www.mobihand.com (tracks fitness programs), www.myphone.com, www.nutribase.com

LOW-FAT RECIPES/COOKING

1. **www.cookinglight.com/cooking; www.eatingwell.com**
2. **www.healthychoice.com**
3. **www.fatfree.com**
4. **www.foodstuff.com**
5. **www.prevention.com/recipes; www.eatbetteramerica.com**
6. **American Heart Association:** www.deliciousdecisions.org
7. **Meals for You:** www.mealsforyou.com (healthy recipes)
8. **All recipes:** www.Allrecipes.com
9. **SPA Finders**: www.spafinders.com (high-nutrition, low-fat recipes made by spa chefs using fruits, vegetables and whole grains)

Appendix C

FAST-FOOD CALORIE INFORMATION

Fast Food "Better" Choices

To help you make better fast food choices, we have listed the top 5-6 recommended items per restaurant, based on these criteria:

- **Goals**:
  Women: 300-400 calories, <15 gm fat per meal
  Men: 500-600 calories, <25 gm fat per meal
  Sides: 50- 200 calories, 0-10 gm fat
- No fried foods
- Sandwiches listed are without mayonnaise or dressings (specify when ordering).
- Salads are without dressings; add ½ pkt dressing of low-fat (LF), reduced-fat (RF), fat-free (FF) or Light (Lt) dressing (unless otherwise noted).
- We listed one choice per category: beef, poultry, salad and breakfast items. Other options may also meet this criteria – check their websites.

Tips • Know what you will order before you go.
- Check websites frequently for new items and updated data.
- Take fruit from home; or baby carrots or grape tomatoes to balance meals.
- Since fast foods are high in sodium, averaging 1000-1500 mg Sodium per meal, balance these meals with home meals that are low in sodium and rich in vegetables, fruit and wholegrains.

LEGEND
Lt = light
FF = fat-free
LF = low fat
RF = reduced-fat
Drsg = dressing
Pkt = packet
Ckn = chicken
Tky = turkey
Rst = roasted
Brst = breast
sm = small
med = medium
pc = piece

300-400 Calories, <15 gm Fat

Arby's
Junior or Regular Roast Beef
Grilled Chicken Fillet Sandwich or SW Ckn Wrap (no sauce)
Ham & Swiss Melt Sandwich
Baked Potato w/ Broccoli & Cheese
Sourdough w/ Egg & Cheese
Salads: Martha's Vineyard or Santa Fe Grilled Chicken
+ ½ Packet Light Buttermilk Ranch or Raspberry Vinaigrette

Boston Market
¼ White Rotiss Ckn (no skin) or Roasted Tky Breast
   + 2 sides (below)
Roasted Sirloin + 1 side (below)
Sides: broccoli w/ garlic butter, fresh steamed vegetables, green beans, green bean casserole, fresh fruit salad, garlic dill new potatoes, butternut squash or Soups: Chicken or Turkey Tortilla Soup (no toppings) or Chicken Noodle
Open faced sandwiches: Ckn, Tky, Sirloin
Salads: Caesar Salad Entrée or Market Chopped Salad w/
   ckn, tky, or sirloin or Oriental Grilled Ckn (no noodles)
   + 1 indiv portion (1.5 oz) Light Ranch

Burger King
Whopper Jr, w/ or w/o Cheese
Tendergrill Chicken Sandwich
BK Veggie Burger (no cheese)
Ham Omelet Sandwich
Salad: Tendergrill Garden + 1 pkt FF Ranch or Ken's Lt Ital

500-600 Calories, <25 gm Fat

(May also choose a 300-400 calorie meal plus 1-2 sides)

Arby's
Roast Turkey Reuben Wrap
Large Roast Beef Sandwich
French Dip & Swiss Toasted Sub

Boston Market
¼ White Rotiss Chicken (no skin) or Rst Turkey Breast
   + 3 sides (below)
Roasted Sirloin + 2 sides (below)
Sides: broccoli w/ garlic butter, fresh steamed vegetables, green beans, green bean casserole, fresh fruit salad, garlic dill new potatoes, butternut squash; soups: Ckn or Tky Tortilla Soup (no toppings) or Chicken Noodle; or side Caesar or Market Chopped salads w/o ckn + 1 indiv portion (1.5 oz) Lt Ranch
Salads: Caesar Salad Entrée, Market Chopped Salad w/
   ckn, tky, or sirloin, or Oriental Grilled Ckn (no noodles)
   + 1 individual portion (1.5 oz) Light Ranch

Burger King
Whopper (no cheese or mayo)

300-400 Calories, <15 gm Fat continued

Chick-Fil-A
Chargrilled *or* Spicy Chicken Cool Wraps (no dressings)
Chick-Fil-A Chicken Sandwich on Wheat Bun
1 small Folded Egg + Multigrain Bagel + med Fruit Cup
Salads: Chargrilled Ckn Garden *or* SW Ckn Salad
  + ½ pkt Lt Italian, FF Honey Mustard *or* RF Raspberry
  Vinaigrette
Side Salad + ½ pkt Lt dressings (above) + Hearty Chicken
  Soup + small Fruit Cup

Jack in the Box
Hamburger or Cheeseburger
Chicken Whole Grain Fajita Pita (no sauce) *or* SW Ckn Pita
Grilled Chicken or Sirloin Tacos
Breakfast Jack
Salads: Acapulco *or* SW *or* Asian w/ Grilled Chicken Salad
  + ½ pkt Asian Sesame, LF Balsamic Vinaigrette or Lt Ranch

Kentucky Fried Chicken
Original Chicken Breast (no skin or breading), 1 pc + 2 sides
Tender Roast Sandwich (no sauce) + 1 side
Sides: green beans; mashed potatoes (no gravy), 3" corn on
  cob, sweet corn, mean greens, 3-bean salad
Salad: Roasted Chicken + ½ pkt FF Ranch or Lt Italian

McDonalds
Hamburger or Cheeseburger + ½ small Fry
Grilled Snack Wraps, any + Honey Mustard
Grilled Chicken Classic Sand (no mayo)
Egg McMuffin
Scrambled Eggs (2) + English Muffin + Low-fat Milk
Salads: any (SW, Asian, Caesar, *or* Bacon Ranch) w/ Grilled
  Ckn + 1 pkt LF Balsamic Vinaigrette, FF Family Italian or
  Lf Sesame Ginger

Pizza Hut
Fit N Delicious *or* Thin N Crispy (any type, *except* Meat
  Lovers), 12" medium, 1 slice
Pan *or* Hand-Tossed (any type *except* Meat Lovers) 12"
  medium, 2 slices

Schlotzsky's Deli
Sandwiches (small) on Wheat Bread: Tuna, Smoked
  Turkey Breast, Ckn Breast, Chipotle Ckn, Dijon Ckn,
  Pesto Ckn, Fresh Veggie, Roast Beef, Corned Beef
Mediterranean Tuna Wrap or Asian Chicken Wrap
Any 8" Pizza, 1/2

cont. pg. 282

500-600 Calories, <25 gm Fat continued

Chick-Fil-A
Chargrilled Chicken + Small Hearty Breast of Chicken Soup
  + Side Salad + ½ pkt Lt Italian, FF Honey Mustard *or* RF
  Raspberry Vinaigrette
Chicken Deluxe Sandwich on Wheat Bun + Fruit Cup
Large Hearty Breast of Chicken Soup + Carrot & Raisin
  Salad

Jack in the Box
Chicken Sandwich + Fruit Cup
Hamburger Deluxe + Side Salad + Light Dressing
Sourdough Breakfast Sandwich + Orange Juice

Kentucky Fried Chicken
Original Chicken Breast (no skin or breading), 2 pc + 2 sides
Original Chicken Breast, 1 pc + 3 sides
Tender Roast Sandwich (no sauce) + 2-3 sides
Oven Roasted Twister Sandwich (no sauce) + Red Beans/Rice
Salad: Roasted Chicken + ½ pkt FF Ranch or Light Italian
Sides: green beans; mashed potatoes (no gravy), 3" corn
  on cob, sweet corn, mean greens, 3-bean salad

McDonalds
Premium Grilled Chicken Classic Sandwich + Fruit N'
  Yogurt Parfait
Hamburger or Cheeseburger + Salad (Southwest, Asian,
  Caesar, or Bacon Ranch) w/o chicken + 1 pkt LF
  Balsamic Vinaigrette, FF Family Italian, LF Sesame
  Ginger
Hamburger + ½ small Fry
Big 'N Tasty + Apple Dippers

Pizza Hut
Thin N Crispy (Cheese, Veggie, Ham & Pineapple), 12"
  medium, 3 slices
Pan or Hand-Tossed Pizza (any except Meat Lovers), 12"
  medium, 2 slices
Personal Pan Pizza, Veggie Lovers or Cheese

Schlotzsky's Deli
Medium Sandwiches on Wheat Bread:
  Albacore Tuna w/ or w/o cheese, Smoked Turkey Breast,
  Chicken Breast, Pesto Chicken, Dijon Ckn, Fresh Veggie,
  Mediterranean Tuna, Corned Beef, Roast Beef + Fresh
  Fruit Salad
Asian Chicken Wrap or Zesty Albacore Tuna Wrap +
  Slaw, Fresh Fruit Salad or Soup
Grilled Chicken Romano Panini
8" Pizzas: Baby Spinach, Vegetarian, Mediterranean, Fresh
  Tomato & Pesto

300-400 Calories, <15 gm Fat continued	500-600 Calories, <25 gm Fat continued

Soups (bowl): Ckn Tortilla, Ckn Gumbo, Ckn Noodle, Minestrone, Ravioli, Hearty Veg Beef, *or* Vegetarian Veg Soup (these are 100-150 cal, 5-6 g fat) + Salads (below)
Salads: Chicken Caesar, Chinese Ckn, Caesar, Smoked Turkey Chef's, Greek, Garden, *or* Ham & Turkey Salad + 1 pkt Lt Italian *or* ½ pkt Lt Spicy Ranch, Greek Balsamic Vinaigrette, or Sesame Ginger Vinaigrette Drsg

Sonic
Jr Burger
Grilled Chicken Wrap
Grilled Chicken on Ciabatta
Salads: Grilled Chicken *or* Sante Fe Ckn + 1 pkt Fat-free Italian or ½ pkt Lt Ranch

Subway
6" Subs with or without cheese:
    Ham, Oven Roasted Ckn, Roast Beef, Subway Club, Sweet Onion Ckn Teriyaki, Tky Brst, Tky Brst & Ham, Veggie Delite + (*optional*) *1 Tbsp of* : FF Honey Mustard, Lt Mayo, Mustard, Red Wine Vinaigrette or FF Sweet Onion dressing
4" Mini Sandwich (Ham, Rst Beef, Tky Brst) + Soup (Roasted Ckn Noodle *or* Garden Veg) *or* 1 pkg Baked Lays Chips *or* yogurt *or* fruit *or* raisins
Western Breakfast Sandwich, no cheese
Salad: "Jared" w/ cheese + 1-2 Tbsp Lt dressing (above)

Taco Bell
(choose **Fresco** items – they contain less fat)
Taco Fresco (2), Soft Taco Fresco (2) or Crunchy Taco Fresco (2), all types
Ranchero Chicken Soft Tacos (2)
Burrito Fresco, Bean or 7-Layer
Chicken Fiesta Burrito
Gordito Baja, Chicken or Steak
Salad: Zesty Chicken Border Bowl (no drsg) + Salsa
May add Fresco Pintos & Cheese to any meals above.

Wendy's
Jr. Hamburger or Cheeseburger or Classic Single (no mayo)
Grilled Chicken Go Wrap
Ultimate or Reg Grilled Chicken Sandwich
Chili (small) + Side Salad or Caesar Salad + 1 pkt Lt Drsg
Salads: Mandarin Chicken Salad + Almonds (no noodles) + ½ Packet Oriental Drsg *or* Chicken Caesar + I pkt Lt Drsg
Lt Dressings: Ancho Chipolte Ranch, Lt Ranch, RF Creamy Ranch, Balsamic Vinaigrette, Italian Vinaigrette, FF French, Lt Honey Dijon

Sonic
Sonic Burger w/ Mustard
Jr. Burger or Cheeseburger + ½ regular Fry
Grilled Chicken Sandwich + ½ regular Fry
Burrito or Burrito Deluxe
Breakfast Bistro (ham, egg, cheese)

Subway
Footlong Sandwich w/ or w/o cheese: Ham, Oven Rst Ckn, Roast Beef, Turkey, Turkey & Ham, Veggie, Subway Club, Sweet Onion Ckn, Ckn Teriyaki
    + (*optional*) 1 Tbsp of : FF Honey Mustard, Lt Mayo, Mustard, Red Wine Vinaigrette or FF Sweet Onion Drsg.
6" Sandwich w/ or w/o cheese: (Ham, Oven Roasted Ckn, Roast Beef, Subway Club, Sweet Onion Ckn Teriyaki, Tky Brst, Tky Brst & Ham, Veggie Delite)
    + (optional) dressing (*above*) + Soup (Roasted Ckn Noodle *or* Garden Veg) *or* 1 pkg Baked Lays Chips *or* yogurt *or* fruit *or* raisins

Taco Bell
(choose **Fresco** items – they contain less fat)
Ranchero Chicken Soft Taco Fresco, 2
Grilled Steak Soft Tacos Fresco (2) + Pintos & Cheese Fresco
Beef Enchirito Fresco + Taco Fresco + Mexican Rice Fresco
Tostada (1) + Crunchy Taco Fresco

Wendy's
Single Hamburger (1/4 lb) + Mandarin Orange Cup
Ultimate Chicken Grill Sandwich + ½ small Fry
Small Chili + Plain Baked Potato + Side Salad + 1 pkt Lt dressing (see below)
Jr. Hamburger or Cheeseburger + ½ small Fry + Side Salad + Lt Dressing (see below)
Lt Dressings: Ancho Chipolte Ranch, Lt Ranch, RF Creamy Ranch, Balsamic Vinaigrette, Italian Vinaigrette, FF French, Lt Honey Dijon

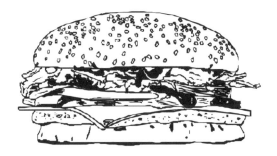

© 2009, *The Cooper Clinic Solution to the Diet Revolution* by Georgia G. Kostas, M.P.H., R.D., L.D., Dallas, Texas

Whataburger

Justaburger or Whataburger Jr (no mayo, no cheese)
Grilled Chicken Sandwich w/ mustard, small bun (special request)
Grilled Chicken Fajita Taco (special request)
Egg Sandwich
Salad: Grilled Chicken or Garden Salad w/ cheese
+ 1 pkt Thous Island *or* ½ pkt RF Ranch or Caesar drsg

Whataburger

Grilled Chicken Sandwich + Garden Salad w/ cheese
+ 1 pkt Thous Island *or* ½ pkt RF Ranch or Caesar drsg
Justaburger or Whataburger Jr. + ½ small Fry

Sides/Others: 50-200 Calories, 0-10 Fat gm

Arbys

Fruit Cup
Kid's Mini Ham & Cheese
Green Beans
Green Bean Casserole
Broccoli w/ Garlic Butter
Chicken Tortilla Soup, no toppings
Fresh Fruit
Garden Fresh Cole Slaw
Cranberry Walnut Relish
Butternut Squash
Sweet Corn
Garden Dill Potatoes
Soups, non-creamy

Jack in the Box

Fruit Cup
1 Regular Beef Taco
Side Salad + ½ pkt Light Dressing

Kentucky Fried Chicken

House Side Salad + ½ pkt fat-free dressing
Seasoned Rice
Red Beans & Rice
Mean Greens
Green Beans
Teddy Grahams
Sweet Life Oatmeal Raisin Cooke

Chick-Filet

Ice Dream Cone
Small Hearty Breast Chicken Soup
Fruit Cup
Side Salad + Lt Drsg

McDonalds

Apple Dippers
Reduced Fat Ice Cream Cone
Southwest or Asian Salad, no Chicken + ½ pkt dressing
English Muffin

Taco Bell

Pintos & Cheese
Mexican Rice

Sonic

Junior Banana Split
12 oz Fruit Slush
Vanilla Cone

Schlotzsky's Deli

Original Baked Crisps
Greek, Garden or Side Salad + ½ pkt Lt dressings
Pasta Salad

Subway

Roasted Ckn Noodle, Vegetable Beef or Tomato Garden
Veg. Soup
Apple Slices
Raisins
Yogurt – Dannon All Nat. Strawberry

Wendy's

Jr. Frosty (Choc. or Vanilla)
Garden Side Salad + ½ pkt Lt dressings

Whataburger

Garden Salad + ½ pkt Lt dressing

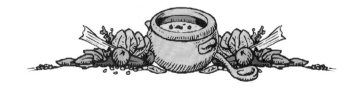

Fast Food Restaurant Websites

Check often for the latest updates.

Fast Food Resources:

www.calorieking.com
www.nutritiondata.com
www.nal.usda.gov
www.fitday.com
www.foodcount.com

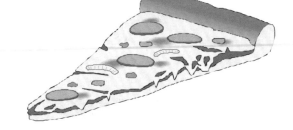

Fast Food General:

www.chowbaby.com

Restaurants:

Arby's	www.arbys.net
Boston Market	www.bostonmarket.com
Burger King	www.burgerking.com
Carl's Junior	www.carlsjr.com
Chick-fil-A	www.chick-fil-a.com
Dairy Queen	www.dairyqueen.com
Dominos Pizza	www.dominos.com
Jack In The Bos	www.jackinthebox.com
Kentucky Fried Chicken	www.kfc.com
Long John Silver's	www.ljsilvers.com
McDonald's	www.mcdonalds.com
Papa John's	www.papajohns.com
Pizza Hut	www.pizzahut.com
Schlotzky's	www.schlotzskys.com
Subway	www.subway.com
Taco Bell	www.tacobell.com
Wendy's	www.wendys.com
Whataburger	www.whataburger.com
White Castle	www.whitecastle.com

Many other restaurants list their foods and nutrient content on their websites. Check out your favorite dishes. Examples:

Applebee's	www.applebees.com
Chili's	www.chilis.com
Luby's Cafeteria	www.lubys.com
Macaroni Grill	www.macaronigrill.com
Peiwei	www.peiwei.com
P.F. Chang's China Bistro	www.pfchangs.com
Red Lobster	www.redlobster.com
Red Robin	www.redrobin.com
Ruby Tuesday	www.rubytuesday.com

Appendix D
RECIPES

- Sole With Parmesan Breadcrumbs
- Molasses-Barbequed Chicken
- Black Beans With Wild Rice With Spicy Mango Salsa
- Gourmet Burritos
- Fetticcine Alfredo With Spring Vegetables
- Tex-Mex Corn Saute
- Ranch Pasta and Vegetable Salad
- Wilted Spinach Salad
- Five Vegetable Primavera
- Roasted Vegetables
- Brownies De-Light

Sole with Parmesan Breadcrumbs

4 (4-ounce) sole fillets
1 cup soft breadcrumbs
½ cup grated Parmesan cheese
2 tablespoons reduced-fat soft margarine, melted
½ cup finely chopped watercress(optional)

Seasonings:
2 tablespoons lemon juice
1 teaspoon all-purpose seasoning or hot sauce
    (such as Tabasco)
¼ teaspoon garlic powder
¼ teaspoon salt

1. Combine lemon juice, hot sauce, garlic powder and salt in a small bowl; brush on both sides of fillets. Broil on rack of a broiler pan 6 to 8 minutes or until fish flakes with a fork.

2. Meanwhile, mix breadcrumbs, Parmesan cheese and margarine; mix well and stir in watercress. Spoon breadcrumb mixture on fish; broil 2 minutes or until mixture is lightly browned.

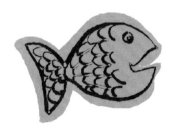

Yield: 4 servings
Per Serving: 215 Calories, 8 g Fat

Molasses-Barbecued Chicken

2 teaspoon olive oil
¾ cup finely chopped onion
½ teaspoon garlic powder
¼ to ½ teaspoon red pepper
½ cup molasses
1/3 cup cider vinegar
¼ cup Dijon mustard
2 tablespoons lemon juice
1 tablespoon reduced-sodium soy sauce
8 (6-ounce) skinned chicken breast halves
salt and pepper

1. Heat oil in a heavy medium saucepan over medium heat. Add onion, garlic powder and red pepper; sauté 3 minutes.
2. Add molasses, vinegar, mustard, lemon juice and soy sauce; bring to a boil. Reduce heat, and simmer uncovered 10 to 15 minutes or until thickened, stirring occasionally. Cool.
3. Pre-heat a broiler or light barbecue coals outside.
4. Sprinkle chicken lightly with salt and pepper. Broil for 5-8 minutes or grill over medium-hot coals (350° to 400°) about 5 to 8 minutes on each side. Baste often with some of the sauce, until chicken is glazed and no longer pink. Serve with remaining sauce.

Yield: 8 servings
Per Serving: 270 Calories, 4 g Fat

All recipes are from "The Guilt-Free Comfort Food Cookbook" by Georgia Kostas. More recipes are available from "What's Cooking at the Cooper Clinic" by the Cooper Clinic nutrition staff available at The Cooper Clinic, 12200 Preston Road, Dallas, Texas 75230, phone 1-800-444-5764, ext. 3129.

Black Beans and Wild Rice With Spicy Mango Salsa

(one-dish dinner)

vegetable cooking spray
2 teaspoons olive oil
2 cloves garlic, minced
1 cup finely chopped red pepper
1/2 cup sliced green onion
3 cups cooked black beans, drained
3 cups cooked wild rice, cooked without salt or fat
2/3 cup minced fresh cilantro
Spicy Mango Relish (recipe follows) or buy
     prepared salsa

1. Coat a large nonstick skillet with cooking spray; add oil, and place over medium-high heat until hot. Add garlic and red pepper; sauté 5 minutes or until tender.
2. Stir in green onion; sauté 1 minute.
3. Stir in beans, rice and cilantro; cook 2 minutes or until hot, stirring frequently.
4. Spoon Spicy Mango Relish over bean mixture to serve.

Spicy Mango Relish (1 ½ cups)

1 cup finely diced mango
1/2 cup finely diced red onion
1/3 cup finely diced poblano chile peppers
1 tablespoon honey
1 tablespoon white wine vinegar
1 tablespoon olive oil
1/2 teaspoon curry powder(optional)
1/4 teaspoon salt
1/4 teaspoon red pepper

1. Combine all ingredients; mix well. Cover and let stand at room temperature 1 hour before serving.

Yield: 6 servings
Per Serving: 275 Calories, 5 g Fat

Gourmet Burritos

(one-dish supper)

1 pound lean ground beef
2 cloves garlic, minced
3 tablespoons ketchup, divided
2 tablespoons reduced-sodium soy sauce
1/3 cup minced green onions
1/3 cup minced fresh cilantro
1 tablespoon grated fresh ginger
1 (15-ounce) can black beans, drained and
     mashed
1/2 teaspoon ground cumin
1/4 teaspoon ground red pepper
6 (8-inch) flour tortillas, heated
12 to 18 spinach leaves, trimmed
vegetable cooking spray

Toppings:
plain nonfat yogurt
diced tomatoes
shredded lettuce
cilantro leaves

1. Cook ground beef and garlic in a large skillet until browned, stirring to crumble. Drain in a colander; pat meat dry with paper towels.
2. Return to skillet, and stir in 2 tablespoons ketchup, soy sauce, green onions, cilantro and ginger; cook over medium heat, stirring frequently, until mixture is hot. Remove from heat; cover to keep warm.
3. Combine beans, remaining ketchup, cumin and red pepper in a small saucepan; cook over medium-low heat, stirring constantly, until hot.
4. To serve, arrange 2 or 3 spinach leaves on each tortilla; spread evenly with bean mixture, and top with ground beef mixture. Roll up and serve immediately with desired toppings.

Yield: 6 servings
Per Serving: 385 Calories, 10 g Fat

Fettuccine Alfredo with Spring Vegetables

vegetable cooking spray
1 1/2 cups sugar snap or snow pea pods
3/4 cup baby carrots, trimmed and cut in half
     lengthwise
1 cup small fresh broccoli flowerets
1 cup sliced fresh mushrooms
Goat Cheese Alfredo Sauce(recipe follows)
12 ounces fettuccine, cooked without salt or fat

1. Coat a large nonstick skillet with cooking spray; place over medium heat until hot.
2. Add sugar snap peas and carrots, and sauté 2 minutes.
3. Add broccoli and mushrooms; sauté just until vegetables are crisp-tender.
4. Stir in Goat Cheese Alfredo Sauce; cook just until hot. Pour over hot, cooked fettuccine, and toss well.

Goat Cheese Alfredo Sauce (2 cups)

1 1/2 cups nonfat cottage cheese
4 ounces goat cheese or feta
2 tablespoons butter-flavored granules
1/2 cup fat-free milk
1 teaspoon dried basil leaves
1/2 teaspoon freshly ground pepper

1. Combine all ingredients in container of an electric blender; process until smooth, scraping sides of blender as necessary.
2. Pour into a small saucepan; cook over low heat, stirring constantly until hot. (Do not boil; mixture will separate. If it separates, return to blender and reprocess or press through a fine-mesh sieve.)

Yield: 6 servings
Per Serving (including sauce):
325 Calories, 5 g Fat

Tex-Mex Corn Saute

vegetable cooking spray
1 tablespoon olive oil
3/4 cup chopped green pepper
3/4 cup chopped onion
1 teaspoon ground cumin
2 1/2 cups fresh corn
2 large ripe tomatoes, peeled
   and chopped
1/2 teaspoon sugar
1/4 teaspoon salt
1/2 to 1 teaspoon hot sauce (such as Tabasco)
1/4 cup minced fresh cilantro or parsley

1. Coat a large heavy skillet with cooking spray; add oil and place over medium-high heat until hot. Add green pepper and onion; sauté until tender.
2. Stir in cumin; add corn and sauté 3 to 5 minutes or until corn is just tender.
3. Stir in tomatoes, sugar, salt and hot sauce; sauté 3 minutes.
4. Remove from heat; stir in cilantro.

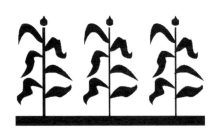

Yield: 6 servings
Per Serving: 100 Calories, 3 g Fat

Ranch Pasta and Vegetable Salad

6 ounces corkscrew pasta, uncooked
1/4 pound fresh snow peas, trimmed (about 1 ½ cups)
1 1/2 cups broccoli flowerets
1 cup sliced fresh mushrooms
1 cup cherry tomato halves
2 medium yellow squash, trimmed and cut into
       2"x ¼" strips
3/4 cup nonfat buttermilk
1/2 cup 1% lowfat cottage cheese
2 teaspoons white wine vinegar
1 clove garlic, chopped
1/4 teaspoon salt
1 green onion, chopped (about 1/3 cup)
1 jalapeno pepper, seeded and chopped (about 2
       Tbsp.)
1/3 cup chopped fresh cilantro or parsley

1. Cook pasta according to package directions, omitting salt and fat. Drain; rinse under cold water, and drain again. Place in a large bowl.
2. Blanch snow peas, broccoli and squash in boiling water 30 seconds; drain and rinse under cold water to stop cooking process. Drain well; add to pasta.
3. Process buttermilk and next 4 ingredients in an electric blender until smooth; add green Onion, jalepeno and cilantro; process until minced. Pour over pasta mixture, and toss. Cover and refrigerate at least 2 hours.

Yield: 8 cups (8 servings)
Per Serving: 125 Calories, 1 g Fat

Wilted Spinach Salad

8 cups torn fresh spinach leaves (about a pound)
1/2 cup fresh orange sections
1/3 cup snipped fresh chives or minced green
       onion
1/4 cup whole-berry cranberry sauce
2 tablespoons balsamic or red wine vinegar
2 tablespoons olive oil
1 tablespoon honey
1 teaspoon dried thyme
1/4 teaspoon salt
1/2 teaspoon freshly ground pepper

1. Combine spinach, oranges and chives in a salad bowl; set aside.
2. Combine remaining ingredients in a small saucepan; bring to a boil. Pour over spinach mixture, and toss. Serve immediately.

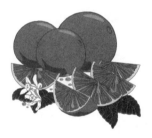

Yield: 6 servings
Per Serving: 95 Calories, 5 g Fat

Five Vegetable Primavera

1/4 cup reduced-sodium chicken broth, divided
2 teaspoons Dijon mustard
2 teaspoons white wine vinegar
vegetable cooking spray
1 tablespoon canola oil
1 1/2 cups sliced yellow squash
1 cup thinly sliced carrots
1 cup diced red peppers
3 cups broccoli flowerets
1/2 cup frozen peas, thawed
1/4 cup minced fresh parsley

1. Combine 2 tablespoons broth, mustard and vinegar; mix well and set aside.
2. Coat a large nonstick skillet with cooking spray; add oil, and place over medium heat until hot. Add squash, carrots and pepper; sauté 5 to 6 minutes or until vegetables are just tender. Add remaining chicken broth to skillet; add broccoli and peas.
3. Cover tightly and cook 4 to 5 minutes or until broccoli is crisp-tender.
4. Stir in mustard mixture; sauté 1 minute. Stir in parsley and serve immediately.

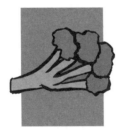

Yield: 5 – 1 cup servings
Per Serving: 80 Calories, 3 g Fat

Roasted Vegetables

Your choice of any combination in any amount:

Zucchini or Summer squash	***Eggplant***
Carrots	***Red Bell Pepper***
Onions	***Green Beans***
Sweet potatoes	***Asparagus***
	Etc.

1. Pre-heat oven to 450 degrees.
2. Slice chosen vegetables about ¼ - ½ inch thick.
3. Lightly "spritz" vegetables with olive oil or 2 – 3 tablespoons of your favorite light Italian dressing.
4. Arrange in a single layer on a cookie sheet or shallow pan.
5. Roast for 10-15 minutes, stirring every 5 minutes.

Yield: Varies
Average serving (per cup): 65 calories, 3 gm fat

Brownies De-light

1 box brownie mix, any brand
4 oz. non-fat plain yogurt
amount of water as shown on box
chocolate packet, if included

1. Omit eggs and 1/2 cup oil from recipe directions on box of brownies. Instead, add yogurt to brownie mix and blend together in a mixing bowl.
2. Pre-heat oven to 350 degrees.
3. Pour mixture into a pan sprayed with non-stick cooking spray; bake about 30 minutes, as directed on the brownie package.

Yield: 24 brownies
Per Serving: 120 Calories, 3 g Fat

Appendix E
TIPS FOR THE HEALTH PROFESSIONAL

I. MOTIVATING MOVEMENT THROUGH THE STAGES OF CHANGE

As a health professional, you can help your clients progress through the stages of change by providing support, education, behavioral strategies, and by promoting realistic and positive thinking. This section discusses in more detail the concept of Stages of Change. Here are several suggestions to help others make positive changes:

1. Help individuals identify their **motivational readiness**. Listen and understand their triumphs and struggles, fears, barriers and expectations. Encourage with facts and optimism.

2. Provide them with practical knowledge and behavioral strategies for changing, based on the **stage of change** they are in.
   For example:
   ◆ Discuss **precontemplators**' concerns and reasons not to start.
   ◆ Show **contemplators** how to get started (see section on Barriers and Solutions, Step 1).
   ◆ Give **preparing** individuals an action plan and tell them how to stay with it.
   ◆ Show **action-ready** persons where slip-ups may occur and how to anticipate and handle these vulnerable situations and succeed.
   ◆ Show **maintainers** what skills they possess to continue no matter what.

3. Help individuals weigh the pros and con's of change and recognize simple, **workable solutions** and backup plans when a primary plan is not workable.

4. **Encourage confidence and optimism**. Be supportive. Be there. Encourage social support and a "buddy system" in the beginning; then community/social involvement to keep one motivated for life.

5. Draw on **motivation** from various sources: self-confidence, social support, a "fun" program, small steps that promote success, lifestyle skills to gain and assure appropriate action, realistic thinking and action, compliments, expanded commitment, community reinforcement, etc.

II. IDENTIFYING ONE'S STAGE OF CHANGE

Prochaska's model of behavioral change states that one must progress through five stages of change in order to build permanent lifestyle changes. Here are the stages and examples:

STAGES	EATING BEHAVIORS	EXERCISE BEHAVIORS
Precontemplation "No. I'm not going to start…	eating better	… exercising."
Contemplation "I'm beginning to think about…	eating better	… starting to exercise."
Preparation "I'm getting ready; I'm buying…	some low-fat foods *(fruit; vegetables; lite dressings, cheese, mayonnaise and margarine; nonfat yogurt)*	… walking shoes and comfortable exercise shorts, socks, T-shirts."
Action "I'm ready…	I'm eating healthier, lighter foods on a daily basis and enjoying them.	… I am consistently exercising 3 times a week."
Maintenance "This is my life!…	I've eaten this way for over 6 months now. I like it and I plan to eat this way always. It's my way of life.	… I'm walking 3 to 5 times a week. I think about fitting in a walk every day. It's a key part of my life."

III. Helping Clients Move Through the Stages of Change

Stage: Precontemplation

1. Provide knowledge—small changes, outcome and value.
2. Discuss benefits of small changes.
3. Identify barriers and solutions. Build confidence.
4. Recognize thinking of change as an important step forward. Attitude about eating well and being more physically active also is significant.
5. Confront.
6. Raise consciousness.

Stage: Contemplation

1. Show ways to make desired changes work and fit into one's life. Let client choose to make first small step.
2. Develop backup plans (weekends, vacations, hectic schedules).
3. Encourage tracking/ feedback system/ accountability.
4. Try one strategy each week; build confidence with each success. Encourage.

Stage: Preparation

1. Create "action plan." Show how/where to begin, to be successful.
2. Solicit commitment.
3. Enlist social support.
4. Establish backup plans to be successful.
5. Encourage, congratulate, build confidence. Provide support. Reassure "perfection" not expected.
6. Set a short-term goal.

Stage: Action

1. Provide ongoing information, encouragement, feedback, solutions.
2. Enlist support.
3. Suggest rewards.
4. Encourage tracking.
5. Discuss backup plans.
6. Encourage, reinforce, praise.

Stage: Maintenance

1. Reinforce, support change. Offer accountability.
2. Encourage goal setting.
3. Reinforce ongoing commitment . . . through visits, phone calls, correspondence, new ideas, etc.
4. Practice backup plans.
5. Reinforce ongoing commitment

IV. Motivating Physical Activity (From Stage to Stage)

Provide clients with both knowledge and behavioral strategies:

1. Present Facts.
Educate about the many benefits of physical activity, the varieties of moderate-intensity activities that count, and how to accumulate moderate-intensity activity.

2. Know Benefits.
Ask the patient to think about the possible <u>personal</u> benefits they might enjoy by becoming and maintaining a physically active lifestyle.

3. Know Risks of Not Changing.
Discuss the risks of an inactive lifestyle such as loss of an active life, increased mortality, loss of quality of life, increased risk of health problems (heart disease, high blood pressure, diabetes, osteoporosis, back and joint problems, immobility, etc.).

4. Care.
Encourage the person to think about how inactivity affects family and friends, as well as self.

5. Discuss Ways to Fit In Fitness.
Ask the person to investigate activities, parks, malls, and recreation centers close to home or work.

6. Enlist Commitment.
Ask the sedentary person to set specific short-term goals to accumulate 2 to 5 minute walks on at least 3 days.

7. Seek Social Support.
Identify friends and family members who might also want to become more active in a joint effort.

8. Seek Exercise Solutions.
Fit exercise to time and place, backups as well as solutions. Find times in each day when moderate-intensity physical activities can replace sedentary activities, such as walking or sit-ups during television commercials, taking 10-minute walks at lunch time, taking stairs 10 times, walking in the mall, or lifting weights at home with bean bag/socks or milk jugs filled with sand or beans in each hand.

9. Reward Achievement.

10. Encourage person to establish appropriate rewards for meeting short and long term goals; praise for meeting commitments; praise for being aware and thinking of activity and making an effort.

11. Have a "Reminders System."
Try different types of self-tracking and use one that works best, e.g., step counters, records of thinking about activity, calendars with steps or minutes of activity, computer calendars, notes on bathroom mirror and in day-timer, scheduled classes, or gym bag in car.

* Adapted from the Cooper Institute © 1999; research by Andrea Dunn, Ph.D.

V. Motivating by Reinforcing the Benefits of Change

Benefits motivate one to make healthier, low-fat food choices and incorporate physical activity into one's lifestyle. Help an individual identify the benefits important to him/her.

Low-Fat Eating

◊ Weight loss
◊ Weight maintenance
◊ Feel better
◊ Reduce risk for heart disease
◊ Increase productivity
◊ Longer life expectancy

◊ Lower blood cholesterol
◊ Lower triglycerides
◊ Reduce risk of cancer
◊ Improve self-image
◊ Better quality of life
◊ Control blood sugar levels

Physical Activity

◊ More stamina/energy
◊ Weight loss
◊ Easier weight maintenance
◊ Lower blood pressure
◊ Improve self-image
◊ Better mood
◊ Better quality of life
◊ Better sleep patterns
◊ Strengthened heart and lungs
◊ Less stress

◊ Lower triglycerides
◊ Feeling great
◊ More muscle tone
◊ Increase productivity
◊ Controlled blood sugar levels
◊ Fewer feelings of depression & anxiety
◊ Longer life expectancy
◊ Healthier bones, muscles and joints

* Adapted from The Cooper Institute © 1999; research by Andrea Dunn, Ph.D.

Index

About the Author

Georgia G. Kostas, M.P.H., R.D., L.D., served for 25 years as Director of Nutrition at the Cooper Clinic, a division of the Cooper Aerobics Center in Dallas, Texas, where she founded the clinic's nutrition program in 1979. Today she continues to design nutrition programs for individuals, teach healthful eating and consult with corporations, food companies and wellness programs for adults and children. A clinical nutritionist and registered and licensed dietitian, her specialties include preventive and cardiovascular medicine, weight management, sports nutrition and nutrition media communications. She is also a public speaker, author and consultant to numerous organizations. As president of Georgia Kostas & Associates, Inc., she also develops educational materials (www.georgiakostas.com).

Kostas has authored *The Balancing Act Nutrition & Weight Guide*, *The Guilt-Free Comfort Food Cookbook* and *What's Cooking at the Cooper Clinic*. In addition, she has contributed to several books by Dr. Kenneth H. Cooper, M.D., M.P.H., including *The Aerobics Program for Total Well-being, Controlling Cholesterol* and *Overcoming Hypertension.* She is quoted frequently in popular publications such as *Reader's Digest, Family Circle, Redbook, Woman's Day, Good Housekeeping, Ladies Home Journal, American Health, Prevention, Shape, Men's Health, Mature Outlook, Living Fit* and others.

Kostas has received several awards including the prestigious "Medallion Award" (2007), one of the American Dietetic Association's highest honors, in recognition of her service, dedication and advancement of the nutrition profession. She was named the "Distinguished Dietitian of the Year" from Texas (2006), and received the "American Dietetic Association's Sports and Cardiovascular Nutritionists Achievement Award" (1990) and "Recognized Young Dietitian of the Year" from Texas (1981). She completed a bachelor's degree in biology from Rice University, a master of public health in nutrition from Tulane University of Public Health and Tropical Medicine, and residency in dietetics from Ochsner Hospital in New Orleans.

As you read *The Cooper Clinic Solution to the Diet Revolution*, Kostas hopes that you and your family will benefit from her practical, realistic approach to healthier eating and weight loss, and find your own best solutions for lifelong weight control.

About The Cooper Aerobics Center

Founded by Dr. Kenneth H. Cooper, M.D., M.P.H., in 1970, the Cooper Aerobics Center emphasizes all aspects of total wellness. The main campus is located on 30 landscaped acres in Dallas, Texas and consists of the divisions listed below. A second, larger campus at Craig Ranch in McKinney, Texas (north of Dallas) includes a world-class clinic and fitness center.

- **Cooper Clinic:** Offers nutrition, weight loss and exercise counseling as part of a comprehensive medical exam that includes cardiovascular risk and fitness assessments and optional ultra-fast CAT Scans (to assess artery disease).

- **The Cooper Institute:** A nonprofit division delivering world-renowned research and education on exercise and its impact on health.

- **Cooper Fitness Center:** Features a one-mile outdoor trail, more than 70 group exercise classes a week, tennis, boxing and state-of-the-art strength training equipment.

- **Cooper Wellness Program:** Offers four-, six- and 13-day programs for individuals wanting to gain healthy eating and exercise habits for a better quality of life.

- **Cooper Concepts:** Provides Dr. Cooper's "Cooper Complete" and other dietary supplements including fish oils, Vitamin D_3 and others.

- **The Guest Lodge:** A full-service, 62-room hotel complete with conference facilities and a heart-healthy restaurant.

- **The Spa at The Cooper Aerobics Center:** A luxurious 3,200-square foot day spa providing massages, facials, manicures, pedicures and other restorative body treatments.

- **Cooper Ventures:** Consults with businesses regarding fitness facilities, programming and staffing.

Order Form for Books & Resources

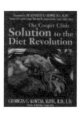

❖ **BOOKS**

The Cooper Clinic Solution to the Diet Revolution: Step up to the Plate!
by Georgia G. Kostas: A step-by-step, no gimmick, realistic approach to healthy eating and weight loss. Call for volume discounts or see www.georgiakostas.com.

❖ **REPRODUCIBLE MASTERS (Handouts for Teaching) - call (214) 587-4241**

Copier-ready pages from *The Cooper Clinic Solution to the Diet Revolution.* Available as hard copies, CD's or e-handouts. Call for details or see www.georgiakostas.com.

❖ **NUTRIENT ANALYSIS by The Cooper Clinic - call (972) 560-2655**

Diet Analysis – of your diet, based on a three-day record you send us.
Recipe Analysis – of your own recipes. Learn the calories, fat and nutrient content.

Call (214) 587-4241 for questions, orders, volume discounts
order online at www.georgiakostas.com, or phone, mail or fax:

ORDER FORM

Please send me:

_____ copies of **The Cooper Clinic Solution to the Diet Revolution** @ $34.95 each = $_____

add Shipping & handling @ $6.00 per book = $_____
Texas residents, please add **$2.90 sales tax** per book = $_____

Total enclosed $_____

Pay by credit card online, by phone or fax (VISA, Mastercard, American Express accepted)

■ Send book to:

Customer Name _____
Address _____
City, State, Zip _____
Daytime phone number _____ Date _____
Email _____

> Order online:
> www.georgiakostas.com
> Fax orders to:
>   (214) 363-0539
> Mail orders to:
>   Good Health Press
>   6702 Park Lane
>   Dallas, TX 75225

■ Payment information: ☐ Check Enclosed. (Make checks payable to "**Good Health Press**")

☐ VISA   ☐ Mastercard   ☐ Am Exp   Purchase Order #_____

Card # _____
Expiration Date _____
Verification Code _____ (3-4 digit # on back of card)
Name on Card _____
Address (where statement is sent):_____
_____

_____
Signature

Let us help you become healthier & better informed about your health. Thank you!

Customers

Angel Medical Center
Baptist Medical Center (AR)
Bay Area Hospital
Berger Hospital
Blount Memorial Hospital
Brainerd Public Schools
Chattanooga Heart Institute
Chimeketa Community College
Christiana Health Care
City Of Dallas
Clay County Medical Center
Columbia Life Care Center
Columbia Athletic Club
Community Medical Center Inc. (NC)
Connecticare
Cooper Wellness Program
County Of Fairfax
Duval County (FL)
The Fitness Nurse
Fitness Center On The River
Foundation Health Hospital (CA)
Frederick Memorial Hospital
General Health System (MD)
HealthNet
Howard University
Humana Hospital
Huntsville Hospital
Institute of Preventive Medicine & Weight Control
(Raleigh, NC)
Jacksonville Cardiovascular Clinic
Lake Charles Memorial Hospital
Las Colinas Medical Center
Lawrence Hospital
University Of Alabama
Linn-Benton Community College
Maryview Medical Center
Mattel Health & Fitness Center
Memorial Health Care Systems (NE)
Memorial Hospital (KS)
Memorial Hospital (MS)
Mercy Hospital (OK)
Meritcare Hospital
Milford-Whitinsvillle Regional Hospital (MA)
Montclair State University
Mood Spa
Motorola Wellness Works
New Hanover Regional Medical Center
New Mexico State University
New York Med Center Of Queens
North Carolina Baptist Hospitals, Inc.
Northport District Community Hospital
Northwest Covenant Medical Center
Northwest Health District

Northwest Health District
Northwestern University
P/Sl Medical Center (Denver)
Pensacola Jr. College
Pomona Valley Hospital
Portland Community College
Presbyterian Healthcare Services
Proctor Hospital
Purdue University
Riverside Hospital
Santa Rosa Junior College
Sharp Healthcare
Shawano Medical Center
Sisters Of Charity
Slender Lady, Inc.
Southeast Community College
Southwest Missouri State Univeristy
Spa Fitness & Wellness Center
St. Joseph's & St. Anthony's Hospital
St. Joseph's Hospital Of Atlanta
St Luke's Hospital (ND)
St. Mary Medical Center – Hobart
St. Mary's-Rogers Hospital
St. Patrick's Hospital
Sumter City Health Dept
Susan Allan Memorial Hospital
Texas Children's Hospital
The Houstonian Fitness Center
The Medical Center, Inc.
The North Carolina Baptist Hospital
Tune Up Your Body
The Woodlands Wellness Center
Union Hospital
University Of Alabama
University Of Alaska - Anchorage
University Of Arizona
University Of Georgia
University Of Kentucky
University Of Minnisota
University Of Missouri
U.S. Army
U.S. Customs
U.S. Navy
Valley Memorial Hospital
Virginia Beach Health Department
Virgiana County Of Fairfax
Wake Forest University Baptist Hospital
Washington Hospital
Waukesha Memorial Hospital
Westwood Health & Fitness Center
Willis-Knighton Hospital
Winter Haven Hospital
Wyoming Valley Health Care Center

The 20 Things You Need to Know About Nutr

As a sports nutritionist who works with professional and competitive athletes, including tennis players, I'm always on the lookout for tips and tricks that give my clients an edge. And in my 10-plus years of practice, not a week goes by that we don't learn more about how particular foods and nutrients help the body operate like a well-oiled machine. Each one of your body's 100 trillion cells relies solely on what you eat and drink to fuel your performance and help you recover. And while sports nutrition isn't an exact science, there are plenty of tried and true techniques every tennis player should know.   *By Cynthia Sass*

tion 2 1

THE RIGHT **BREAKFAST** FIGHTS HUNGER ALL DAY

A recent study published in the journal *Obesity* finds that eating breakfast, especially one with a healthy dose of protein, may be the key to controlling appetite all day long. For three weeks, the subjects either skipped breakfast or munched on breakfast meals containing cereal and milk (which contained normal quantities of protein) or higher protein options. Brain scans showed that the regions of the brain that trigger the desire to eat were less stimulated later in the day, and even more so by the higher protein breakfasts. Eating anything is better than nothing, but if you tend to find yourself raiding the snack drawer in the afternoon or overeating at night, bolster your breakfast with such lean protein as non-fat Greek yogurt, non-fat cottage cheese, egg whites, or an on-the-go option like soy nuts.

YOUR DIET IMPACTS YOUR BRAIN FUNCTION

A new study has confirmed what nutritionists have long suspected—your diet can impact how your brain functions. The animal study conducted by scientists at the University of Washington in Seattle looked at the short- and long-term effects on the brains of rodents fed a typical American diet. Within the first three days, the rats downed nearly double their usual daily calorie intakes, and not only did the animals gain weight, they also developed inflammation in the hypothalamus, the part of the brain that regulates body weight. They experienced changes typically associated with brain injuries such as stroke and multiple sclerosis. Scientists say the study points to the notion that the overconsumption of a classic western diet can lead to brain changes that create a domino effect that may impact weight regulation. Ditch the processed stuff loaded with refined carbs, added sugar and salt, fried stuff and fatty animal products, and load up on fruits veggies, whole grains, lean proteins and plant based fats. Even if you don't eat less, it's quality that counts.

FOOD for THOUGHT

#3

FOOD CAN **FIGHT** PAIN

When inflammation occurs in the joints, it creates a cascade of problems—the loss of cartilage, a painful grating sensation, and reduced flexibility. But anti-inflammatory foods like ginger quell the flames. In a study of more than 250 people with osteoarthritis of the knee, those who received ginger extract twice a day experienced less pain and needed fewer pain-killers compared to those who received a placebo. Ginger has been shown to share the same pharmacological properties as ibuprofen and naproxen. Other potent anti-inflammatory foods include tart cherries, berries, extra virgin olive oil and turmeric.

5 | **SLEEP** Matters . . . A LOT

It may not seem like a nutrition-related issue, but I ask all of my clients about the quantity and quality of their sleep because it's so vital to metabolism and recovery. Healing and repair from the wear and tear of exercise largely occurs during sleep, and getting too little shut has been shown to rev up hunger hormones, increase inflammation, up the risk of obesity, depression, type 2 diabetes and heart disease, and negatively impact productivity and performance. To get the most out of your workouts and healthy eating regime, you absolutely must make sleep a priority. Establish a regular sleep and wake time schedule, even on the weekends, and create a sleep-conducive environment. Ideal sleep conditions include a dark, quiet room between 54 and 75 degrees Fahrenheit.

4 | DON'T RUN ON EMPTY

You may have heard that you'll burn more body fat by exercising on an empty stomach. We don't know for sure, but we do know that it's impossible to burn pure body fat. During aerobic exercise you burn a combination of carbs and fat. When carbs aren't readily available, your body is forced to break down its own muscle mass and convert it into carbohydrate. By skipping, you end up eating away at your own muscle rather than building it. A recent study found that for cyclists who trained with nothing in their stomachs, 10 percent of what they burned was protein. If you don't feel like eating, grab a sports drink—it will protect you from tapping into your lean tissue.

N°6

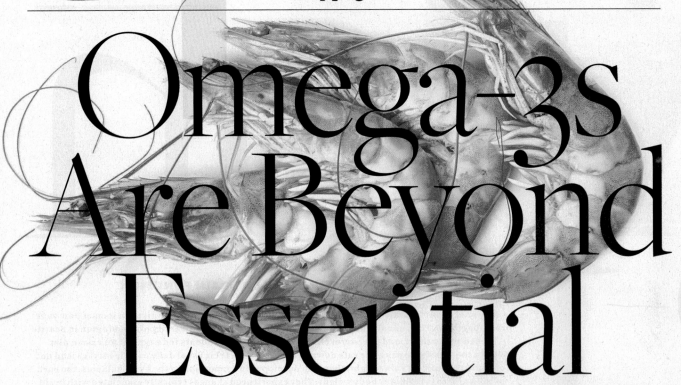

Omega-3s Are Beyond Essential

Omega-3 fatty acids have been linked to a laundry list of benefits, from fighting heart disease and Alzheimer's to staving off type 2 diabetes. But a recent study published in the *Journal of Physiology* found that they also influence protein metabolism. In a study on steer, researchers added supplements of either omega-3s from fish oil or a mixture of cottonseed and olive oils without omega-3s to the regular diet of the animals. After five weeks, those receiving fish oil showed increased sensitivity to insulin, which in turn, improved muscle development. Twice the amount of amino acids were used by their bodies to build new protein tissues, especially in skeletal muscles. If you don't eat enough seafood or you're concerned with mercury, consider taking a daily omega-3 supplement that supplies about 1,000 mg of DHA and EPA combined.

Milk
Does More Than Double Duty

Milk has been touted as a simple way to burn more body fat. A study published in the *American Journal of Clinical Nutrition* confirms that, but also finds that milk-drinkers gain more muscle mass. Researchers took three groups of young men 18-to-30 years of age and gave them a five-days-per-week strength-training program over 12 weeks. After each session, the volunteers drank either two cups of skim milk, a soy alternative with an equivalent amount of protein and calories, or a carbohydrate beverage with an equal amount of calories. Milk drinkers lost nearly twice as much fat—two pounds—and gained 63 percent or 3.3 pounds more muscle mass than the carbohydrate drinkers. Keep in mind, organic milk packs 75 percent more beta-carotene, as much as a serving of Brussels sprouts, and 50 percent more vitamin E, a powerful antioxidant.

8 | DON'T GET FOOLED BY THE AFTERBURN MYTH

While it's true that you do torch more calories in the hours after a workout, it may be far less than you think. In fact, it can account for as few as 50 calories. If your goal is to lean down, you can eat more on the days you train hard, but use what I call the 50/50 principle—add about half the calories you burn during exercise to your usual intake, preferably about 50 percent before to help fuel the activity, and 50 percent after, for recovery. For example, an hour of singles burns 500 calories (for 150-pound person), which means you can "spend" an extra 125 calories both before and after your court time. That's the amount in one slice of whole grain bread spread with one tablespoon of natural peanut butter before, and a half cup each of non-fat Greek yogurt and sliced strawberries topped with a tablespoon of sliced almonds after.

9 | ORGANIC FOOD is worth the extra money

There is no doubt that organic food is better for the environment, but it's also better for your physique. Organic foods contain more antioxidants, which not only protect your cells from aging, inflammation and disease, but may also make you leaner. In a recent study, University of Florida researchers found that people who consumed more antioxidants had lower body mass indices, smaller waistlines, and lower body fat percentages than those with lower intakes, even though both groups consumed about the same number of daily calories. In addition, research shows that pesticide residues from conventionally grown foods may be a factor in rising obesity rates. If you can't go 100 percent, buy organic versions of the staple foods you eat most often, particularly such animal-based foods as milk, eggs and meat.

10 | ALCOHOL may weaken muscle

Recent research in the *Journal of Science and Medicine in Sport* found that alcohol accelerates post-exercise muscle loss. Healthy males engaged in strength training followed by a cocktail—either vodka and orange juice or OJ alone. Vodka didn't trigger more soreness, but did impact a loss of muscle strength by as much as 40 percent. Alcohol has also been shown to interfere with replenishing glycogen, your body's carbohydrate 'piggy bank' after exercise, which leads to a lack of endurance the next day. In one study when carbs were displaced by alcohol, glycogen stores plummeted by 50 percent, even eight hours later.

11
RELYING ON THE SUN FOR VITAMIN D MAY BE A MISTAKE

Vitamin D's nickname is the "sunshine vitamin" because exposure to the sun's ultraviolet rays triggers its production in the body. But recent research found that Hawaiians who spend more than 20 hours a week in the sun, including half of the time without sunscreen, still had low vitamin D levels. And a study published in the *Journal of Clinical Endocrinology and Metabolism* found that nearly 60 percent of Americans have too little Vitamin D in their blood and nearly a quarter had serious deficiencies. Not getting enough has been linked to autoimmune disorders, certain cancers, increased body fat and decreased muscle strength. In healthy, young Californians, researchers found an inverse relationship between blood Vitamin D levels and muscle fat. Ask your doctor to test your blood vitamin D level to determine if you need a supplement.

FOOD for THOUGHT

12

SPICES ARE A SECRET WEAPON

A Penn State University study found that adding such herbs and spices as oregano, cinnamon, turmeric, black pepper, cloves and garlic powder to meals significantly upped post- meal blood levels of antioxidants, lowered insulin levels and reduced unhealthy blood fats by a 30 percent. Other research shows that such natural seasonings can also boost satiety and rev up metabolism. Many herbs and spices are even more potent sources of antioxidants than fruits and vegetables. To harness their power, sprinkle a little into each meal.

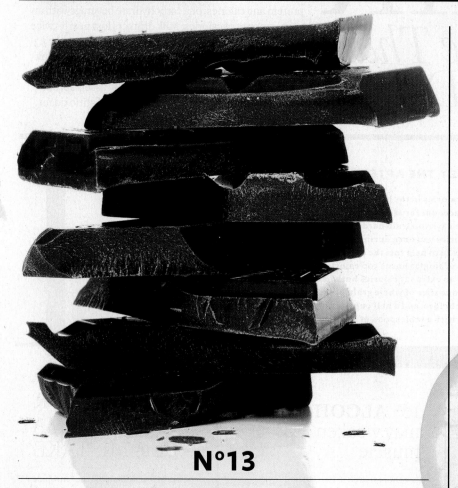

N°13

Chocolate
IS A KEY SUPERFOOD

In addition to being a feel-good food, dark chocolate may be life-saving. One study found that heart-attack survivors who ate chocolate just twice a week over a two-year period cut their risk of dying from heart disease threefold. Another reported that when women ate dark chocolate daily for just seven days, their levels of "bad" cholesterol, LDL, dropped by six percent, and their levels of HDL, the "good" kind, rose by nine percent. Dark chocolate is also linked to a reduction in the risk of stroke, reduced inflammation and better blood pressure control. Indulge in a small amount each day, up to an ounce. Look for 70 percent dark or greater for the most antioxidants.

14 | Buyer beware when it comes to SUPPLEMENTS

Some consumers believe that supplements are as highly regulated as medications, but the guidelines are complex. A law passed in 1994 called the Dietary Supplement Health and Education Act or DSHEA prevents the Food and Drug Administration from regulating supplements in the same way as prescription drugs. That means no product is required to be tested for safety or effectiveness before it gets into your hands. There is also no guarantee that a bottle contains exactly what it states or that it's not contaminated with additives that shouldn't be there. Supplements can also interact with each other as well as prescription drugs. For these reasons, it's always best to use supplements under the guidance of your doctor or dietitian. Before you put anything into your body ask him or her about brands they trust and which formulas and amounts are right for you.

15 | A little VITAMIN C makes a big difference

Researchers at Arizona State University discovered that vitamin C's role goes beyond fending off sniffles. This powerhouse nutrient can build stamina and squash a spare tire because the amount in your blood stream is related to your body's ability to burn fat for fuel, both at rest and during exercise. Men in the study with low vitamin C levels burned 25 percent less fat during a treadmill test compared to those with adequate vitamin C. The link: C is essential for the production of carnitine, a nutrient that helps turn fat into a useable fuel source. This domino effect delays fatigue—each gram of fat packs nine calories, compared to four in carbohydrate. Vitamin C-rich foods include peppers, broccoli and citrus fruits.

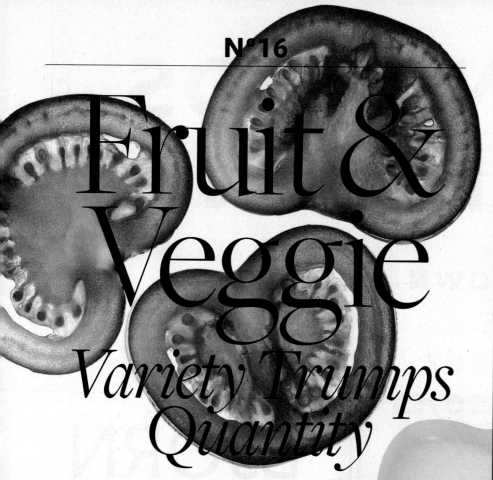

Fruit & Veggie
Variety Trumps Quantity

Researchers at Colorado State University fed more than 100 subjects one of two diets: one with produce from five distinct plant families, and the other with fruits and vegetables from 18 distinct plant families. Both diets were consumed for two weeks at a time and provided identical amounts of produce. But blood samples revealed that the more varied diet significantly reduced oxidation in the body, a marker for disease protection. Aim for a wide array of colors and types of produce.

17
DRINKING MORE **WATER** MAY HELP YOU **LOSE WEIGHT**

A recent study found that adults who simply gulped two cups of water before meals enjoyed a major weight-loss benefit—they shed 40 percent more weight over a 12-week period while following a low-cal plan identical to a second group of dieters. The same group of scientists previously found that subjects who drank two cups before meals naturally consumed 75-90 fewer calories, an amount that could snowball day after day. According to the Institute of Medicine, women 19 and over need 2.7 liters of total fluid per day (about 11 8-oz cups) and men need 3.7 (about 15 8-oz cups). But that's total fluid, not just water. Foods provide about 20 percent of your needs, which still leaves nearly nine cups of fluid to go, so if water is the only beverage you drink, eight glasses a day is a smart strategy.

18 | **BACTERIA** are critical to your health

A recent study published in the *European Journal of Clinical Nutrition* found that a probiotic supplement, specifically Lactobacillus gasseri, helped adults with obese tendencies achieve weight-loss success. The study assigned 87 overweight people to receive a daily dose of fermented milk, with or without added probiotics, for a 12-week period. The supplemented group had a 4.6 percent reduction in belly fat and a 1.4 percent reduction in body weight, compared to no changes among those who didn't receive the "good" bacteria. Probiotics also fight arthritic inflammation and boost immunity—a Swedish study found that employees given Lactobacillus got sick less often and missed far fewer days of work. The best food sources are yogurt, kefir, miso, sauerkraut and Kimchi.

19 | CALCIUM ISN'T JUST FOR STRONG BONES

In a study published in the British Journal of Nutrition, obese women who consumed less than 600 mg of calcium per day, 60 percent of the daily recommended intake, followed a low-calorie diet for 15 weeks. The women were instructed to take either 1,200 mg of calcium or a placebo. The calcium group lost nearly 12 pounds over the course of the program, compared to just two pounds in the control group. Nearly 55 percent of men and 78 percent of women aged 20 and up fall short of the recommended 1,000 mg of calcium, which ramps up to 1,200 mg after age 50. If you supplement your intake don't take more than 500 mg at once, as absorption decreases as the dose increases. And look for calcium citrate, which is well tolerated and absorbed efficiently.

20 | LET AN **EXPERT** PERSONALIZE YOUR PLAN

As with many things in life there is no one size fits all. That's why many competitive and recreational athletes opt to enlist the help of a dietitian or sports nutritionist to craft an individualized meal plan that matches their performance and recovery needs. If you're not sure where to find one, hop online. You can search for a registered dietitian in your area who specializes in sports nutrition at www.eatright.org. The initials CSSD after an expert's name means he or she is Board Certified as a Specialist in Sports Dietetics.

STANDARDS *of* EXCELLENCE

A COUNTDOWN OF THE 10 GREATEST MEN'S SEASONS OF THE OPEN ERA

10 BJÖRN BORG
— 1979 —

It's often said that men's tennis is deeper and more competitive than it has ever been. And it's true; the sport has never been played at a higher level. But over the last five years, it hasn't been the excellence of the ATP as a whole that's been most impressive. It has been the dominance of the top players despite that depth. Since 2006, we've seen three players—Roger Federer, Rafael Nadal and Novak Djokovic—put together seasons that rank among the most gloriously accomplished of the Open era.

Now that the third and perhaps finest of those seasons, Djokovic's remarkable 2011, is complete, it seems like a good time to look back at where it—as well as Federer's and Nadal's best years—fits among the greatest single seasons of the Open era. There's no right answer, and that's what makes this parlor game so much fun. Here we present our countdown of the 10 best men's seasons since the Open era began in 1968.

BY STEPHEN TIGNOR

The Viking God is known for his body of work rather than for a singular season, which is understandable considering that none of them featured a US Open title. But it's also unfair to a player who had a winning percentage of 90 or higher in four different years. His highest was 93.3 percent (84-6) in 1979. By then, Sweden's Teen Angel, tennis' first matinee idol, had evolved into the scarier and scruffier Angelic Assassin. At 23, already with three Wimbledon titles and three French Opens, Borg was at the height of his powers. In '79, he would add a fourth French and fourth Wimbledon, win his first year-end Masters, and finish No. 1 for the first time. Borg's only loss of note that year came, under the lights he hated at Flushing Meadows, to a bullet-serving Roscoe Tanner. The next season would bring a new challenger in John McEnroe, but in '79, Borg left an old one behind. In what may have been his most satisfying achievement, he beat his former nemesis Jimmy Connors all six times they played.

✛ READ MORE ABOUT THE GREATEST SEASONS IN TENNIS HISTORY ONLINE AT TENNIS.COM